The Juice Lady's Guide to Juicing for Health

Revised Edition

The Juice Lady's Guide to Juicing for Health

Unleashing the Healing Power of
Whole Fruits and Vegetables

CHERIE CALBOM, M.S.

AVERY

a member of

Penguin Group (USA) Inc.

New York

Published by the Penguin Group
Penguin Group (USA) Inc., 375 Hudson Street, New York, New York 10014, USA
Penguin Group (Canada), 90 Eglinton Avenue East, Suite 700, Toronto, Ontario M4P 2Y3,
Canada (a division of Pearson Canada Inc.) · Penguin Books Ltd,
80 Strand, London WC2R 0RL, England · Penguin Ireland, 25 St Stephen's Green,
Dublin 2, Ireland (a division of Penguin Books Ltd) · Penguin Group (Australia),
250 Camberwell Road, Camberwell, Victoria 3124, Australia (a division of Pearson
Australia Group Pty Ltd) · Penguin Books India Pvt Ltd, 11 Community Centre,
Panchsheel Park, New Delhi–110 017, India · Penguin Group (NZ), 67 Apollo Drive,
Rosedale, North Shore 0632, New Zealand (a division of Pearson New Zealand Ltd) ·
Penguin Books (South Africa) (Pty) Ltd, 24 Sturdee Avenue,
Rosebank, Johannesburg 2196, South Africa

Penguin Books Ltd, Registered Offices: 80 Strand, London WC2R 0RL, England

Most Avery books are available at special quantity discounts for bulk purchase for sales promotions, premiums,
fund-raising, and educational needs. Special books or book excerpts also can be created to fit specific needs.
For details, write Penguin Group (USA) Inc. Special Markets, 375 Hudson Street, New York, NY 10014.

Library of Congress Cataloging-in-Publication Data

Calbom, Cherie.
The juice lady's guide to juicing for health : unleashing the healing power of whole
fruits and vegetables / Cherie Calbom.—Rev. ed.
p.   cm.
Includes bibliographical references and index.
ISBN 978-1-58333-317-4
1. Fruit juices—Therapeutic use.   2. Vegetable juices—Therapeutic use.   I. Title.
RM255.C35   2008   2008028355
613.2'6—dc22

Printed in the United States of America
3 5 7 9 10 8 6 4

BOOK DESIGN BY TANYA MAIBORODA

Acknowledgments

To those who have assisted me with this book, I am forever grateful.

Thank you, Michele Libin, who assisted in researching and writing this book; I am so very appreciative. You are a dear friend and a valued writer with a wonderful future ahead; thank you for your great contribution to this project.

To my editor, Miriam Rich, you've added valuable input.

To my literary agent, Pamela Harty, you once again helped me find a home for my work.

Lastly, I wish to express my deep and lasting appreciation to all the people, the Holy Trinity, and the angels who have assisted me with this book. To my dear heavenly Father, Jesus Christ, and Holy Spirit, thank you for guiding me throughout this project. You showed me Your ways of wisdom and truth as to how to care for the human body. You have guided me to the fountain of life in the juicing and cleansing programs I've embraced. Thank you for health and the awesome responsibility of guiding those who have lost their health, their peace of mind, or their way concerning the care of their bodies. For the healing You've given and Your unconditional love, I am so very grateful.

—Cherie Calbom

Contents

Introduction

Do you want to lose weight? Get rid of cellulite? Look years younger? How about improving your health? Do you want to do your part to recover from a disease or illness? Countless scientific studies have proven that a diet rich in fruits and vegetables can vastly improve your fitness and vitality, promote weight loss, boost your energy levels, fight the effects of aging, and enhance your general well-being. Now, you can tap into the power of juicing to achieve the best health possible with this revised edition of *The Juice Lady's Guide to Juicing for Health.*

If you have one or more of the ailments covered in the pages that follow, this can be your opportunity to discover not only what contributes to your ill health, but also what will enable you to get well and become healthier than ever. Even if you don't have any particular ailments, you can experience more energy and greater vitality and prevent disease by using the delicious juice recipes and the great programs such as juicing, short juice fasts, and periodic detoxes for various organs of the body. You can use the A-to-Z guide to look up an illness whenever the need arises, such as a cold or flu, and find out what juices and diet will help you recover faster.

Since 1990, I have appeared on television, hosted infomercials, written books and articles, and conducted seminars all across America on the healing power of juicing. Why am I so passionate about juicing? The energy I enjoy today is something I didn't experience for a good portion of my life. What I've learned from years of juicing and detoxing is that supplying the body with superior nutrition

1

and removing toxicity that undermines our health enables us to experience a high level of wellness.

✳ Sickness Became a Way of Life

I can't remember ever being particularly healthy and energetic, even as a child. My grandmother told me that I was sick a great deal of the time in childhood, often sidelined because of colds and flu. I'm convinced that my problems began before I was born. My maternal heritage was not one of good health. My mother had not been well most of her life. She died at the age of forty-five of breast cancer; I was six years old.

The surprising part of my health history was that not one doctor ever figured out why I was so tired and why I kept getting sick so often. Once a doctor suggested that I might have an allergy to dairy products, and when I stopped eating them, my health improved somewhat.

Maybe I should have seen a veterinarian. Growing up in Iowa, and with relatives who farmed in Minnesota, I often heard people question what the cattle or other farmyard animals had been eating when they got sick. No one ever asked me what I'd been eating.

What I'd been eating might have killed a strong athlete. I loved junk food, candy, soft drinks, cinnamon rolls, cookies, ice cream, chips, buttered popcorn—anything sweet or salty. Sweets were my preferred food. I have since discovered that sweet cravings (on an emotional level) can be triggered because a person is trying to bring sweetness into her life. I certainly needed sweetness after losing my mother when I was so young.

Never having considered the connection between a healthy diet and a healthy body, I rarely thought twice about what I put in my mouth. I can't remember eating fresh green vegetables in the winter. Though my father and I lived with my maternal grandparents, and my grandmother grew a bountiful organic garden each year and prepared lots of vegetables for summertime meals, I didn't think most vegetables were particularly appealing. I liked eating sweet peas and baby carrots right out of the garden, corn off the cob with lots of butter, and berries and grapes picked fresh off the vine, but that was about it. For the most part, my interest centered on my grandmother's homemade bread with plenty of butter plus her mouthwatering cinnamon rolls, date bread, pies, and cookies.

Through junior high I continued to catch nearly every cold and flu bug that circulated in school, and I was often home due to illness and fatigue. There were many mornings when I was so exhausted I could barely drag myself from bed. Feeling tired and unwell became a natural state of being—one I accepted without question for many years.

My health fluctuated through high school and my twenties. In order to stay thin, I started avoiding sweets, which helped my health to a degree, but I also put myself on a number of crash or starvation diets. Lacking the nutrients it needed, my body was crying for help. Once an aunt convinced me to take vitamin and mineral supplements. I noticed an increase in energy almost immediately when I took them, but I still suffered from bouts of fatigue, colds, and flu. Whatever good I was doing by taking nutritional supplements was nearly canceled out by my poor diet and occasional binges on sweets.

✳ My Journey Toward Health

My real health crisis came when I turned thirty. I developed a devastating case of chronic fatigue syndrome. I felt as though I had never-ending flu and was perennially lethargic. In constant pain, I suffered as though I'd been bounced around in a washing machine. That, coupled with a diagnosis of hypoglycemia and an infection with *Candida albicans* (a systemic yeast infection), caused me to feel hopeless. I visited a holistic doctor who tested me for food allergies, and I left his office with a list of allergens longer than my arm. It was one of the most discouraging times of my life.

Not finding any clear answers from the medical profession as to how to heal my physical condition, I finally went to a health food store. I talked with employees and browsed the bookshelves. There I found answers. Clearly, I was eating poorly, not providing my body with the nutrients it needed to heal and gain energy. Most important, I learned about the energizing benefits of juicing fresh vegetables and fruit, and the healing, restorative power of juice fasting. I learned that my body was toxic and in need of detoxification. The information I'd gathered offered me the first rays of hope I'd had. There was something *I could do* to restore my health.

Too tired to work, but armed with a juicer, I moved from California to my father's home in Colorado and made it a full-time job to get healthy. I embarked on a self-designed program, kicking it off with a five-day juice fast of mostly vegetable juices.

I then turned to vegan eating, along with drinking lots of vegetable juices every day for the following three months. But instead of feeling better, I felt a little worse. What I didn't realize was that I was detoxing. Though my father was pessimistic about my program, based on the results, I was determined to get well. In desperation, I saw a reflexologist (a therapist who uses a form of massage with applied pressure to certain parts of the feet). He determined that I needed a gallbladder cleanse based on painful areas of my feet. The gallbladder detox produced amazing results. And I felt a little better. But I still had plenty of "not so good" days.

But one morning, without warning, I woke up early feeling brand-new, with so much energy I wanted to go jogging. I felt as if someone had given me a new body. I thought, "Wow! That was the best cure on earth." I realized that freshly made vegetable juices, veggie smoothies, lots of raw foods, periodic cleansing, and a nutritious, whole-foods diet was a lifestyle I could follow to produce the health I wanted. I also realized that there were foods I needed to let go of—like sweets, refined-flour products such as bread and pasta, and dairy products—so I could maintain my high level of health.

With my juicer in tow, a new lifestyle fully embraced, and an exciting set of goals, I returned to Southern California and my friends. For nearly a year, it was "ten steps forward" with renewed, vibrant health and more energy and stamina than I'd ever remembered.

Then, all of a sudden, I took a giant step back.

✳ A New Health Crisis

I was house-sitting in a lovely Southern California neighborhood for vacationing family friends and working on my first book. A burglar broke into their home one night. I was shocked to wake up around 3 a.m. and see a strange young man crouched in the corner of the bedroom. Instead of running, he leaped off the floor and attacked, beating me repeatedly with a pipe, yelling, "Now you are dead!" and then choking me unconscious. I knew I was dying. I felt my spirit leave, floating up and out of my body. Then all was peaceful and still. I sensed that I was traveling, at what seemed like the speed of light, through black space, with twinkling lights in the distance. Suddenly, however, I was back in my body, outside the house, clinging to a fence at the end of the dog run, and screaming for help. I don't know how I got there. A neighbor heard me screaming and sent her husband to help. Within minutes, I was on my way to the hospital. I suffered serious injuries to my head, neck, back, and right hand, with multiple head wounds and part of my scalp torn from my head.

This time, it took every ounce of my will, faith, and trust in God; deep spiritual work; alternative medical help; extra vitamins and minerals; juicing; emotional release; healing prayer; and numerous detox programs to heal physically, mentally, and emotionally. I met a nutritionally minded physician who had healed his own slow-mending broken bones with lots of vitamins and minerals; he gave me vitamin cocktail IVs. Juicing, cleansing, nutritional supplements, a nearly perfect diet, and prayer, along with physical therapy, helped my bones and other injuries heal.

After following this regimen for about nine months, what my hand surgeon said would be impossible became real—a fully restored, fully functional hand. He had told me that I'd never use my right hand again, and that it wasn't even possible to put in plastic knuckles because of its poor condition. But my knuckles did indeed re-form, and function of my hand returned. A day came when he told me I was completely healed, and though the doctor admitted he didn't believe in miracles, he did say, "You're the closest thing I've seen to one."

Equally important in the restorative process was the healing of my soul—a place in which no one could determine the degree of injury. I experienced healing from the painful memories and trauma of the attack through prayer, laying on of hands, and deep emotional healing work. It seemed as if endless buckets of tears had been stored up in my soul from new and old wounds, such as my mother's death when I was six, my maternal grandfather's death when I was nine, a tragedy concerning my father when I was thirteen, and the emotional pain of the attack—all of which needed release. Forgiveness and letting go came in stages, and were an integral part of my total healing. I had to be honest about what I really felt and willing to face the pain and toxic emotions pent up inside and let them go. I felt as though I cried buckets of tears. But finally one day, after a long healing journey, I was free. A time came when I could celebrate the Fourth of July (the anniversary of the attack) without fear.

At last, I knew more peace and health than I had ever thought would be possible. I experienced what it was to feel whole—complete, not damaged, broken, wounded, or impaired, but truly healed and restored to wholeness in body, soul, and spirit. And I knew there was a purpose for my life—a reason I had lived. I could help others find their way to wholeness.

✳ From Tragedy to Purpose

I became so passionate about what had brought about my health, healing, and vitality—not once, but twice—that I decided to attend graduate school and pursue a master's degree in nutrition. I wanted to be a credible source of information when I told people what juicing, detoxing, and eating whole organic foods could do for them. I enrolled at Bastyr University in Seattle—a school of natural medicine dedicated to improving the health of the human community. It was there, before I graduated, that I met the owners of the Juiceman company, who were looking for a couple of graduate students to write a little booklet containing juice recipes and nutrition information to accompany the Juiceman juicer. I was one of the people chosen for the project. (That booklet is still included with the Juiceman juicer.)

One thing leads to another. By the time I had graduated with my master's degree, I was the company's Juice Lady. I traveled around the country almost weekly teaching people about health and nutrition, and what juicing could do for them. In 1992, my first juice book was released. *Juicing for Life* became an international best seller and has helped millions of people experience better health though the power of juicing. One day my husband summed it up: "You truly are living your purpose," he said. "All the tragedy of your life has shaped a passion inside your soul to help others find their path to wholeness."

✳ You Can Experience Vibrant Health

Juicing can help you achieve the abundant health you long for. The programs in this new edition of *The Juice Lady's Guide to Juicing for Health* go far beyond salads and V8 juice. In fact, juices that are canned, frozen, or bottled have been pasteurized, which means that many of their life-giving nutrients, such as enzymes and vitamins, have been killed in the process. And while these processed options are better than soda, they are a poor substitute when compared with freshly made juice. Raw juices offer an abundance of nutrients. They make your body feel alive!

I want you to discover how easy juicing can be. I hope you look forward to drinking the fresh juices you make each day so you can experience their life-giving benefits as I did. I'm thrilled to pass on to you the knowledge about juicing, delicious recipes, and dietary choices that I've discovered are effective, on my own journey toward health, through what my clients have taught me, and through the dedicated scientific research of others.

One of the greatest gifts I can give you is knowledge about the life-promoting power of juicing, along with the healing power of detoxification programs and an understanding of the cause and prevention of disease. To that end, I've written a revised edition of *The Juice Lady's Guide to Juicing for Health.* It offers you a comprehensive plan for incorporating juice therapy, diet, and supplements into a holistic wellness plan for a variety of ailments and health challenges. Following the A-to-Z guide of ailments are the cleansing programs.

You'll learn how the cleansing programs can help you naturally and safely eliminate toxins from your body so your organs can function more efficiently. This will help you experience more energy and a higher level of wellness. Best of all, you'll discover a way of life that will help you feel and look alive and vibrant each and every day of your life. A healthier life truly does await you!

All About Juice

ARE YOU EATING ENOUGH vegetables and fruit every day? Well, just when we thought we had the five-a-day down, the guidelines changed. The latest nutritional guidelines indicate that we need between nine and thirteen servings of vegetables and fruit each and every day to stay healthy, depending on age and activity level, with an emphasis on dark green leafy vegetables and red and yellow vegetables and fruit.

* * *

To determine a serving size, the following equals one serving: one-half cup of raw or cooked vegetables, three-quarters cup of vegetable juice, or one cup of raw leafy vegetables.

If you're going to get the minimum of nine servings daily, you'll need something like two cups of green leafy vegetables (that's about one good-size salad) and four cups of fruit and vegetables. Wow! That's not so easy to do on most days. That's where juicing can really help you fill in the gaps. When you drink a glass or two of fresh vegetable juice, eat a piece or two of fresh fruit, have a salad and a steamed vegetable or two, you'll reach the recommended goal.

It is very easy to incorporate juicing into your life. Fresh juice is a great way to start the day, and it's far more energizing than a cup of coffee. Make some extra juice and take it to work in an insulated container for a midmorning pick-me-up.

Before dinner, start with a "salad in a glass" instead of a cocktail or a glass of wine—all the nutrients fresh juice offers are far more calming, and you'll sleep better at night. Once you start experiencing the benefits of fresh juice, juicing each day will become a habit for life.

If you have a health problem, it's even more important to juice fresh vegetables. Fresh juice offers increased energy and strengthened immunity, plus the raw materials that help your body heal more quickly and completely. If you want to prevent disease, the surest path to a disease-free life begins with a diet rich in plant foods. Juicing provides the nutritional advantages of plants in a concentrated form that is easy to absorb. It is a delicious, simple way to increase your consumption of these life-giving foods.

In this section, you'll learn why juicing is important for good health. You'll also find answers to several commonly asked questions about juicing. I'll show you how to find the juicer that best meets your needs. And I'll explain why organic produce is always the best choice.

✳ A Look at What Fresh Juice Offers

If you want a vitamin-mineral cocktail with an abundance of the nutrients you need, fresh juice is your answer. Juice provides your body with water and easily absorbed protein, carbohydrates, essential fatty acids, vitamins, minerals, enzymes, and phytochemicals. Researchers are continuing to explore how the nutrients found in juice can ease specific disorders, as you'll see in The Science-Based Juice Pharmacy on page 11.

Water. Juice provides a great deal of water, which is the most abundant component in the body, accounting for about 70 to 75 percent of the body's composition. About two-thirds of the body's water supply is in the cells, while the rest is used to transport nutrients. Water lubricates joints, assists in maintaining a constant body temperature, creates chemical reactions in a process called hydrolysis, generates energy, helps form the structure of cell membranes, and regulates all bodily functions.

Protein. Protein is the next most plentiful component in the body. We use protein to form muscles, ligaments, tendons, hair, nails, and skin. Protein is needed to create enzymes, which direct chemical reactions, and hormones, which direct bodily processes. Fruits and vegetables contain lower quantities of protein than animal

The Science-Based Juice Pharmacy

Scientific research supports the fact that fresh juice is good for you. Many studies on the benefits of the various nutrients found in fruits and vegetables have been published in some of the most prestigious medical journals, and a number of studies attest to the health benefits of specific juices such as the ones that follow:

Beetroot juice. Volunteers recruited for a study at St. Bartholomew's Hospital in London were asked to drink approximately one British pint, equivalent to about twenty ounces in U.S. measurements, of beetroot juice or water. Those who had the beetroot juice started to show reductions in blood pressure after one hour. At about 2.5 hours, participants who had the juice began to show significant reductions in both their systolic and diastolic readings. The effect was linked to the nitrate found in the beetroot, which reacted with bacteria in the mouth and resulted in blood vessels dilating. (Andrew J. Webb, et al. "Acute Blood Pressure Lowering, Vasoprotective and Anti-Platelet Properties of Dietary Nitrate via Bioconversion to Nitrite," *Hypertension—Journal of the American Heart Association*, published online 4 February 2008, doi: 10.1161/HYPERTENSIONAHA.107.103523.)

Cabbage juice. Dr. Garnet Cheney from Stanford University's School of Medicine performed several studies with cabbage juice, and found it was extremely effective in treating peptic ulcers. (Cheney, G., et al. "Anti-Peptic Ulcer Dietary Factor [Vitamin "U"] in the Treatment of Peptic Ulcers," *Journal of the American Dietetic Association* 25:668–672, 1950.)

Cherry juice. Cherry juice has been shown to be effective in easing attacks of gout and gouty arthritis, with patients reporting greater freedom of movement in their fingers and toes. Keracyanin, the pigment found in cherries, is believed to be the beneficial agent. (Blau, L. W. "Cherry Diet Control for Gout and Arthritis," *Texas Report on Biology and Medicine* 8:309–312, 1950.)

Citrus juice. One study showed that drinking citrus juices regularly, along with reducing dietary sodium, helped prevent kidney stones. ("Keeping Kidneys Stone-Free: Hold the Salt and Pass the OJ," *Modern Medicine* 63:15, January 1995.)

Cranberry juice has been shown effective in the treatment and prevention of urinary tract infections. (Kuzminskik, L. N. "Cranberry Juice and Urinary Tract Infections: Is There a Beneficial Relationship?" *Nutrition News* II:S87–S90, November 1996.)

Tomato juice. A Harvard study showed that men who eat at least ten servings a week of tomato-based foods are up to 45 percent less likely to develop prostate cancer, while men who eat four to seven servings a week show a 20 percent reduction in prostate cancer rates. Tomatoes and tomato juice contain large amounts of lycopene, which is a powerful antioxidant. ("Cancer and Tomatoes," *Nutrition Week* 7, 15 December 1995; taken from 6 December 1995 issue of *Journal of the National Cancer Institute*.)

Another study showed that feeding tomato juice to mice kept them from developing emphysema after cigarette smoke exposure that was long enough to induce emphysema in a control group. ("Tomato Juice Keeps Emphysema from Developing In New Model; Lycopene," *American Journal of Physiology–Lung Cellular and Molecular Physiology* in *Science Daily* Jan. 25, 2006.)

Vegetable juices. In a study conducted at Norway's Oslo Rheumatism Hospital, rheumatoid arthritis patients drank fresh carrot, celery, and beetroot juices as part of a special dietary program. Doctors found a substantial reduction in disease activity among these patients. (Kjeldsen-Kragh, J., et al. "Controlled Trial of Fasting and One-Year Vegetarian Diet in Rheumatoid Arthritis," *The Lancet* 338:899–902, 12 October 1991.)

Juice (fruit and vegetable). The Kame Project showed that those who drank juices more than three times per week compared to less than once a week were 76 percent less likely to develop Alzheimer's disease. (Dai, Q., Borenstein, et al. "Fruit and vegetable juices and Alzheimer's disease: the Kame Project." *The American Journal of Medicine* 119 (9): 751–759. PMID 16945610, 2006).

foods such as meat and dairy products. Therefore, they are thought of as poor protein sources. However, juices are concentrated forms of fruits and vegetables, and so provide an abundance of easily absorbed amino acids, the building blocks that make up protein. For example, sixteen ounces of carrot juice (two to three pounds of carrots) provides about 5 grams of protein (the equivalent of about one chicken wing or two ounces of tofu). Vegetable protein does not provide all the amino acids your body needs. You will want to add other protein sources, such as legumes (beans, lentils, and split peas), nuts, seeds, and whole grains, and/or organic, free-range muscle meats and wild-caught fish to your daily diet (see Basic Guidelines for the Juice Lady's Health and Healing Diet, page 290).

Carbohydrates. The third most plentiful substance in the body is carbohydrates. They provide fuel for the body to be used for movement, heat production, and chemical reactions. The chemical bonds of carbohydrates lock in the energy a plant takes in from the sun, and this energy is released when the body burns plant food as fuel. There are three categories of carbohydrates: simple (sugars), complex (starches and fiber), and fiber. Choose more complex carbohydrates in your diet than simple carbs. There are more simple sugars in fruit juice than vegetable juice, which is why you should juice more vegetables and in most cases drink no more than four ounces of fruit juice a day. Both insoluble and soluble fibers are found in whole fruits and vegetables, and both types are needed for good health. Who said juice doesn't have fiber? Soluble fiber is in juice in the form of pectin, gums, and mucilage, which are excellent for the digestive tract. This fiber also helps to lower blood cholesterol levels, stabilize blood sugar, and improve good bowel bacteria.

Essential fatty acids. There is very little fat in fruit and vegetable juices, but the fats these juices do contain are essential to your health. The essential fatty acids (EFAs)—linoleic and alpha-linolenic acids, in particular—found in fresh juice function as components of nerve cells, cellular membranes, and hormonelike substances called prostaglandins. They are also required for energy production.

Vitamins. There are more than a dozen major vitamins—vitamins A, C, D, E, and K, along with the B complex—and they are all essential to your good health. Vitamins take part, along with minerals and enzymes, in chemical reactions. For example, vitamin C participates with iron, facilitating iron absorption. Fresh juices are excellent sources of water-soluble vitamins (many of the B vitamins and vitamin C), some fat-soluble vitamins (the carotenes, known as provitamin A, which are converted to vitamin A as needed by the body), and vitamins E and K.

Minerals. Your body needs about two dozen minerals to function normally. Minerals, along with vitamins, are components of enzymes. Minerals also make up part of bone and blood tissue, and help maintain normal cell function. The major minerals include calcium, chloride, magnesium, phosphorus, potassium, sodium, and sulfur. Trace minerals are those needed in very small amounts, which include boron, chromium, cobalt, copper, fluoride, manganese, nickel, selenium, vanadium, and zinc. Plants incorporate minerals, which occur in inorganic forms in the soil, into their tissues. As a part of this process, the minerals are combined with organic molecules into easily absorbable forms, which makes plant food an excellent dietary source of minerals. Juicing is believed to provide even better mineral absorption than eating whole fruits and vegetables because the process of juicing liberates minerals into a highly absorbable form.

Enzymes. Fresh juices are chock-full of enzymes—those "living" molecules that work, often with vitamins and minerals, to speed up reactions necessary for the human body to function. Without enzymes, we would not have life in our cells. Enzymes are prevalent in raw foods, but heat, such as is used in cooking and pasteurization, destroys them. Fresh juice contains enzymes that help break down food in the digestive tract, thereby sparing the body's enzyme producers from overwork. This sparing action is known as the "law of adaptive secretion of digestive enzymes." According to this law, when a portion of the food you eat is digested by enzymes present in the food itself, the body will secrete less of its own enzymes. This allows the body's energy to be shifted from digestion to other functions such as repair and rejuvenation. Fresh juices require very little energy expenditure to digest. And that is one reason people who start drinking fresh juice regularly often report that they feel better and are more energized right away.

Phytochemicals. Plants contain substances that protect them from disease, injury, and pollution. These substances are known as phytochemicals; "phyto" means plant and "chemical" in this context means nutrient. There are tens of thousands of phytochemicals in the foods we eat. For example, the average tomato may contain up to ten thousand different types of phytochemicals, the most famous being lycopene. Phytochemicals give plants their color, odor, and flavor. (Unlike vitamins and enzymes, they are heat stable, meaning that they can withstand cooking.) Researchers have found that the people who eat the most fruits and vegetables, which are the best sources of phytochemicals, have the lowest incidence of cancer and other diseases. Drinking vegetable juices gives you these vital substances in a concentrated form. Here are just a few of these plant heroes and what they do for us:

- Allyl sulfides, in garlic and onions, have been found to lower the risk of stomach cancer.
- Curcumins, present in gingerroot and the spice turmeric, stimulate the activity of chemicals called glutathione S-transferase, which are thought to be cancer inhibitors.
- Ellagic acid, found in grapes and strawberries, neutralizes cancer-causing agents and prevents these agents from altering the DNA in cells (a first step in the process by which cancer develops).

- Gingerol, found in gingerroot, has been shown to help reduce inflammation, lower cholesterol levels, and heal ulcers.
- Indoles, isothiocyanates, and sulforaphanes, which are found in the cruciferous vegetable family (broccoli, cabbage, and cauliflower), are thought to lower the risk of breast, lung, and stomach cancer.
- Limonene, found in citrus fruits, stimulates enzymes that break down carcinogens.
- Lycopene, abundant in tomatoes, has been shown to lower the risk of stomach and prostate cancer.
- Monoterpenes, found in cherries, have been shown to lower the risk of breast, skin, liver, lung, stomach, and pancreatic cancer.

✳ Some Commonly Asked Questions About Juicing

Now that you know why juice is so good for your health, you may have some questions about juicing. Following are some of the most commonly asked questions:

✳ *Isn't it better to eat whole fruits and vegetables for the fiber?*

Of course we need to eat whole vegetables and fruits for fiber. Whole fruits and vegetables have insoluble and soluble fiber. Both fibers are very important for colon health. However, soluble fiber in the form of pectin, gums, and mucilage is found in juice. That is a fact proven by research. These soluble fibers are excellent for the digestive tract. They also help to lower blood cholesterol levels, stabilize blood sugar, and improve good bowel bacteria.

✳ *Does a significant percentage of the nutrients get lost because they're attached to the insoluble fiber?*

In the past, some people thought that a significant amount of nutrients remained with the insoluble fiber after juicing, but that theory has been disproved. The Department of Agriculture analyzed twelve fruits and found that 90 percent of the antioxidant activity was in the juice rather than the ejected fiber. That is why juice makes such a great supplement to a high-fiber diet.

✳ *Is fresh juice better than commercially processed juice?*

Fresh juice is "live food" with its full complement of vitamins, minerals, phytochemicals, and enzymes. It also contains that living ingredient—*light energy*—that revitalizes the body. You feel different when you drink it. In contrast, commercially processed canned, bottled, frozen, or packaged juices have been pasteurized, which means the juice has been heated to high temperatures, and many of the vitamins and enzymes have been killed or removed. This means the juice will have longer shelf life, but it won't give your body the kind of life you'll get from raw juice. Making your own juice also allows you to use a wider variety of vegetables, stems, and leaves you might not get otherwise. For example, some of the recipes in this book include Jerusalem artichokes and jicama, beetroot leaves, green cabbage, celery leaves, and parsley. These sweet, crisp tubers and healthy greens are not found in most processed juices.

✳ *How long can fresh juice be stored?*

The sooner you drink juice after you make it, the more nutrients you'll get. However, you can store juice and not lose too many nutrients by keeping it cold and covered, such as in an airtight container, in the refrigerator, or in a thermos.

On a personal note: When I had chronic fatigue syndrome, I would juice in the afternoons, when I had the most energy, store the juice covered in the refrigerator, and drink it for the next twenty-four hours until I juiced my next batch.

✳ *How much produce do you need to make a glass of juice?*

People often ask me if it takes a bushel basket of produce to make a glass of juice. Actually, if you're using a good juicer, it takes a surprisingly small amount of produce. For example, all of the following items, each weighing roughly a pound, yield about one eight-ounce glass of juice: three medium apples, five to seven carrots, or one large cucumber. The following each yield about four ounces of juice: three large (thirteen-inch) stalks of celery or one orange. Juicing is actually economical as well as nutritious.

✳ Choosing the Right Juicer

To gain the greatest benefits of juicing, choose the juicer that is right for you. It can make the difference between juicing daily and never juicing again.

First, I need to distinguish between a blender and a juicer. A juicer separates the liquid from the pulp (insoluble fiber). A blender liquefies everything that is placed in it; it doesn't separate the pulp from the juice. If you think it might be a good idea to have carrot, beetroot, parsley, or celery pulp in your juice for added fiber, I can tell you from experience that it tastes like juicy sawdust. For the most flavorful vegetable juice, which is juice you'll drink every day, I recommend using a juicer. Look for the following features:

- *Choose a machine with adequate horsepower (hp).* I recommend a juicer with 0.5 hp. Weak machines with low horsepower ratings must run at extremely high rpm (revolutions per minute). A machine's rpm does not accurately reflect its ability to perform effectively because rpm is calculated when the juicer is running idle, not while it is juicing. When you feed produce into a low-power machine, the rpm will be reduced dramatically, and sometimes the juicer will come to a full stop. I have "killed" some machines on the first carrot I juiced.
- *Sustained blade speed during juicing.* Look for a machine that has electronic circuitry that sustains blade speed during juicing.
- *Able to juice all types of produce.* Pick a machine that can juice tough, hard vegetables and fruits, such as carrots and beetroot, as well as delicate greens, such as parsley, lettuce, and herbs. Make sure it does not need a special citrus attachment. For wheatgrass juice, you'll need a wheatgrass juicer. The machines that juice wheatgrass along with other vegetables are very time-consuming to clean and use.
- *Large feed tube.* Look for a large feed tube so that you don't have to cut your produce into very small pieces before juicing. This saves a lot of time.
- *Ejects pulp.* Choose a juicer that ejects pulp into a receptacle. This design is far better than one in which all the pulp stays inside the machine, and so has to be scooped out frequently. Juicers that keep the pulp in the center basket rather than ejecting it cannot juice continuously. You'll need to stop the machine often to wash it out. Plus, you can line the pulp catcher with a free plastic bag from the grocery store produce section and you won't have to wash the receptacle each time. When you're done juicing, you can either toss the pulp or use it in cooking or composting.
- *Only a few parts to clean.* Look for a juicer with only a few parts to clean. The more parts a juicer has, and the more complicated the parts are to wash, the longer it will take to clean your juicer and put it back together. That makes it less likely you will use your machine daily. Also, make sure the parts are dishwasher-safe.

- *Tool that loosens blade not recommended.* There are popular juicers that need a tool to loosen the blade. I've had such juicers and found this to be a hassle. Plus, if you lose the tool, you can't use your juicer until you order a new one.

✳ Getting the Most from Your Juicer

Juicing is a very simple process, though it helps to keep a few guidelines in mind to get the best possible results:

- *Wash all produce before juicing.* Fruit and vegetable washes are available at many grocery and health food stores. Cut away all moldy, bruised, or damaged areas.
- *Always peel oranges, tangerines, and grapefruits* before juicing because the skins of these citrus fruits contain bitter-tasting oils that can cause digestive problems. (Lemon and lime peels can be juiced, if organic, but they also add a distinct flavor that is not one of my favorites in most recipes. I usually peel them.) Leave as much of the white pithy part on the citrus fruit as possible, since it contains the most vitamin C and bioflavonoids. Always peel mangoes and papayas, since their skins contain an irritant that is harmful when eaten in quantity. Also, I recommend that you peel all produce that is not labeled organic, even though the largest concentration of nutrients is in and next to the skin. The peels and skins of sprayed fruits and vegetables also contain the largest concentration of pesticides.
- *Remove pits, stones, and hard seeds* from such fruits as peaches, plums, apricots, cherries, and mangoes. Softer seeds from oranges, lemons, watermelons, cantaloupes, cucumbers, grapes, and apples can be juiced without a problem. Because of their chemical composition, apple seeds should not be juiced in large quantities for young children, but usually don't cause problems for adults.
- *You can juice the stems and leaves* of most produce—for example, beetroot stems and leaves, strawberry caps, celery leaves, and small grape stems—since they offer valuable nutrients. Discard larger grape stems, as they can dull the juicer blade. Also remove carrot and rhubarb greens because they contain toxic substances.
- *Cut fruits and vegetables* into sections or chunks that will fit your juicer's feed tube. You'll learn from experience what size works best for your machine. If you have a large feed tube, you won't have to cut up a lot of produce.

- *Some fruits and vegetables don't juice well.* Most produce contains a lot of water, which is ideal for juicing. Those vegetables and fruits that contain less water, such as bananas, mangoes, papayas, and avocados, will not juice well. They can be used in smoothies and cold soups by first juicing any other produce and then pouring the juice into a blender and adding the avocado, for example, to make a cold soup.
- *Drink your juice as soon as it's made, if possible.* If you can't drink it right away, store it in an insulated container such as a thermos or an airtight, opaque container in the refrigerator for up to twenty-four hours. Light, heat, and air destroy nutrients quickly. Be aware that the longer juice sits before you drink it, the more nutrients it loses. If juice turns brown, it has oxidized and lost a large amount of its nutritional value. After twenty-four hours, it may become spoiled. Melon and cabbage juices do not store well; drink them soon after they've been made.

✳ Choose Organic Produce

The best way to get the healthiest juice possible is to use organic produce whenever available. The popularity of organic foods has increased dramatically in recent years, and continues to grow. Sales of organic foods reach into the billions of dollars each year and have been growing annually. It appears that a large number of people want to avoid the billion pounds or more of pesticides and herbicides sprayed onto or added to our crops yearly. And for good reason. It is estimated that only about 2 percent of this amount actually fights insects and weeds, while the rest is absorbed into our air, soil, and water. These pesticide residues pose long-term health risks, such as cancer and birth defects, and immediate health risks from acute intoxication, such as vomiting, diarrhea, blurred vision, tremors, convulsions, and nerve damage. If pesticides and herbicides do not (as we're told) pose a risk to our health, then why is there a greater incidence of cancer—lymphoma, leukemia, and cancer of the brain, skin, stomach, and prostate—among farmers and their families when compared with cancer rates among the general public?

I'm often asked if organic produce is more nutritious than conventionally grown produce. Studies have shown that it is. According to results from a $25 million study of organic food—the largest of its kind to date—organic completely outshines conventional produce. A four-year European Union–funded study found that organic fruits and vegetables contain up to 40 percent more antioxidants. They have higher levels of beneficial minerals like iron and zinc. Milk from organic herds contains up to 90 percent more antioxidants. The researchers obtained their results after growing fruits and vegetables, and raising cattle, on adjacent organic and nonorganic sites. They say that eating organic foods can even help to increase the nutrient intake of people who don't eat nine to thirteen servings of fruits and vegetables a day (*New York Times* online, October 28, 2007).

Additionally, a 2001 study done as part of a doctoral dissertation at Johns Hopkins University looked at forty-one studies involving field trials, greenhouse pot experiments, market basket surveys, and surveys of farmers. The most-studied nutrients across those surveys included calcium, copper, iron, magnesium, manganese, phosphorus, potassium, sodium, zinc, beta-carotene, and vitamin C. According to the study, there was significantly more vitamin C (27 percent), iron (21 percent), magnesium (29 percent), and phosphorus (13 percent) in the organic produce than in the conventionally grown vegetables. The vegetables that had the biggest increases in nutrients between organic and conventional production were lettuce, spinach, carrots, potatoes, and cabbage. Couple that with fewer chemical residues and you can see that buying organically grown food is well worth the effort and the additional cost.

When choosing organically grown foods, look for labels marked "certified organic." This means the produce has been cultivated according to strict uniform standards that are verified by independent state or private organizations. Certification includes inspection of farms and processing facilities, detailed record keeping, and pesticide testing of soil and water to ensure that growers and handlers are meeting government standards. You may occasionally see a label that says "transitional organic." This means the food was grown on a farm that recently converted, or is in the process of converting, from chemical to organic farming.

You may not be able to afford to purchase everything organic. When that's the case, choose wisely. According to the Environmental Working Group, a non-profit research organization, commercially farmed fruits and vegetables vary in their levels of pesticide residue. Some vegetables, like broccoli, asparagus, and onions, as well as foods with peels, such as avocados, bananas, and oranges, have relatively low levels of pesticides compared to other fruits and vegetables. However, some vegetables and fruit contain large amounts of pesticide.

Four Foods That Are a Must-Buy Organic

Potatoes: Potatoes are a staple of the American diet. One survey found that they account for 30 percent of our overall vegetable consumption. A simple switch to organic potatoes has the potential to have a big impact because commercially farmed potatoes are some of the most pesticide-contaminated vegetables. A 2006 USDA test found that 81 percent of potatoes tested still contained pesticides after being washed and peeled, and the potato has one of the highest pesticide contents of forty-three fruits and vegetables tested, according to the Environmental Working Group.

Peanut butter: Go organic with kid favorites like peanut butter. More acres are devoted to growing peanuts than any other legume, fruit, vegetable, or nut, according to the USDA. More than 99 percent of peanut farms use conventional farming practices, including the use of fungicide to treat mold, a common problem in peanut crops. Given that some kids eat peanut butter almost every day, this seems like a simple and practical switch. Organic brands are readily available in regular grocery stores.

Ketchup: For some families, ketchup accounts for a large part of the household vegetable intake. About 75 percent of tomato consumption is in the form of processed tomatoes, including juice, tomato paste, and ketchup. Notably, recent research has shown that organic ketchup has about double the antioxidants of conventional ketchup.

Apples: Apples are the second most commonly eaten fresh fruit, after bananas. Apple juice is the second most popular, after orange juice. But apples are also one of the most pesticide-contaminated fruits. The good news is that organic apples are easy to find in regular grocery stores.

When organic vegetables or fruits that you want are not available, ask your grocer to get them. You can also look for small-operation farmers in your area and check out farmers' markets in season. Many small farms can't afford to use as many chemicals in farming as large commercial farms. Another option is to order organic produce by mail (see Sources, page 347).

Avoid the "Dirty Dozen"

Though I strongly suggest that you buy all organically grown produce, I recommend that you especially avoid buying conventionally grown foods on the "dirty dozen" list. And if you can't afford to purchase all organic, you could still fare

* * *

The Dirty Dozen List	The Cleanest Food List
• Peaches	• Papaya
• Apples	• Kiwifruit
• Bell peppers	• Bananas
• Celery	• Broccoli
• Nectarines	• Onions
• Strawberries	• Asparagus
• Cherries	• Sweet peas
• Pears	• Mangos
• Grapes (especially imported varieties)	• Cauliflower
• Spinach	• Pineapples
• Lettuce	• Avocados
• Potatoes	• Sweet corn

quite well when buying conventionally grown produce on the "cleanest food" list. The Environmental Working Group reports periodically on health risks posed by pesticides in produce. The group says you can cut your pesticide exposure by almost 90 percent simply by avoiding the twelve conventionally grown fruits and vegetables that have been found to be the most contaminated. It has been discovered that eating these contaminated produce items will expose a person to about fourteen pesticides per day, on average. Eating the twelve least contaminated will expose a person to fewer than two pesticides per day. This list changes year to year, based on testing. You can keep updated at www.foodnews.org.

What About Irradiated Food?

Stay away from irradiated fruits and vegetables. Some food producers use gamma-ray radiation to kill pests and germs in stored food, and to increase the food's shelf life. Although the Food and Drug Administration (FDA) has approved the practice, eating irradiated food is not a wise choice. The average dose of radiation used to decontaminate most foods can be up to 5 million times that of a typical chest X-ray. This practice destroys vitamins, phytochemicals, and enzymes. It also generates harmful by-products such as free radicals, which are toxins that can damage cells, and harmful chemicals known as radiolytic products, including formaldehyde and benzene.

Irradiation of fruits and vegetables poses an even greater problem than irradiation of other foods because the large quantities of water found in produce allow for greater free-radical production. The answer to food-borne illnesses is not irradiation, but stopping the overuse of pesticides, transforming overcrowded factory-farm animal lots, and ensuring more sanitary conditions in food-processing plants.

Say No to GMO

Whenever possible, avoid genetically modified foods, also known as GMs or GMOs. Scientists, doctors, and educators in many sectors of the health industry have long warned about the possible deleterious effects of GM crops on the health of animals and humans. An Australian project to develop genetically modified peas with built-in pest resistance had to be abandoned after tests showed they caused allergic lung damage in mice. A similar situation occurred in the early 1990s when a strain of bioengineered soybeans was found to cause an allergic response in people with Brazil nut allergies.

A March 2007 article in the journal *Archives of Environmental Contamination and Toxicology* reported on a study that was commissioned by the environmental group Greenpeace in which rats were fed for ninety days on GM maize (corn) developed by the chemical giant Monsanto. The rats showed signs of toxicity in the liver and kidneys. In reporting on this study, *Scientific American* quoted a statement by Greenpeace spokesman Arnaud Apoteker: "It is the first time that independent research, published in a peer-reviewed journal, has proved that a GMO authorized for human consumption presents signs of toxicity."

A genetically modified organism (GMO) is an organism whose genetic material has been altered using bioengineering techniques. These GMO foods have raised concerns because they force genetic information across the protective species barrier in an unnatural way. In other words, nature does not sustain them. These new organisms are in many cases untested, yet they are on grocery store shelves everywhere without protective labeling. We may not know we are buying them.

The United States is the main supplier of GMO seeds worldwide, and the crops are virtually uncontrolled in this country. On the other hand, many countries around the world have banned their use, including many in the European Union that are fighting to keep crops pure in their countries. Hungary, one of Europe's biggest grain producers, became the first country in Eastern Europe to ban GMO crops or foods when it outlawed the planting of maize seeds marketed by Monsanto in January 2005. As it stands now, we have about a 70 to 75 percent chance of picking a product with GMO ingredients without even realizing it. This is astounding! We need to take notice when we're selecting food to build our health and to remove toxins. We can each make it known that we don't want GMO crops grown in the United States by voting with our dollars, with the food we buy, signing petitions whenever possible, and making our voices heard with Congress.

We can avoid GMO foods by becoming aware of which foods are most prone to genetic engineering and what products are made from them. The biggest GM crops are soybeans, corn, and sugar beets, from which thousands of processed foods are made. Look at the labels to see if they contain corn flour or cornmeal, soy flour, cornstarch, textured vegetable protein, corn syrup, or modified food starch. Check labels of soy sauce, tofu, soy beverages, soy protein isolate, soymilk, soy ice cream, margarine, and soy lecithin, among dozens of other products. If it doesn't say organic for these foods, the chances are strong that they are GMOs, so don't buy it.

It's particularly important to choose organic soy and corn products to ensure that they are not GMO. Aside from corn and soy, other GMO foods grown in the United States include cotton, canola, squash, and papaya. Purchase only products labeled organic, especially when it comes to foods and by-products of food that are likely to be grown from GMO crops.

Become an informed consumer, since the FDA has refused to require labeling of genetically engineered foods, despite overwhelming American support for mandatory labeling. Since the agency has refused to protect us, some food companies are now taking action by labeling certain products or ingredients "non-GMO," which means "made without genetically modified organisms." The United States may soon be the only country in the world that does *not* require labeling of genetically engineered food.

Diseases are crises of purification,
of toxic elimination. Symptoms are
natural defenses of the body. We
call them diseases, but in fact they
are the cure of diseases.

—HIPPOCRATES

Using Juices for Healing

PEOPLE ALL OVER THE WORLD have found healing from ailments such as cancer, chronic fatigue syndrome, fibromyalgia, high blood pressure, heart disease, arthritis, and many other conditions by juicing and making dietary changes. The body was made to heal itself. When you provide it with the materials it needs for repair and rejuvenation, and remove irritating substances that contribute to disease and illness, the healing process begins. Therefore, make sure you add fresh juice and a healthy diet to whatever treatment plan your health-care provider recommends.

There is a large and growing body of scientific research that shows a firsthand connection between diet and the recovery process. Most of the diet and juice recommendations for the disorders covered in this section are based on such research, much of it done in recent years. I want you to benefit from the latest information. In addition, I have included remedies that are time-honored traditions, meaning people have used them for years and passed them down for generations because they worked. I have also included nutritional supplement and herb recommendations. And finally, I've made some lifestyle recommendations because I want you to have a well-rounded health plan. My desire is that this book can be your resource guide for ailments. I don't want you to have to search, as I did for such a long time, to find answers to your health questions. I want you to find what you need in an easily accessible format.

There are a few tips you should be aware of before using this section. While using organic produce is always a good idea, it is especially important for some fruits and vegetables (see "Avoid the Dirty Dozen," page 21). If you have more than one ailment, you may sometimes find conflicting advice, such as the recommendation to add fruit juice under one disorder and the caution to omit all fruit under another. In this case, always omit the items as advised.

Be aware that getting well can be like unraveling a tangled ball of yarn; sometimes the situation gets worse before it gets better. Such "healing crises" are often a sign that the body is ridding itself of toxins. This is known as the Herxheimer reaction, and during the process you might get headaches, chills, skin eruptions, diarrhea, rashes, or cold or flulike symptoms as your body releases toxic substances. The important point is for you not to give up on your recovery efforts.

Finally, if your health professional has prescribed nutritional supplements for your condition, note that supplements work best when taken with juices that are high in those nutrients. Nature has combined vitamins, minerals, enzymes, phytochemicals, and many other compounds that act as cofactors (helpers) to make your vitamins and minerals more effectively absorbed and utilized. You will get the maximum healing possible when you incorporate freshly made juices, especially vegetable juices, into your health and healing recovery plan.

✳ Juicing for a Life of Vibrant Health

Juicing is an easy, delicious way to add the goodness of fruits and vegetables to your daily diet. A good juicer and fresh produce will allow you to enjoy a wealth of nutrients every day, which is important even if your health is good. If your health is not good, juicing is even more vital. In the next section, I'll show you how to use juicing in the treatment of various disorders to regain your health and enjoy energy and high-level wellness. You may never know how good you can feel until you make juicing fresh organic vegetables a way of life.

Allergies

AIRBORNE ALLERGENS such as pollen, dander, and dust mites can cause what is popularly called hay fever (allergic rhinitis). Hay fever is marked by watery nasal discharge, sneezing, and itchy eyes, nose, and skin. It occurs when the immune system overreacts to the allergen(s), causing the release of an inflammatory chemical called histamine. Allergies occur when certain cells in an individual's body become too sensitive to a foreign particle (allergen), thus causing a variety of symptoms. Up to one-third of people with seasonal allergies may suffer oral *allergy* syndrome (OAS), which results from a cross-reactivity between seasonal airborne pollen proteins from weeds, grass, and trees and similar proteins in some fresh fruits, vegetables, nuts, seeds, certain sweeteners, and herbs. For example, people with ragweed pollen allergies might experience symptoms if they eat foods such as bananas, cucumbers, melons, zucchini, sunflower seeds, chamomile tea, and echinacea. People with birch tree pollen allergies may experience OAS symptoms if they eat foods such as peaches, apples, pears, cherries, carrots, hazelnuts, kiwifruit, or almonds. In most cases, cooking these foods will reduce or prevent an allergic reaction.

Food allergy is a reaction of the body's immune system to something in a food or an ingredient in a food—usually a protein. The number of people suffering from food allergies and other adverse reactions to food has gone up dramatically in recent years. Symptoms of food allergy differ greatly among individuals. They can also differ in the same person during different exposures. Celiac disease is sometimes considered a food allergy because it is the result of an adverse immune response to gluten, a protein in wheat, barley, rye, and oats. Common symptoms of food allergy include skin irritations such as rashes, hives, and eczema, and gastrointestinal symptoms such as nausea, diarrhea, and vomiting. Sneezing, runny nose, and shortness of breath can also result from food allergy, as can dizziness, fatigue, headaches, panic attacks, dark circles or puffiness under the eyes, chronic fluid retention, and swollen glands. Some individuals may experience a more severe reaction called anaphylaxis. Food allergy causes roughly thirty thousand episodes of anaphylaxis yearly and one hundred to two hundred deaths per year in the United States. Nuts and peanuts are the leading causes of deadly allergic reactions.

Some people are sensitive but not allergic to naturally occurring substances found in a variety of foods, including dairy, wheat, corn, eggs, fish, nuts, soy, chocolate, peanuts, shellfish, preservatives, and colorings. Food intolerances often get confused with food allergies. Symptoms can include adverse reactions to a food substance that involves digestion or metabolism. Lactose intolerance is one of the most common types of food intolerance. It occurs when a person lacks an enzyme needed to digest milk sugar, and symptoms include gas, bloating, and abdominal pain. Fewer people have true food allergy involving the immune system than have food intolerances.

The primary cause of the increase in food allergies in recent years appears to be genetically modified (GM) foods. In June 2007, the Institute for Responsible Technology reported on studies (twenty-eight references cited) that point out the effects of GM foods on the rise in food allergies. GM crops resist pests because their genetic makeup contains pesticides that destroy the digestive system of the bugs that eat the crop. The foods are supposedly safe for humans, but research contends that they cause extensive allergic reactions, particularly in susceptible individuals. Soy, a leading GM crop in this country, is the foremost allergenic food for children. Other contributors include frequent consumption of such food additives as dyes, stabilizers, preservatives, and flavorings (items often found in commercially prepared foods), and eating the same foods over and over, such as wheat, sugar, and dairy products. Other causes are linked to heredity, stress, infection, low nutritional status, introducing solid foods too early to infants, and impaired digestion.

❋ Avoid the "Dirty Dozen"

Though I recommend that you buy all organically grown produce, it is especially important to avoid conventionally grown foods on the "dirty dozen" list (see page 22).

❋ Lifestyle Recommendations

For airborne allergies, eliminate allergens to the extent possible. Clean (often and well) carpets, rugs, upholstered furniture, and other surfaces where allergens can collect. Allergy-proof your bedroom. Encase the mattress, box spring, and pillows in allergen-proof covers, and wash bedding, towels, curtains, and clothing in environmentally friendly, fragrance-free detergent. Install an air purifier with a HEPA filter (a special filter that can trap tiny particles). Use a vacuum cleaner that has a HEPA filter. Have your furnace and air ducts cleaned yearly. Dust can build up in these places and make your allergy symptoms worse.

Reduce stress levels as much as possible. Stress weakens the immune system, which increases susceptibility to, and magnitude of, an allergic response. To learn more, see Stress, page 261.

❋ Diet Recommendations

For food allergies, identify the offending food(s). The Elimination Diet (see page 301) can help you pinpoint the offenders. Keep in mind that a food allergy or intolerance may be something you like and eat often, since people frequently develop cravings for foods to which they are allergic (see Cravings, page 118). Once allergenic or intolerant foods are identified, the next step is to rotate foods, both to control preexisting allergies or intolerances and to prevent the development of new ones. As much as possible, continue to avoid all foods to which you are sensitive.

Consume more raw fruits, vegetables, and fresh vegetable juices. Strengthening the immune system and cleansing the liver are at the root of improving the body's response to all allergens. This requires high-level nutrition and specialized cleansing programs (see pages 303–325). At least 50 percent of your diet should consist of raw fruits, vegetables, vegetable juices, sprouts, nuts, and seeds. Eating junk foods, along with too many cooked and commercially prepared foods, strains the digestive system. The organs that produce digestive juices are then overburdened because enzymes are missing in these "nutritionally empty" foods. This leads to deficiencies in important enzymes that are needed to break down foods properly and provide nutrients for the cells. In addition, constant stimulation of the digestive organs can result in excess acidity within the body and an overstressed enzymatic system, which leads to allergies. Raw foods and freshly made vegetable juices alkalinize the body and provide an abundance of enzymes that help the digestive system return to balance. After one eats raw foods freely for a period of time, many allergies subside, as confirmed by Dr. John Douglas, who has worked extensively with allergy patients at the Kaiser Permanente Medical Center in Los Angeles. (For more information, see Basic Guidelines for the Juice Lady's Health and Healing Diet, page 290).

Avoid sugar and alcohol. Sugar and alcohol produce an acidic condition in the body that can accentuate allergic reactions, especially those to airborne allergens. (Alcohol acts like sugar in the body.)

✳ Nutrient Recommendations

Bioflavonoids, especially quercetin, have been shown to both reduce histamine levels and relieve allergy symptoms. Quercetin inhibits the release of an inflammatory chemical called arachidonic acid and reduces histamine release. Yellow onions and shallots are particularly rich sources of quercetin. In addition, bioflavonoids, along with molybdenum and selenium, enhance the actions of vitamin C. *Best juice sources of bioflavonoids:* bell peppers, berries (blueberry, blackberry, and cranberry), broccoli, cabbage, lemons, limes, parsley, and tomatoes.

Gamma-linolenic acid (GLA) is a fatty acid the body uses to make inflammation-inhibiting substances called prostaglandins. GLA is found in evening primrose oil, which is best taken in supplement form.

Vitamin C benefits allergy sufferers by providing an important cellular defense against oxidizing agents, tissue-damaging substances that are produced in increased amounts during allergic reactions. *Best juice sources of vitamin C:* kale, parsley, broccoli, Brussels sprouts, watercress, cauliflower, cabbage, strawberries, spinach, lemons, limes, turnips, and asparagus. Carotenes enhance vitamin C's effectiveness, and are found abundantly in most fruits and vegetables that are high in vitamin C.

✳ Help for Seasonal Airborne Allergies

The supplements for seasonal airborne allergies should be taken from early spring to the time of the first frost. Try substituting quercetin for over-the-counter medications. It inhibits histamine release without side effects, in direct contrast to many medications that simply block the effect of histamine during an allergic reaction. When combined with the herb nettle, it's quite effective against sneezing, itching, and swollen nasal passages. Nasal congestion may be reduced with pantothenic acid, a B vitamin.

Dosages

- Nettle: 250–300 mg on an empty stomach three times daily. Standardized to contain at least one percent of the herb silica.
- Vitamin C: 1,000 mg three times daily. If diarrhea develops, reduce the dose.
- Quercetin: 500 mg two times daily. Take about twenty minutes before meals.
- Pantothenic acid: 500 mg three times daily. Take with food.

✳ Herb Recommendations

Astragalus can help build overall health and strengthen the body. You should take one dose daily one month before hay fever season. As a precautionary step, do not take it if signs of an infection or fever exist. Children who have chronic allergies can be given a dose two to three times daily for a week.

Licorice inhibits phospholipase A, an enzyme that, like platelet-activating factor, starts inflammatory reactions. Use a medicinal form of the herb, not licorice candy. Avoid licorice if you have high blood pressure, and do not use for prolonged periods of time.

✳ Juice Therapy

Alfalfa sprout and celery juices especially raise blood alkalinity, which helps reduce allergic reactions.

Parsley juice helps stop allergy attacks, and ounce for ounce has more than three times the vitamin C of oranges. Drink parsley juice immediately after an allergic reaction; this may help ease the symptoms. (If it's a serious anaphylactic reaction, seek medical help immediately.) A safe, therapeutic dose is one-half to one cup of parsley juice per day. Parsley can be toxic in overdose, and should be especially avoided by pregnant women.

✳ Juice Recipes

Pure Green Sprout Drink (*pg 340*)   **Allergy Relief** (*pg 326*)   **Waldorf Twist** (*pg 345*)
Ginger Twist (*pg 322*)   **Morning Energizer** (*pg 337*)   **Antiviral Cocktail** (*pg 327*)
Beet-Cucumber Cleansing Cocktail (*pg 328*)   **Healthy-Sinus Solution** (*pg 334*)
Immune Builder (*pg 335*)   **Liver Life Tonic** (*pg 336*)   **Peppy Parsley** (*pg 339*)
Wheatgrass Light (*pg 345*)

Alzheimer's Disease and Dementia

ALZHEIMER'S DISEASE (AD) is marked by tissue atrophy within the frontal and temporal parts of the brain, resulting in the loss of mental capacity. It leads to nerve cell death and tissue loss throughout the brain. Over time, the brain shrinks dramatically, affecting nearly all its functions. The cortex shrivels up, damaging areas involved in thinking, planning, and remembering. AD is characterized by a loss of cognitive function and memory, and typically interferes with daily activities until the person loses all ability to care for him or herself. Symptoms can include depression, incontinence, delusions, hallucinations, aggression, rage, combativeness, wandering, binge eating, and lack of sexual constraint. Symptoms usually worsen with time.

Dementia is the progressive loss of mental function, including short- and long-term memory. This condition is characterized by mental disorientation and impaired judgment; it typically has an adverse effect on emotions and learning capabilities, and it may cause functional incontinence.

Today more than 5 million Americans have AD. That includes 10 percent of those over sixty-five years of age, and nearly 50 percent of those over eighty-five. By 2050 that number may reach 16 million. The likelihood of developing AD doubles every five years after age sixty-five. After age eighty-five, the risk is approximately 50 percent.

AD occurs when protein-based plaques are deposited in the brain. Doctors believe that the plaques and tangles seen in this disease cause the brain damage. Family history is an important risk factor. If a parent or sibling has AD, you could be two to three times more likely to develop it. Serious head injury is thought to be a risk factor, along with smoking. Latinos and African Americans seem to have a greater risk.

Adults with damaged blood vessels in their brain or atrophy in their temporal lobe are more likely to develop AD. It is known that blood vessel damage in the brain is more likely to occur in patients with high blood pressure, high cholesterol, or diabetes. Therefore, prevention of these conditions can lower risk of developing Alzheimer's, as well as preventing heart attack and stroke.

One encouraging finding is that researchers have discovered that one-third of those with an average age of eighty-five did not experience signs of cognitive decline, despite the fact that half of them had significant Alzheimer's disease pathology and close to one-quarter had cerebral vascular disease. Researchers believe these people have a sort of "reserve capacity" that allows them to stay cognitively sharp even though their brains showed signs of disease.

✳ Lifestyle Recommendations

There are several lifestyle factors that could help prevent and/or reverse AD, which include:

- Get intellectual stimulation (e.g., playing chess, cards, or games, or doing crossword puzzles).
- Get regular physical exercise.
- Engage in regular social interaction. Lonely individuals may be twice as likely to develop the type of dementia linked to AD in later stages of life as those who are not lonely.

- Don't worry; worry accelerates your risk of AD.
- Drink purified water. Fluoridated water has been implicated as a contributing factor in AD. Fluoride's ability to damage the brain represents one of the most active areas of research on fluoride toxicity today.
- Eat less food. No plaque development occurred in mice that were fed a restricted diet (meaning they couldn't eat all they wanted). The restricted diet activated pathways responsible for breaking down beta-amyloid peptides in the brain before they were able to form plaques.
- Based on data from the Women's Health Initiative, female hormone-replacement therapy is no longer thought to prevent dementia, and it poses other health risks.

✳ Diet Recommendations

Eat a Mediterranean-type diet with an emphasis on whole foods and plenty of fresh fruits and vegetables, as well as being low in animal fat.

Cook with curry. In India, the rate of AD is more than four times less than that in the United States. Some researchers believe this is due partly to curcumin, the yellow pigment in curry. Curcumin is more effective in inhibiting the formation of protein fragments than many other potential AD treatments. The structure of curcumin allows it to penetrate the blood–brain barrier effectively and bind to beta-amyloid (the main constituent of amyloid plaques in the brains of Alzheimer's disease patients).

Drink fresh vegetable juice. Drink a minimum of one glass of fresh vegetable juice at least four days a week. The KAME project (*The American Journal of Medicine,* 2006) showed that those who drank such juices more than three times per week compared to less than once a week were 76 percent less likely to develop AD. These juices are rich in polyphenols, which offer even stronger protection than antioxidants against hydrogen peroxide, which causes oxidative damage in the brain. Fresh vegetable juice can play an important role in delaying or preventing the onset of AD. And if you have AD, it just might help improve your symptoms.

On a personal note: One woman who contacted me was caring for an AD patient. When she started giving the lady fresh vegetable juice every day, she noticed a striking improvement in the lady's health and cognitive abilities. She said that even the neighbors began commenting on the improvement in the patient's condition.

Avoid all sweeteners. A research study found that drinking sugary beverages like soda may increase the risk of AD. Although the exact mechanisms aren't known, obesity and diabetes are both associated with higher incidences of AD. Researchers have tested whether high sugar consumption in an otherwise normal diet would affect AD progression. They used a genetic mouse model that develops Alzheimer's-like symptoms in adulthood, and over a twenty-five-week period supplemented the regular, balanced diet of half the animals with 10 percent sugar water. Afterward, they compared the metabolism, memory skills (by means of various mazes), and brain composition of the regular and sugar-fed mice. The sugar-fed mice gained about 17 percent more weight than controls, had higher cholesterol levels, and developed insulin resistance. These mice also had worse learning and memory retention, and their brains contained more than twice as many amyloid acidic plaque deposits, an anatomical hallmark of AD. The only sweeteners I recommend using (and only in small amounts) are stevia (found at health food stores) and agave syrup.

Avoid the excitotoxins MSG and aspartame. These two substances are called excitotoxins because they "excite" brain neurons due to their chemical similarity to neurotransmitters found in the body. Because of this, these chemicals turn into dangerous and addictive compounds that kill brain cells. It has been demonstrated that high concentrations of blood glutamate and aspartame from foods can enter the so-called "protected brain" by seeping through the unprotected areas, such as the hypothalamus. When you consume excitotoxins from foods that contain MSG and aspartame (NutraSweet), chronic elevations of blood glutamate and aspartame can even seep through the normal blood–brain barrier when these high concentrations are maintained over a long period of time. Glutamate functions as a very excitatory neurotransmitter and is caustic to the brain in large quantities. Experiments show that fifteen to thirty minutes after neurons suspended in tissue culture are exposed to high levels of glutamate, they swell up like balloons. The chemical process going on within the cell releases free radicals that kill brain cells. Glutamate is often thought to play a role in AD, senile dementia, and adult mental illness.

Both MSG and aspartame are found in milk products, soft drinks, candy, chewing gum, health drink powders, some medications, and binders for nutritional supplements, and both prescription and over-the-counter medicines. Food manufacturers skillfully hide MSG behind many ingredient names that are printed on food packages, including gelatin, calcium caseinate, textured vegetable protein, sodium caseinate, yeast nutrient, autolyzed yeast, hydrolyzed protein, carrageenan, maltodextrin, malt extract, natural food flavoring, bouillon, natural chicken flavoring, natural beef flavoring, soy sauce extract, whey protein concentrate, and anything protein fortified, containing flavorings, or enzyme modified. Some of the products known to contain aspartame include sugar-free foods, chewing gum, beverages, gelatin desserts, packaged sweeteners, ice cream, breath mints, cereals, cocoa mixes, coffee beverages, frozen desserts, juice drinks, multivitamins, pharmaceuticals, health supplements, instant tea and coffee, topping mixes, wine coolers, and yogurt.

✳ Nutrient Recommendations

Amino acids. Patients with properly diagnosed Alzheimer's or Parkinson's disease typically have inefficient dopamine (a chemical compound found in the brain). When neurotransmitters are tested in urine, they can be either too elevated or too low. Either is reflective of inefficient levels of dopamine for focus and memory. Balancing neurotransmitters allows for improving the brain's response to stress. If we are able to handle stress well we are less likely to have anxiety and worry or sleep cycle problems, which are a causal factor in adrenal fatigue; and depletions in dopamine (responsible for short- and long-term memory). Alzheimer's patients who utilize amino acid therapy typically have more energy, less depression, and less rage and combativeness. (For more information on amino acid testing, see Sources, page 347).

Antioxidants can neutralize free radicals, and an increase in free-radical damage and fat damage has been seen in people with AD. Antioxidants protect autonomic nerve cells (those involved in automatic bodily functions) from being destroyed. Be sure you get plenty of the following nutrients:

- **Beta-carotene** is a powerful antioxidant. *Best juice sources of beta-carotene*: carrots, kale, parsley, spinach, Swiss chard, beetroot greens, watercress, broccoli, and romaine lettuce.
- **Selenium** helps activate glutathione peroxidase, an enzyme that serves as an antioxidant. *Best juice sources of selenium:* Swiss chard, turnips, garlic, radishes, carrots, and cabbage.

- **Vitamin C** helps protect brain cells from free-radical attack. *Best juice sources of vitamin C:* kale, parsley, broccoli, Brussels sprouts, watercress, cauliflower, cabbage, strawberries, spinach, lemons, limes, turnips, and asparagus.

Omega-3 fats, which are often deficient in a typical Western diet, are essential for the creation of strong cell membranes. Faulty cell membranes play a role in degenerative diseases such as AD. In comparing the brain cell membranes of AD patients with those of other individuals, scientists found a dramatic reduction in the essential fatty acid (EFA) content and an increase in the saturated fat content. A report in the April 2006 *Nature* described the first direct evidence for how omega-3s might have a helpful effect on nerve cells (neurons). Working with laboratory cell cultures, the researchers found that omega-3s stimulate growth of the branches that connect one cell to another. Rich branching creates a dense "neuron forest," which provides the basis of the brain's capacity to process, store, and retrieve information. Omega-3s are abundant in such cold-water fish as salmon, trout, tuna, mackerel, halibut, and sardines, and fish oils like cod-liver oil. They are also plentiful in flaxseed, hemp seeds, and walnuts.

Vitamin B$_{12}$ (cobalamin) deficiency and **folate** deficiency are common among AD patients. Elderly people with low blood levels of vitamin B$_{12}$ and folate may face an increased risk of developing AD. Some researchers have linked low blood levels of these vitamins to AD and mental decline. Prolonged B$_{12}$ deficiency may lead to irreversible changes in mental function. Vitamin B$_{12}$ is not found in fruits and vegetables. The best food sources of this vitamin are meat, poultry, and fish. One reason many older people are B$_{12}$ deficient is because they have low levels of intrinsic factor, a substance in gastric juice that increases absorption of B$_{12}$. As people age, secretion of gastric juices declines. Supplementation with betaine HCl, available at most health food stores, may aid protein digestion, and increase vitamin B$_{12}$ absorption. B complex supplements may be helpful. Metagenics has a form of intrinsic factor folic acid called Intrinsic B$_{12}$ Folate (5-tetrahydrofolate). Folic acid is found in kale, spinach, and beetroot greens; it's also in foods such as beans, lentils, dried peas, nuts, and oatmeal.

Zinc deficiency is a major problem in older people, and has been implicated as a factor in AD. Patients with AD who have received zinc supplementation have shown improvement in memory, understanding, socialization, and communication.

Best juice sources of zinc: gingerroot, turnips, parsley, garlic, carrots, spinach, cabbage, lettuce, and cucumbers.

✳ Herb Recommendations

Ginkgo biloba is a plant extract containing several compounds that may have positive effects on cells within the brain. It's known to increase blood flow to the brain. In a study published in the *Journal of the American Medical Association* (1997), researchers observed a modest improvement in cognition, activities of daily living such as eating and dressing, and social behavior with the use of gingko biloba.

Huperzine A (pronounced HOOP-ur-zeen) is a moss extract that has been used in traditional Chinese medicine for centuries. It has properties similar to those of cholinesterase inhibitors, one class of FDA-approved Alzheimer medications. As a result, it is promoted as a treatment for AD. Evidence from small studies shows that the effectiveness of huperzine A may be comparable to that of approved drugs. In 2004, the National Institute on Aging (NIA) launched the first large U.S. clinical trial of huperzine A as a treatment for mild to moderate AD.

✳ Juice Therapy

Juices help flush out toxins from the brain and bring vital nutrients to brain cells. Though studies have proven that fruit and vegetable juices can keep AD at bay, to date we don't know which juices are the most effective. Therefore, I recommend that you drink a wide variety of vegetable juices and a small amount of fruit juice. The KAME Project (2006) showed that those who drank juices more than three times per week compared to less than once a week were 76 percent less likely to develop AD.

✳ Juice Recipes

Tomato Florentine *(pg 343)*   Spinach Power *(pg 341)*   Wheatgrass Light *(pg 345)* Memory Mender *(pg 336)*   Sweet Dreams Nightcap *(pg 342)*   Bladder Tonic *(pg 329)* Calcium-Rich Cocktail *(pg 329)*   Afternoon Refresher *(pg 326)*   Cranberry-Apple Cocktail *(pg 331)*   Happy Morning *(pg 333)*   Immune Builder *(pg 335)*   Liver Life Tonic *(pg 336)*   Magnesium-Rich Cocktail *(pg 336)*   Mood Mender *(pg 337)*   Orient Express *(pg 338)*

Anemia

A NEMIA is a condition marked by a deficiency either of red blood cells or of hemoglobin, the oxygen-carrying substance found in red blood cells. A nutritional deficiency often underlies anemia, usually a deficiency of one of three nutrients—iron, vitamin B_{12} (cobalamin), or folic acid.

In menstruating women, dietary iron deficiency is a common cause of deficient red blood cell production. It is important to know which nutrient(s) is deficient in order to treat anemia effectively. Iron-deficiency anemia is characterized by small red blood cells and low levels of circulating hemoglobin. Symptoms of iron deficiency include impaired intellectual performance, pale skin, a light pink color (rather than red) inside the lower eyelids, canker sores, irritability, weakness, dizziness, and headaches. It is also marked by extreme fatigue; red, even burning, tongue; inflammation of the lips; and a spoonlike deformity of the fingernails.

Vitamin B_{12} deficiency, known as pernicious anemia, is characterized by large, immature red blood cells. Symptoms include weight loss, problems with sensation and muscle control, and yellow-blue color blindness. Vitamin B_{12} absorption requires a sufficient amount of intrinsic factor, a substance found in gastric juice. Gastrointestinal problems, such as bacterial or parasitic infection, can lead to B_{12} anemia (see Parasitic Infections, page 238).

Folic acid–deficiency anemia, also called macrosydia anemia, is characterized by red blood cells that are improperly formed. This form of anemia can produce sleeping disorders and a sore, red tongue.

Most anemia results from not having enough iron. But there are also other causes, especially those frequently seen in strict vegetarians. Macrocytic anemia ("macrocytic" means large red blood cells) can be a sign of vitamin B_{12} deficiency, which may be due to low intrinsic factor. It may also be caused by folate deficiency. This deficiency is not common because folate is in most raw vegetables, but some drugs (methotrexate and trimethoprim) and alcohol can cause folate deficiency, as can intolerance to wheat (celiac disease).

Most commonly, people with anemia report a feeling of weakness or fatigue, general malaise, and sometimes poor concentration. People with more severe anemia often report dyspnea (shortness of breath) on exertion. Very severe anemia prompts the body to compensate by increasing cardiac output, leading to palpitations and sweatiness, and eventually to heart failure. Pallor (pale skin, mucosal linings, and nail beds) is often a useful diagnostic sign in moderate or severe anemia, but it is not always apparent. Pica is the consumption of nonfood such as dirt, paper, wax, grass, and hair. It is a rare but characteristic sign of iron-deficiency anemia.

Left untreated, anemia can be very dangerous, even fatal. If you have a number of these symptoms, it's important to get a diagnosis and treatment, especially if you are a menstruating woman or are taking aspirin or any nonsteroidal anti-inflammatory drug (NSAID) that can cause blood loss from chronic bleeding in your stomach. Keep in mind that one should not rely on measuring serum iron to determine iron levels. To diagnose iron problems such as anemia or hemochromatosis, you need to have a measure of your serum ferritin level in conjunction with a total iron binding level.

✳ Diet Recommendations

If you have iron-deficiency anemia, eat an iron-rich diet. There are two types of iron in the foods we eat: heme and nonheme. Heme iron is the type primarily found in animal foods. Nonheme iron makes up the remainder, and is the only iron present in plant foods. The absorption rate of heme iron is considerably higher than that of nonheme iron. *Best food sources for heme iron:* meat (especially liver), poultry, and fish. For best iron absorption, always combine an iron-rich food with a vitamin C–rich choice. *Best juice sources of nonheme iron:* parsley, dandelion greens, broccoli, cauliflower, strawberries, asparagus, Swiss chard, blackberries, cabbage, beetroot with greens, carrots, and prunes.

Eat and juice dark green vegetables. These foods contain generous amounts of nonheme iron and folic acid, as well as vitamin C and chlorophyll. The best green vegetables are broccoli, kale, parsley, Jerusalem artichoke, beetroot with greens, Swiss chard, dandelion greens, and bok choy.

Avoid high-fructose corn syrup. It's in many processed foods. The consumption of high-fructose corn syrup not only exacerbates the obesity epidemic, it also harms the way primary organs like the liver and pancreas function, leading to anemia, bone loss, and heart problems.

✳ Nutrient Recommendations

Copper in food is necessary to help your body absorb and use iron properly. *Best juice sources of copper:* carrots, garlic, gingerroot, and turnips.

* * *

The amount of iron absorbed from the diet depends on many factors:

- Iron from meat, poultry, and fish (heme iron) is absorbed two to three times more efficiently than iron from plants (nonheme).
- The amount of iron absorbed from plants depends on the other types of foods eaten at the same meal. For example:
  - Foods containing heme iron (meat, poultry, and fish) enhance iron absorption from foods that contain nonheme iron (e.g., beans and spinach).
  - Foods containing vitamin C enhance iron absorption when eaten at the same meal. A good example would be a glass of tomato juice and a dark green vegetable with a serving of animal protein.
  - Substances like polyphenols, phytates, and calcium that are part of certain foods or drinks such as tea, coffee, whole grains, legumes, and milk and other dairy products can decrease the amount of nonheme iron that is absorbed at a meal. However, for healthy individuals who consume a varied diet of nutritious whole foods, the amount of iron inhibition from these substances is usually not of concern.
  - Certain foods have been found to interfere with iron absorption in the gastrointestinal tract and should be avoided by people with established iron deficiency. They include: tannins (tea and coffee), phytates (wheat bran and other grains, legumes, and seeds), oxalates (spinach, kale, rhubarb, and chocolate), chewing gum, red wine, phosphates (large amounts in soft drinks), EDTA (food preservative), beer, and dairy products.
- Vegetarian diets are often low in heme iron; it takes careful meal planning to increase the amount of nonheme iron absorbed.
- Other factors: Taking antacids can reduce the amount of acid in the stomach and, consequently, the iron absorbed, which causes iron deficiency. For people age forty and over, betaine HCL is recommended with meals to aid digestion of protein.

Folic acid can be obtained from food although if you have folic acid–deficiency anemia, you may also need to take a folic acid supplement. *Best juice sources of folic acid:* asparagus, spinach, kale, broccoli, cabbage, and blackberries. *Other foods rich in folic acid:* dried beans, peas, avocados, and nuts.

Iron supplementation; be aware. Anemia is often associated with low levels of iron. But be careful of trying to increase your iron intake with supplemental iron.

There is a much more common condition that stems from exactly the opposite problem—iron overload (or iron toxicity), also called hemochromatosis. If your body has excess iron, deposits of iron can appear in practically every major organ, particularly the liver, pancreas, and heart, resulting in complete and widespread organ failure. This is particularly common in women who are not menstruating and in many men. It's best to get your iron from food.

Vitamin B$_{12}$ (cobalamin) is generally found in small amounts in animal foods, and is not available in fruits and vegetables. Strict vegans—people who eat no animal products at all—are particularly susceptible to vitamin B$_{12}$ deficiency. *Best food sources of vitamin B$_{12}$:* beef, poultry, eggs, lamb, sardines, oysters, and fish. You may need to take a B$_{12}$ supplement; see your doctor about whether the oral or injectable form would be best in your case. You can also try using a digestive aid called betaine HCl, a supplement available in most health food stores that can help improve vitamin B$_{12}$ absorption.

Vitamin C significantly enhances iron absorption. *Best juice sources of vitamin C:* kale, parsley, broccoli, Brussels sprouts, watercress, cauliflower, cabbage, strawberries, spinach, lemons, limes, turnips, and asparagus.

Zinc in excess can cause anemia. Zinc has the potential to be toxic if too much is taken. Excess zinc can result in copper deficiency, which is associated with anemia.

✳ Herb Recommendations

Anise tea enhances iron absorption. Mint, caraway, cumin, and licorice teas are also effective, but anise is the best.

Chinese wild yam increases the assimilation of iron, as do carrots, tomatoes, and most green vegetables.

Gentian is used in the treatment of anemia. It stimulates the secretion of digestive juices, thereby enhancing iron absorption.

Linden flowers improve iron absorption. German researchers were so impressed with how linden flowers worked in studies, they suggested that anyone with an iron deficiency drink linden flower tea.

Seaweed and **dulse** are rich in iron.

Yellow dock is rich in iron, and its absorption rate is excellent.

✳ Juice Therapy

Beetroot with greens juice is a good source of iron.

Dandelion greens juice is commonly used in treating anemia. It is a good source of iron, and also contains significant amounts of folic acid, calcium, and potassium, as well as many trace minerals.

Parsley juice is a good source of both iron and vitamin C. Intake should be limited to a safe, therapeutic dose of one-half to one cup per day. Parsley can be toxic in overdose, and should be especially avoided by pregnant women.

Spinach, cabbage, wheatgrass, and **nettle** juices are used to treat anemia, as are other dark green juices, which are rich in chlorophyll.

✳ Juice Recipes

Liver Life Tonic *(pg 336)* Spinach Power *(pg 341)* Triple C *(pg 344)* Morning Energizer *(pg 337)* The Ginger Hopper *(pg 332)* Calcium-Rich Cocktail *(pg 329)* Wheatgrass Light *(pg 345)* Beet-Cucumber Cleansing Cocktail *(pg 328)* Immune Builder *(pg 335)* Icy Spicy Tomato *(pg 335)* Peppy Parsley *(pg 339)* Salsa in a Glass *(pg 340)*

Anxiety and Panic Attacks

PEOPLE WITH GENERALIZED ANXIETY often feel apprehension, uneasiness, or nervousness. They may be easily startled, and may experience a vague, nagging uncertainty about future personal or job-related matters. This constant state of tension often leads to irritability, sleeplessness, fatigue, and difficulty concentrating. They may also suffer from depression, headaches, trembling, twitching, sweating, and muscular tension, which often results in muscle pain and soreness. Because they tighten their abdominal muscles when anxious, they may also experience constipation or diarrhea.

Acute anxiety shows itself as intense dread or terror for no objective reason, and it is often characterized by such symptoms as a pounding or racing heart, trembling, shaking, sweating, shortness of breath, smothering sensations, chest pain, and light-headedness. Many of these symptoms are similar to that of a heart attack and should be taken seriously, and a heart attack should be ruled out.

Panic attacks, characterized by a sudden overwhelming fright without reasonable cause, can be caused by environmental sensitivities, such as those to dust, molds, chemicals, and certain foods. These items can cause allergic reactions that can dramatically influence conditions such as anxiety, panic, and depression. Those who suffer from panic disorder are at almost double the risk for coronary heart disease.

✳ Lifestyle Recommendations

Eliminate respiratory allergies. Reducing any allergic reactions you may have to airborne irritants may reduce your anxiety or panic attacks (see Allergies, page 27).

Prayer and spirituality. Research in behavioral medicine suggests that the interactions of the mind, body, and spirit can have powerful effects on our peace of mind and our health. Only a few published scientific studies have examined the effects of prayer and spirituality on the mind and emotions, but those few show that they are powerfully effective. Adding to or deepening the spiritual aspects in your life through prayer and meditation can be very good for your soul and body. Also, watch the "lies" that can enter your mind. They are usually lies about you such as thoughts of abandonment, insecurity, failure to perform to your expectations, or rejection from others. Be aware of these thoughts, and start intercepting them and rejecting them. Each time one of these negative thoughts enters your mind, tell yourself something good about yourself that counteracts each false premise. You may be surprised how much your life changes as you transform your thought life.

✳ Diet Recommendations

Eat a calming diet. Consuming foods high in tryptophan such as turkey or almonds is worthwhile because they help bolster the nervous system. Dark green leafy vegetables and celery are other calming foods. The better your nutritional status, the better your body can cope with stressful situations that can cause anxiety. (For more information, see Basic Guidelines for the Juice Lady's Health and Healing Diet, page 290.)

Foods that help reduce anxiety and maintain a calm state

- Almonds
- Asparagus
- Garlic
- Eggs
- Fish
- Turkey

- Wheat germ
- Brewer's yeast
- Carrots
- Onions
- Beetroot

- Spinach
- Lettuce
- Celery
- Stone fruit
- Avocados

Eat smaller meals more frequently. Hypoglycemia (low blood sugar) may play a role in anxiety or panic attacks for some people. Therefore, it is important to keep your blood-sugar levels even throughout the day by eating smaller, more frequent meals that include protein, or by eating protein snacks between meals and avoiding sweets and refined carbs (see Hypoglycemia, page 180).

Drink fresh vegetable juices, and try short vegetable juice fasts. Multiple chemical sensitivities have been implicated in anxiety disorder. Fresh vegetable juices and short vegetable juice fasts will help to cleanse the body of toxins. People who juice-fast for short periods of time say they experience a greater sense of well-being (see the Juice Fast, page 304).

Identify food allergies and intolerances. Avoid foods you are allergic to or don't tolerate well, since food allergies are known to cause anxiety and fatigue (see Allergies, page 27; also see the Elimination Diet, page 301).

Detoxify your body. Anxiety can also be attributed to the negative effects of high levels of heavy metals commonly found in the body. Aluminum, mercury, lead, and copper can make the body toxic, interfering with brain function and contributing to anxiety (see the Cleansing Programs, pages 303–325 and Heavy Metal and Toxic Compound, Cleanse Products, page 349).

Avoid sweets and refined foods such as baked goods made with white flour. Reducing your intake of sweets and refined foods can be very helpful in reducing anxiety and panic attacks. These foods affect the blood sugar, causing it to swing high and low, which can lead to anxiety and mood swings.

Avoid stimulants. Stimulant usage will exacerbate anxiety and panic because serotonin must be excreted to help "sweep up" the effects of a stimulating factor on the brain. Low serotonin is implicated in anxiety and panic attacks. Be aware that prescription drugs, amphetamines, and recreational drugs such as cocaine contain caffeine, which can increase anxiety and panic attacks. Also, several studies have implicated caffeine as a contributing factor in anxiety and panic disorders. Caffeine use can lead to a stress response characterized by depression, anxiety, nervousness, irritability, recurrent headaches, heart palpitations, and insomnia. The recommended safe caffeine dosage is less than 100 mg per day, which is no more than one cup of coffee (about 80 mg). Less than 50 mg per day is preferable; black tea contains about 40 mg; green and white teas have even less. Caffeine is found in coffee; black, white, and green teas; cola; chocolate; and some drugs. Even decaffeinated coffee has some caffeine.

Stop smoking. Nicotine stimulates increased physiological arousal and vasoconstriction, and makes your heart work harder. Smokers tend to be more anxious than nonsmokers and also tend to experience sleep disturbances.

Avoid food additives. Food additives such as dyes, preservatives, stabilizers, and fillers have been implicated in hyperactivity and attention deficit disorder in children. They should not be overlooked as contributing factors to adult anxiety. Choose fresh, whole foods, and avoid packaged and processed foods as much as possible. Choose only freshly made fruit and vegetable juices whenever possible, since bottled juices often contain additives. (Even the commercial "fresh" juices have been pasteurized, which means some of the vitamins and enzymes have been destroyed.)

✳ Nutrient Recommendations

Alpha-linolenic acid (ALA) is an essential fatty acid. Some scientists believe that people who suffer from panic attacks may be deficient in ALA. In one study, individuals suffering from panic attacks for more than ten years experienced a significant improvement within two or three months of consuming increased amounts of ALA. Supplements may be advised. *Best food sources:* leafy greens, walnuts, chia seeds, and oils such as flaxseed, hemp, and black currant.

Amino acids. Anxiety, panic, and depression may be the result of shortages of key brain chemicals that can be restored naturally. Give the brain the amino acids it needs and your mind can glow again. Mood, behavior, and brain biochemistry are intricately linked. Anxiety may be the result of flawed message transmission in the brain, flawed because key brain chemicals known as neurotransmitters are in short supply. They're in short supply because the body's amino acid pool from which they're made is itself low.

Anxiety and panic attacks are exacerbated by low serotonin. Low serotonin may also be the causal factor in anxiety, panic, and stress. Anxiety and panic often increase over time because it is very difficult to make adequate quantities of the neurotransmitter serotonin from our diet. Gamma-aminobutyric acid (GABA) is an amino acid that can be taken for temporary relief, but most GABA only crosses the blood–brain barrier at a rate of 10 percent. Beta phenyl gamma–aminobutyric acid, however, crosses at a 90 percent rate.

B vitamins, omega-3 fatty acids, and varied protein consumption is imperative with the amino acid program. Get three to four servings of protein a day; include nuts, seeds, beans, eggs, and muscle meats such as fish, chicken, turkey, and beef. (Choose organically fed, free-range / cage-free, and no hormones or antibiotics.)

Testing neurotransmitters is the best way to quantify your depletion in brain chemicals. Testing can be completed whether you are taking medications or not. What you never knew was how good you could feel. For more information on the amino acid program, see Sources (page 347).

B vitamins can help reduce the effects of anxiety. In fact, vitamin B–complex deficiencies can cause anxiety. The best juice sources of B vitamins overall are green leafy vegetables. In addition, several specific B vitamins are especially beneficial. **Note:** When taking B vitamin supplements, it's usually best to take them as a complex, since they work together.

- **Biotin** is important during times of anxiety and panic because it plays a special role in helping the body to use glucose and promotes overall equilibrium. *Best food sources:* cauliflower, peanuts, eggs, and cheese.
- **Folic acid** is required when the body is dealing with anxiety or panic. Also, research suggests that folic acid may help relieve depression, which is often associated with anxiety and panic. *Best juice sources:* asparagus, beetroot, Brussels sprouts, bok choy, cabbage, savoy cabbage, spinach, and broccoli. *Best food sources:* avocados, peas (fresh), beans (dried), chickpeas, lentils, oranges, and turkey.
- **Inositol** can help alleviate panic disorders. *Best juice sources of inositol:* grapefruit, cabbage, strawberries, and tomatoes.

- **Pantothenic acid** (vitamin B) is known as the antistress vitamin because it helps the body resist stress. *Best juice sources of pantothenic acid:* broccoli, cauliflower, and kale. *Other sources include:* avocados, salmon, mushrooms, sunflower seeds, and yogurt.
- **Vitamin B$_3$ (niacin)** has been found to reduce anxiety because of its effect on the brain, which is similar to such benzodiazepine tranquilizers as Valium. Because of its calming effects, this vitamin can also help reduce the effects of benzodiazapine withdrawal, which include anxiety. Vitamin B$_3$ is not found in appreciable amounts in fruits and vegetables. *Best food sources of vitamin B$_3$:* brewer's yeast, rice, wheat bran, peanuts, turkey, chicken, lamb, and fish.
- **Vitamin B$_6$ (pyridoxine)** helps the body manufacture brain chemicals (neurotransmitters) such as serotonin, which are essential to cope with anxiety and panic. It can also help boost the immune system during times of stress. *Best juice sources of vitamin B$_6$:* kale, spinach, turnip greens, bell peppers, and prunes. *Best food sources:* sweet potatoes, avocados, bananas, sunflower seeds, tuna, chickpeas, salmon, potatoes, turkey, chicken, bok choy, brown rice, and barley.

Magnesium deficiency can trigger or cause anxiety and panic attacks. The introduction of magnesium either by a high-magnesium diet with green drinks and/or magnesium supplements can help alleviate these conditions. In general, to get as much magnesium as possible in your diet, eat plenty of organic leafy green vegetables and green juices, nuts, and seeds every day. Adding green juices and green smoothies to your menu will help you achieve a higher magnesium status. *Best juice sources of magnesium:* beetroot greens, spinach, parsley, dandelion greens, garlic, blackberries, beets, broccoli, cauliflower, carrots, and celery.

❋ Herb Recommendations

Ginkgo biloba has demonstrated antistress and antianxiety activity in animal studies.

Hops is used as a traditional remedy for insomnia caused by anxiety. To use this herb, fill a small sachet-size pillow with hops and place it near your pillow or inside the pillowcase at night.

Kava kava relaxes both the central nervous system and the muscles. Studies show that kava kava has proven long-term effectiveness in helping persons with anxiety, with none of the tolerance problems of antidepressant drugs.

✳ Juice Therapy

Celery juice has a calming effect and is helpful for insomnia.

Fennel juice helps calm the mind.

Parsley juice helps produce an overall sense of well-being. Intake should be limited to a safe, therapeutic dose of one-half to one cup per day. Parsley can be toxic in overdose, and should be especially avoided by pregnant women.

✳ Juice Recipes

Sweet Dreams Nightcap *(pg 342)*   Mood Mender *(pg 337)*   Waldorf Twist *(pg 345)* Magnesium-Rich Cocktail *(pg 336)*   Spinach Power *(pg 341)*   Morning Energizer *(pg 337)*   Liver Life Tonic *(pg 336)*   Happy Morning *(pg 333)*   Memory Mender *(pg 336)*   Spring Tonic *(pg 342)*   Super Green Sprout Drink *(pg 342)* Wheatgrass Light *(pg 345)*

Asthma

Asthma is a chronic disease in which the small air passages, or bronchi, in the lungs are inflamed and constricted, and there is excess mucus secretion. A variety of stimuli can provoke an asthma episode, which is marked by wheezing, coughing, and shortness of breath.

Asthma comes in two forms, extrinsic and intrinsic. Extrinsic asthma is generally considered an allergic condition. It occurs when particles to which a person has become sensitized trigger the release of an inflammatory chemical called histamine. Intrinsic asthma is set off by such nonimmune factors as exercise, emotional upset, heat or cold, stress, chemical irritants, infection, aspirin, and allergens. (The most common foods allergens include fish, eggs, peanuts, nuts, cow's milk, wheat, and soy, along with additives, such as sulfites.)

Increased levels of air pollution, such as those produced by cigarette smoke or a wood-burning stove, can increase the frequency and severity of asthma attacks. Wood smoke contains tiny, irritating particles, and cigarette smoke contains nitrogen oxides and toxic free radicals that are present in the tar. New research suggests that being exposed to tobacco smoke, infections, and some allergens early in your life may increase your chances of developing asthma. Asthma is closely linked to allergies. Most, but not all, people with asthma have allergies.

The rate of asthma in the United States is rising rapidly, especially among children. The reasons include greater stress on the immune system caused by environmental pollutants, earlier weaning and introduction of solid food, and increased use of food additives.

✳ Diet Recommendations

Eat a Mediterranean diet with an emphasis on vegetables and fruit. A study was completed in Crete to determine whether diet was associated with asthma. It was found that asthma is rare in this area and that 80 percent of the children there ate fresh fruit and 68 percent ate vegetables at least twice a day. The intake of grapes, oranges, apples, and fresh tomatoes, the main local produce in Crete, along with a high consumption of nuts, was shown to be protective against wheezing and rhinitis (runny nose). The researchers concluded that this type of diet protects children from asthma. That study is corroborated by a long-term study of twenty-five asthma patients who switched to a vegetarian diet; 92 percent of the participants showed a significant improvement. Adding cold-water fish such as salmon, tuna, halibut, herring, and mackerel, which are rich in omega-3 fatty acids, also provides nutrients that are beneficial for individuals with asthma. Epidemiological studies in children have also shown less asthma with a higher intake of fruits, vegetables, dairy, whole-grain products, and fish. But getting children, or yourself for that matter, to eat lots of vegetables may not be that easy. That's where juicing comes in. You can juice a lot of vegetables and drink a cornucopia of asthma-fighting nutrients.

Eat more apples. European researchers discovered the connection with apples while tracking the diets of some two thousand pregnant women and more than 1,250 of their children for five years. Of that group, more than 11 percent were diagnosed with asthma and nearly 13 percent suffered from wheezing over the previous year. Among all the foods listed by expectant moms during their pregnancies, scientists were surprised to learn that women who ate more than four apples every week reduced their baby's chances of being diagnosed with asthma by 53 percent and wheezing by 37 percent. Be sure to choose organic, since apples are among the most heavily sprayed of the fruits and vegetables.

Avoid fast food; choose whole foods. A study was done on asthma in Saudi Arabia. It was found that eating at fast-food outlets created significant risk factors for wheezy illness. That, coupled with the lowest intake of vegetables, fiber, vitamin E, calcium, magnesium, sodium, and potassium, posed the greatest risk for asthma.

Eliminate all food additives. Dyes and preservatives can contribute to asthma attacks in susceptible individuals.

Eliminate mucus-forming foods. These include dairy products, refined foods (such as white flour), and sugar (including all sweets).

Identify and eliminate all food allergens and sensitivities. Food allergies may play a role in asthma attacks. The most common allergenic foods are dairy products, shellfish, fish, eggs, nuts, peanuts, wheat, chocolate, citrus fruit, and food colorings (see Allergies, page 27; see also the Elimination Diet, page 301).

✳ Nutrient Recommendations

Antioxidants including vitamins C and E, beta-carotene, and selenium are important in the prevention of bronchial reactivity. One study provides evidence that a diet rich in antioxidants may help prevent asthma attacks. It is consistent with the hypothesis that the reduction in antioxidant intake in the British diet over the last twenty-five years has been a factor in the increase in incidence of asthma over this same period. Yellow, orange, red, and dark green vegetables and fruit provide the most antioxidants.

Essential fatty acids (EFAs), especially eicosapentaenoic acid (EPA) and docosahexaenoic acid (DHA), two omega-3 fatty acids found in cold-water fish, are beneficial. Studies have shown that a diet high in EPA and DHA correlates with a low incidence of asthma. You can supplement your diet daily with unrefined flaxseed or hemp oil, since the body can manufacture EPA and DHA from these plant-based oils. (For more information, see the fats and oils section in Basic Guidelines for the Juice Lady's Health and Healing Diet, page 290.)

Magnesium relaxes the smooth muscles and may encourage airway dilation. Decreased levels of magnesium have been associated with an increased risk of bronchial hypersensitivity. *Best juice sources of magnesium:* beetroot greens, spinach, parsley, dandelion greens, garlic, blackberries, beetroot, broccoli, cauliflower, carrots, and celery.

Vitamin B$_{12}$ (cobalamin) has been used as a successful asthma therapy, especially in children. It also appears to be especially helpful for individuals who are sensitive to food additives like sulfites. Vitamin B$_{12}$ is not available in fruits and vegetables. The best food sources of vitamin B$_{12}$ are meat, poultry, and fish. See your doctor about taking B$_{12}$ supplements in either oral or injectable form. In addition, you may want to try using a digestive aid called betaine HCl, which may improve vitamin B$_{12}$ absorption; it's available in most health food stores.

Vitamin C has been shown in studies to cause an immediate decrease in airway constriction by acting against one of the substances in the lungs that induces such constriction. Patients with asthma have been shown to have lower blood concentrations of vitamin C than other individuals. Several studies have concluded that consumption of vitamin C–rich foods can reduce wheezing symptoms in childhood, especially among already susceptible individuals. *Best juice sources of vitamin C:* kale, parsley, broccoli, Brussels sprouts, watercress, cauliflower, cabbage, strawberries, spinach, lemons, limes, turnips, and asparagus.

Vitamin E deficiency has been related to the onset of asthma in adult women. Vitamin E can relax the smooth muscles of the airway by inhibiting the effects of histamine and by modifying formation of inflammation-controlling substances called prostaglandins. *Best juice sources of vitamin E:* spinach, watercress, asparagus, carrots, and tomatoes.

✳ Juice Therapy

Onion juice helps eliminate mucus in the upper respiratory tract.

Parsley juice is a traditional remedy for asthma and allergies. A safe, therapeutic dose is one-half to one cup of parsley juice per day. Parsley can be toxic in overdose, and should be especially avoided by pregnant women.

Radish juice is a traditional remedy for asthma.

✳ Juice Recipes

The Pink Onion *(pg 339)* **Allergy Relief** *(pg 326)* **Sinus Solution** *(pg 341)*
Calcium-Rich Cocktail *(pg 329)* **Tomato Florentine** *(pg 343)* **Spring Tonic**
(pg 342) **Magnesium-Rich Cocktail** *(pg 336)* **Spinach Power** *(pg 341)*

ADD (Attention Deficit Disorder) and ADHD (Attention Deficit Hyperactivity Disorder)

ATTENTION DEFICIT DISORDER (ADD) is defined as a learning disability marked by inappropriately brief attention span and poor concentration.

Attention deficit hyperactivity disorder (ADHD) is a neurobiological disorder resulting from problems in the dopamine neurotransmitter systems in the brain, characterized by pervasive inattention and/or hyperactivity-impulsivity and resulting in significant functional impairment. The prevalence of ADHD in adults is thought to be around 4.4 percent. The CDC estimates that 4.4 million youths ages four to seventeen have been diagnosed with ADHD by a health-care professional, and as of 2003, 2.5 million youths ages four to seventeen are currently receiving medication for the disorder. The CDC states that a diagnosis of ADD/ADHD should be made only by trained health-care providers, as many of the symptoms may also be part of other conditions such as hyperthyroidism.

In looking for causes or aggravating factors of ADD/ADHD, scientists have focused on food additives, food allergies, sugar consumption, frequent ear infections (these conditions may be related to dairy or wheat sensitivity), and thyroid dysfunction. These factors may cause problems in the brain's use of neurotransmitters, the chemical messengers that carry impulses from one brain cell to another.

Roughly one-fifth of all ADHD cases are thought to be acquired after conception due to brain injury caused by either toxins or physical trauma pre- or postnatally, which can include in utero alcohol or tobacco smoke, or lead exposure. It has been observed that women who smoke while pregnant are more likely to have children with ADHD. Complications during pregnancy and birth— including premature birth—could also play a role.

The most common stimulants prescribed for treatment are methylphenidate and amphetamines (Ritalin, Dexedrine, and Adderall), which stimulate the brain to release a greater amount of neurochemicals. Doctors prescribe these drugs to about 2 million children with symptoms every month, according to Yale New Haven Children's Hospital. Ritalin is not a weak stimulant. "It is actually more potent than cocaine," says Dr. Joseph Mercola, D.O. Researchers at the Brookhaven National Laboratory (Upton, New York) found that when Ritalin was given to cocaine users, they couldn't distinguish the Ritalin high from a cocaine high. One study at the University of California at Berkeley found that Ritalin users were three times more likely to develop a taste for cocaine. And other ADHD drugs have been linked to a host of side effects, including hallucinations and cardiovascular problems. The last thing children need when they're just starting out in life is a barrage of drug side effects to overcome, particularly when ADHD often improves dramatically with natural lifestyle changes such as those noted below.

✳ Lifestyle Recommendations

Behavioral interventions using positive reinforcement are an excellent choice, alongside nutritional changes. A five-year study of 135 preschool children ages three to five with symptoms of ADHD found that nonmedicinal interventions work effectively to prevent the related behavioral and academic problems. The study—the largest of its kind to date—evaluated early-intervention techniques and their ability to decrease aggressiveness and behavior problems, while improving academic and social skills. The interventions, which included individualized programs that emphasized positive support to reinforce behavior at home and school, were highly effective.

✳ Diet Recommendations

Eat only fresh, whole foods; increase protein; and reduce carbohydrates. In several studies children have been noted to behave and concentrate better when the ratio of protein was increased and that of carbohydrates decreased. This diet is especially helpful if the person is prone to mood swings. In this case, it is especially important to keep the blood sugar stable by eliminating all sugar, refined carbohydrates (such as white-flour products, including bread, rolls, pasta, and pizza), and alcohol.

Avoid all additives. Dr. Benjamin Feingold, author of *The Feingold Diet*, was the first doctor to propose that food-additive sensitivity, along with sensitivity to several naturally occurring compounds, causes hyperactivity in about half of people with ADD/ADHD. A study published in *The Lancet* (September 2007) has confirmed that common food additives and colorings can increase hyperactive behavior in a broad range of children. Read labels. The best rule is: if you can't pronounce it, don't buy it. In the United States, thousands of additives are used, including bleaches, colorings, flavor enhancers, preservatives, thickeners, fillers, anticaking agents, and vegetable gums. The best choice is to prepare food from scratch. Premade and packaged food will usually have additives.

Especially avoid all sugar (refined and artificial), along with all refined and high-carbohydrate foods. Studies have found a correlation between consumption of sugar and behavior that is aggressive, destructive, and restless. Sugar consumption leads, oddly enough, to low blood-sugar levels, or hypoglycemia, which can promote hyperactivity and aggression (see Hypoglycemia, page 180). Normally, when people ingest sugar, the pancreas releases insulin, which stops blood sugar from rising too high. At the same time, adrenal glands release certain hormones (the catecholamines) to keep the insulin from driving blood-sugar levels too low. According to research, children with ADHD release only about half the amount of these hormones as normal children. It was found that this uncontrolled drop in blood sugar significantly decreased brain activity in these children. It was also found that children with ADHD unconsciously become physically hyperactive in an effort to force their adrenal glands to release more of these hormones. These children are unconsciously placing their bodies under stress by trying to "squeeze" more hormones from their already weakened adrenal glands. As a solution, it is recommended that anyone with ADD/ADHD avoid all sugar and high-carbohydrate foods, while at the same time strengthening the adrenal glands.

Drink plenty of fresh vegetable juice; limit fruit juice to no more than four ounces per day and completely avoid soda. It is important to greatly limit the sugar in the diet, including fruit juice, even though it's natural. Especially avoid the sugars and additives in soda, including diet soda. Fresh vegetable juice is chock-full of vitamins and minerals, and provides the brain with nutrients that will help it function properly. Many cases of ADD/ADHD may be the result of poor nutritional status. Raw juice offers nutrients that are easily absorbed and can greatly improve mental performance.

Identify and avoid all food allergens and sensitivities. Research has shown remarkable improvement in a large percentage of children with severe hyperactivity when underlying food allergies or sensitivities were addressed, and dyes and preservatives were eliminated. These children usually have many characteristics associated with a condition called allergic tension fatigue syndrome (ATFS) such as headache, irritability, and behavior disorders; they may also have dark circles under the eyes. Milk and other dairy products, wheat, yeast, corn, chocolate, peanuts, eggs, soy, and apple and orange juice are common allergens. Pay particular attention to dairy products if recurrent ear infections are a problem. Usually it is the child's favorite food(s) that is the most problematic (see Allergies, page 27; see also the Elimination Diet, page 301). I recommend two books: *Is This Your Child?* and *Is This Your Child's World?* by Dr. Doris Rapp (see Sources, page 350).

Use cleansing programs to help remove heavy metals. A number of studies have shown a relationship between heavy metal toxicity, especially lead, and learning disabilities, behavior disorders, and criminal behavior. Children should not be put on a strict juice fast unless supervised by a health-care specialist. However, consuming fresh vegetable juices and a high-fiber diet, along with plenty of antioxidants, will help cleanse the body of heavy metals. You can also try the Liver Cleanse (see page 310). In addition, choose organically grown foods, since pesticides and chemical fertilizers could be contributing to a toxic overload.

✳ Nutrient Recommendations

Specific nutrient deficiencies found in children with ADD/ADHD include zinc, magnesium, calcium, and essential fatty acids. Also, note that antioxidants fight the toxic effects of free radicals that damage cells, and they can also help with mental performance and overall health.

Amino acid support. There is a direct relationship between ADD/ADHD and neurotransmitter imbalances. Attention issues are very complicated. Neurotransmitter excretion can be elevated, causing the focus issue, or there could be a genetic component that causes dopamine to be inefficient—either too high or too low in urinary excretion. Whatever the situation, focus issues occur. Balancing the brain with good proteins and complex carbohydrates is imperative when these issues occur. Quantifying imbalances let you know which amino acids are needed for focus issues. Without testing, it is very difficult to determine which amino acids should be used.

While medications will allow for improved focus, they often cause sleep problems and weight loss. When an excitatory neurotransmitter is pushed into the synapse for improved focus, the brain also releases serotonin to help buffer these effects. In many situations, when a stimulant medication is used, within three years the patient is also on an antidepressant due to these effects. Serotonin must be supported if the weight-loss and sleep-cycle effects are to be avoided.

An amino acid supplement program tailored to your or your child's specific needs could make a significant difference in rebalancing dopamine, serotonin, and other neurotransmitters that affect mood, behavior, sleep, and carbohydrate cravings. For more information, see Sources (page 350).

Beta-carotene is an antioxidant that helps protect brain cells from free radical attack. *Best juice sources of beta-carotene:* carrots, kale, parsley, spinach, Swiss chard, beetroot greens, watercress, broccoli, and romaine lettuce.

Calcium deficiency has been found in children with ADD/ADHD; 1,000 mg of calcium at bedtime is recommended. *Best juice sources:* parsley, beetroot greens, spinach, broccoli, romaine lettuce, cabbage, celery, carrots, lemons, and beetroot.

Essential fatty acids (EFAs). According to one study, EFAs taken as a supplement may be able to correct fatty-acid imbalances that contribute to attention deficit problems. The standard American diet is quite deficient in EFAs. Unrefined flaxseed and hemp oil, and especially krill oil, are rich sources of EFAs.

Iron deficiency, which is the most common nutrient deficiency in children, may contribute to ADD/ADHD. However, researchers have found that iron supplementation may also help children with these disorders even when they are not iron deficient. (**Note:** Food sources are the best source of iron. Iron tablets are not recommended.) *Best juice sources of nonheme iron, the type found in plant foods:* parsley, dandelion greens, broccoli, cauliflower, strawberries, asparagus, Swiss chard, blackberries, cabbage, beetroot with greens, and carrots. Meat, chicken, and fish are good sources of heme iron.

Magnesium deficiency has been found in children with ADD/ADHD; 500 mg daily of magnesium is recommended, especially if the child (or adult) is ticklish or craves chocolate. *Best juice sources in order of effectiveness:* beetroot greens, spinach, Swiss chard, parsley, blackberries, beetroot, broccoli, cauliflower, carrots, celery, and tomatoes.

Pycnogenol. A European study shows that an antioxidant plant extract called pycnogenol from the bark of a French pine tree may reduce ADHD symptoms. According to the study, pycnogenol works by buffering acidic stress hormones, which in turn lowers the acids of adrenaline and dopamine, thereby improving attention and reducing hyperactivity.

Selenium helps activate glutathione peroxidase, an enzyme that has antioxidant activity. *Best juice sources of selenium:* Swiss chard, turnips, garlic, radishes, carrots, and cabbage.

Vitamin B$_6$ is especially important for people who can't remember their dreams. The recommendation is 50 mg at bedtime. It may be best to combine this in a B complex since the various B vitamins work synergistically.

Vitamin C helps protect brain cells from free-radical attack. *Best juice sources of vitamin C:* kale, parsley, broccoli, Brussels sprouts, watercress, cauliflower, cabbage, spinach, lemons, limes, turnips, and asparagus.

Vitamin E helps protect cell membranes. *Best juice sources of vitamin E:* spinach, watercress, asparagus, carrots, and tomatoes.

Zinc deficiency has been found in children with ADD/ADHD. *Best juice sources of zinc:* gingerroot, parsley, carrots, and spinach.

✳ Juice Therapy

Celery juice has a calming effect.

Fennel juice has been used as a traditional tonic that has been found to help release endorphins into the bloodstream. These feel-good chemicals create a mood of euphoria, and dampen anxiety and fear.

Parsley juice is a rich source of beta-carotene, iron, and vitamin C. Intake should be limited to a safe, therapeutic dose of one-half to one cup per day. Parsley can be toxic in overdose, and should be especially avoided by pregnant women.

Pear can by substituted for apple in any of the juice recipes if apple sensitivity is a problem.

✳ Juice Recipes

Waldorf Twist *(pg 345)*   **Spinach Power** *(pg 341)*   **The Ginger Hopper** *(pg 332)*
Happy Morning *(pg 333)*   **Mood Mender** *(pg 337)*   **Allergy Relief** *(pg 326)*
Mint Refresher *(pg 337)*   **Morning Energizer** *(pg 337)*

Bladder Infections

BLADDER INFECTION, also known as cystitis, occurs when bacteria attack the lining of the bladder, causing inflammation and irritation. Symptoms include urinary urgency, feeling the need to urinate frequently, increased urination at night, burning or other pain with urination, and tenderness in the lower abdomen, just above the pubic bone. The urine may have an unusual odor, and may be cloudy or contain blood. Fever and chills may also occur. But a fever may mean that the infection has reached the kidneys. Other symptoms of a kidney infection include pain in the back or side below the ribs, nausea, or vomiting.

Bladder infections are more common in women than in men. One woman in five develops an infection during her lifetime. That's because the urethra, the tube that carries the urine out of the body, is shorter in women, which gives bacteria a shorter route to the bladder. Menopause and pregnancy are both associated with a greater chance of bladder infection, as is prostate infection in men. Infections can recur, especially if there is a blockage in the urinary tract or if nerve dysfunction prevents the bladder from emptying properly. Recurrent bladder infections can lead to an increased risk of kidney infection, which is a serious health condition. Studies show that antibiotic treatment often does not successfully kill all the bacteria participating in a bladder infection and may, in fact, encourage many of the bacteria to persist in a resting state. This is all the more reason to strengthen the immune system. If the infection persists, it can be very serious. Always see a doctor if you have an infection.

✳ Lifestyle Recommendations

- Do not drink fluids that irritate the bladder, such as alcohol and caffeine.
- Drink unsweetened cranberry juice or use cranberry tablets, but not if you have a personal or family history of kidney stones.
- Drink plenty of fluids.
- Keep your genital area clean.
- Urinate after sexual intercourse.
- Wear cotton undergarments; avoid synthetic undergarments.
- Wipe from front to back.

✳ Diet Recommendations

Avoid sugar and refined carbohydrates (white flour). Sugar can depress the immune response for up to five hours after it is consumed. It doesn't matter if the sugar is in refined or natural form; sucrose (table sugar), fructose (fruit sugar), honey, and maple syrup should all be avoided. Even full-strength fruit juice contains too much sugar when you are fighting an infection. Drink no more than four ounces daily and dilute by half with water, mineral water, or vegetable juice. Avoid artificial sweeteners, which also depress the immune response. Eating white-flour products leads to a surge in blood-sugar levels; therefore, they should be avoided.

Eat an alkaline-rich diet. An alkaline-rich diet contains plenty of vegetables and vegetable juices. It will help reduce the chances that bacteria will grow in your system. **Note:** The blood and interstitial tissues function best in an alkaline environment; however, the bladder needs to be acidic.

Identify food allergies and intolerances. Avoid any foods you are allergic or sensitive to, as these will further tax your immune system (see Allergies, page 27; see also the Elimination Diet, page 301).

Go on juice fasts. Bladder infections can be exacerbated by eating too much food. Therefore, vegetable juices, vegetable broths, and herbal teas are recommended for a short fast when you have an infection (see the Juice Fast, page 304). They can be especially helpful to alkalinze the body, which helps fight infection. Include vegetable broths made from adzuki beans, lima beans, celery, carrots, winter squash, potatoes with skins, and asparagus. Add garlic and onions for their antimicrobial and immune-stimulating properties.

Drink plenty of water. This means at least eight to twelve eight-ounce glasses of pure water every day when you have a bladder infection. Drinking extra water not only helps to flush bacteria out of the urinary tract but also will dilute the urine so that it is less uncomfortable to urinate.

Avoid caffeine and alcohol. Caffeine is in coffee and black, green, and white teas, sodas, cola, and chocolate; it's a bladder irritant and should be avoided when you have an infection. Alcohol also irritates the bladder.

Avoid dairy and citrus fruits. Dairy contains lactose, which is a natural sugar that can feed the bacteria, hence making them harder to eliminate. Citrus causes your urine to become alkaline (base), which helps to encourage bacterial growth.

✳ Nutrient Recommendations

L-methionine is an essential amino acid that helps regulate the formation of ammonia, and is thought to aid in creating ammonia-free urine, leading to reduction of bladder irritation. A study published in 1997 suggested that L-methionine may prevent bacteria from sticking to urinary tract cells. Supplemental L-methionine is recommended.

Vitamin A and **carotenes** are important for good bladder health. Vitamin A deficiency has been shown to increase susceptibility to infection. This vitamin is important for the regeneration and repair of mucous membranes, such as that which lines the bladder. Certain carotenes, such as beta-carotene, can be converted to vitamin A as needed by the body, and both vitamin A and beta-carotene help fight infections. *Best juice sources of carotenes:* carrots, kale, parsley, spinach, Swiss chard, beetroot greens, watercress, broccoli, and romaine lettuce.

Vitamin C and **bioflavonoids** have been shown to be helpful in battling many types of infections. *Vitamin C* helps to increase the activity of white blood cells, the primary cells of the immune system. It is also important for keeping tissues strong and healthy. *Bioflavonoids* are the chemical compounds found in brightly colored fruits and vegetables. They work with vitamin C, making the vitamin's infection-fighting activity more effective. *Best juice sources of vitamin C:* kale, parsley, broccoli, Brussels sprouts, watercress, cauliflower, cabbage, spinach, lemons, limes, turnips, and asparagus. *Best juice sources of bioflavonoids:* bell peppers, broccoli, cabbage, parsley, lemons, limes, and tomatoes.

Zinc is a potent infection fighter. *Best juice sources of zinc:* gingerroot, turnips, parsley, garlic, carrots, spinach, cabbage, lettuce, and cucumbers.

✳ Herb Recommendations

Garlic has natural antibiotic qualities, along with acidophilus to help restore friendly bacteria, which will go a long way toward helping you heal.

✳ Juice Therapy

Asparagus juice is a good diuretic and a traditional remedy for kidney and bladder problems.

Berry juices, particularly those of cranberries (see next entry), blueberries, lingonberries, and huckleberries, are helpful in healing and preventing bladder infections.

Cranberry juice. The most research has been done on cranberry juice, which has been shown to prevent E. coli (the microbe that is the most common bacterial cause of bladder infection) from adhering to the bladder wall. New findings by scientists at Worcester Polytechnic Institute (WPI) present a detailed picture of the biochemical mechanisms that may underlie a number of the beneficial health effects of cranberry juice. A group of tannins found primarily in cranberries can transform E. coli bacteria, making it difficult for bacteria to make contact with cells in the bladder. Also, quality cranberry juice produces hippuric acid in the urine, which acidifies it and prevents bacteria from sticking to the walls of the bladder. If pure cranberry juice is not available, cranberry capsules can be substituted. They can be found in most health food stores. Always take these with a large glass of water. Don't use the kind of cranberry juice that says "juice cocktail" on the label. That has too much sugar and is not concentrated enough with cranberries. Make sure the cranberry juice is 100 percent cranberry juice, as many brands now are. You can use unsweetened cranberry concentrate (available at most health food stores) and mix it with water or unsweetened apple juice.

Parsley juice is a diuretic that also helps decrease inflammation and irritation in the bladder and urethra. A safe, therapeutic dose is one-half to one cup of parsley juice per day. Parsley can be toxic in overdose, and should be especially avoided by pregnant women.

✳ Juice Recipes

Bladder Tonic *(pg 329)*   **Cranberry-Apple Cocktail** *(pg 331)*   **Allergy Relief** *(pg 326)*   **Calcium-Rich Cocktail** *(pg 329)*   **Spinach Power** *(pg 341)* **Morning Energizer** *(pg 337)*   **The Ginger Hopper** *(pg 332)*

Bruises

A BRUISE is an injury that does not break the skin, but does rupture underlying capillaries. This hemorrhaging causes the superficial skin discoloration seen in bruises. If the injury is severe enough, fluid gathers in the affected area, causing swelling, pain, and tenderness.

Easy bruising that occurs with no apparent injury is due to fragile capillaries. These tiny blood vessels can break if their walls are not strong and healthy. While the tendency to bruise easily runs in some families, many people become more prone to this problem as they age or become nutrient deficient.

Purpura is a reddish-purple patch on the skin caused by the bursting of blood vessels in the skin. Older people frequently develop purpura senilis, which are bruises on the hands, arms, and sometimes legs that occur from the slightest contact and take months to heal.

✳ Diet Recommendations

Make dietary changes to help stop easy bruising and to recover from injury. If your skin bruises easily, or if you are recovering from injuries, eat foods rich in vitamin C, bioflavonoids, and vitamin K. These nutrients are highest in the yellow, orange, red, and dark green vegetables. Juicing plenty of these vegetables can make a big difference in preventing bruising.

✳ Nutrient Recommendations

Bioflavonoids are plant pigments responsible for the bright colors of many fruits and vegetables. Two types of bioflavonoids—proanthocyanidins and procyanidolic oligomers (PCOs, which are large, linked proanthocyanidin molecules)—have been studied for their ability to decrease capillary permeability and fragility. PCOs are considered the most effective bioflavonoid in this regard. Citrus bioflavonoids, including rutin, hesperidin, quercetin, and naringin, have also been found effective in treating easy bruising, capillary fragility, and bruising after sports injuries. In addition, bioflavonoids enhance the actions of vitamin C (see the vitamin C entry in this list). *Best juice sources of bioflavonoids:* apricots, bell peppers, berries (blueberries, blackberries, and cranberries), broccoli, cabbage, lemons, limes, parsley, and tomatoes.

Essential fatty acids (EFAs) are recommended for people who bruise easily or are recovering from bruises caused by injury. EFAs must be obtained from the diet. Flaxseed, hemp, and cod-liver oils are excellent sources of EFAs; one tablespoon of any of these per day can be very helpful. (For more information, see the fats and oils section in Basic Guidelines for the Juice Lady's Health and Healing Diet, page 290.)

Vitamin C strengthens capillary walls by playing a role in the formation and maintenance of collagen, the basis of connective tissue. Healthy collagen is important in maintaining the integrity of blood vessels. *Best juice sources of vitamin C:* kale, parsley, broccoli, Brussels sprouts, watercress, cauliflower, cabbage, strawberries, spinach, lemons, limes, turnips, and asparagus.

Vitamin E helps repair tissues. *Best juice sources of vitamin E:* spinach, watercress, asparagus, carrots, and tomatoes.

Vitamin K, research shows, when applied topically, can cause bruises to fade, even those occurring from purpura senilis. In a study of twelve people with significant bruising, vitamin K cream was applied to one arm of each patient and an identical cream without vitamin K was applied to the other. After one month, the arms treated with vitamin K had significantly fewer bruises than those treated with plain ointment. Vitamin K strengthens blood vessel walls, and makes you less prone to bruising. You should consume a minimum of 80 micrograms of vitamin K daily. *Best juice sources of vitamin K:* turnip greens, broccoli, lettuce, cabbage, green beans, and tomatoes.

✳ Herb Recommendations

Arnica, in tincture, salve, or oil form, can be applied externally to a bruised area. Arnica helps stimulate and dilate blood vessels, thereby helping tissues recover from injury. In stimulating good blood flow, arnica helps remove waste products from a bruised area.

Bleeding heart helps deaden the pain associated with bruises, sprains, and contusions. Apply externally and cover the injured area with a hot, moist towel.

Marigold helps heal wounds, bruises, and strains. Use externally as an ointment, salve, poultice, or compress.

Pearly everlasting, applied externally, helps ease the pain, redness, and swelling associated with bruises.

✳ Traditional Remedies for a Bruise

The treatment for a bruise is most effective right after the injury while the bruise is still reddish.

Apply a cold compress such as an ice pack or a bag of frozen peas to the affected area for twenty to thirty minutes in order to speed healing and reduce swelling. Do not apply ice directly to the skin. Wrap the ice pack in a towel. In addition, other remedies may speed healing. Choose from the list below:

Aloe vera: Apply the fresh juice from the fleshy inner part of the leaf. Aloe vera has many healing properties, such as preventing infection, so you can also apply it to minor skin irritations and small wounds to speed up healing.

Apple cider vinegar: Apply a hot or cold poultice of apple cider vinegar to the bruise.

Cabbage leaves: Wash the outer leaves of an organically grown green cabbage. Then remove and discard the main stems, flatten the leaves with a rolling pin to soften, and apply to the bruise. For facial bruises, take the large outer leaves of white cabbage, break the ridges of the leaves, and dip them into very hot water. Then apply to the bruise (but make sure they're not scalding hot as you put them on your face). Cabbage leaves have long been used in folk medicine to speed healing of bruises.

Calendula: To make a salve, heat one ounce of dried calendula flowers or leaves (or one-quarter teaspoon of fresh juice from the herb) with one tablespoon of coconut oil. Once the mixture has cooled, apply it to the bruise. This mixture is also good for sprains, pulled muscles, sores, and boils.

Fenugreek: To make a poultice, put two teaspoons of crushed fenugreek seeds in a small cloth bag and boil it in water for a few minutes. Remove the bag and apply the "tea water" to the area. Make it as hot as you can stand, but make sure it's not scalding.

Garden thyme: Put the green parts of the plant in water and boil for three to four minutes. Turn off the heat, cover the pot, and leave it for another two to three minutes. Strain the mixture, and add the decoction to your bath water. Soak in it for about twenty minutes.

Onion: Apply it raw, directly to the bruise.

Saint-John's-wort: Put ten to fifteen drops of Saint-John's-wort oil in water and apply the mixture to the bruised area. Early Greek herbalists considered Saint-John's-wort an effective herb for healing wounds. It was used to dress sword cuts in the Middle Ages. Modern analysis has shown it to have antibacterial and astringent properties, both qualities useful in the speedy healing of bruises, cuts, and wounds.

Note: Don't smoke or use other tobacco products or allow anyone to smoke around you. Smoking slows healing because it decreases blood supply and delays tissue repair.

☀ Juice Therapy

Parsley juice is an excellent source of bioflavonoids and vitamin C. Intake should be limited to a safe, therapeutic dose of one-half to one cup per day. Parsley can be toxic in overdose, and should be especially avoided by pregnant women.

☀ Juice Recipes

Spinach Power *(pg 341)*   **Icy Spicy Tomato** *(pg 335)*   **Ginger Twist** *(pg 332)*
Peppy Parsley *(pg 339)*   **Beautiful-Skin Cocktail** *(pg 328)*   **Immune Builder** *(pg 335)*   **Turnip Time** *(pg 346)*   **Wheatgrass Light** *(pg 345)*

Bursitis and Tendinitis

BURSITIS is the inflammation of a bursa, which is a small, fluid-filled cavity found in connective tissues, usually in places where friction occurs. (We have about 160 bursae.) Bursae rest at the points where muscles and tendons slide across bone. Healthy bursae create a smooth and almost frictionless gliding surface. The most common bursitis locations are the shoulders, elbows, hips, and knees. When inflammation takes hold, movement that relies on the inflamed bursa becomes rough and painful, and causes the bursa to become more inflamed, perpetuating the problem. Symptoms include pain, swelling, and tenderness, along with restricted range of motion. These symptoms can be experienced particularly when stretching or exercising.

Common causes of bursitis are overuse, stress, or direct trauma to a joint, such as with repeated bumping or prolonged pressure from kneeling. If you work in a profession or have a hobby that requires repetitive motion, you're at increased risk of developing bursitis. The occurrence of bursitis also increases with age. In addition, certain diseases and conditions, such as arthritis, gout, staphylococcal infection, and tuberculosis, increase your risk of developing bursitis. Bursitis can also occur as a result of rheumatoid arthritis (see Rheumatoid Arthritis, page 255). However, many times, the cause is unknown.

Tendinitis is the inflammation of a tendon, the fibrous cord that attaches a muscle to a bone. The condition is painful, and there may be either swelling or a dry, grating sensation. The tendons most often affected are those of the biceps, thumb, knee, inside of the foot, rotator cuff (shoulder), and Achilles tendon in the heel.

The most common causes of tendinitis are injury, overuse, or sudden excessive tension on a tendon. Tendinitis can occur because of poor conditioning, bad posture, or working in an awkward position. It can become chronic, with the formation of calcium deposits in the affected areas.

Conventional medicine treats bursitis or tendinitis with high doses of nonsteroidal anti-inflammatory drugs (NSAIDs), such as ibuprofen. But these drugs can irritate the gastrointestinal tract. Another common approach is to inject cortisone into the affected area. Dr. Jacob Rozbruch of the Mayo Clinic says these injections will not eliminate the mechanical problem, though they will temporarily relieve the pain. He suggests taking a more holistic approach by identifying the underlying cause of the condition, and designing a treatment plan accordingly. This usually involves resting and immobilizing the affected area, and applying ice to reduce swelling.

✳ Lifestyle Recommendations

Rest the affected area. This is the most important treatment for bursitis or tendinitis. Most often, if you rest the affected area, the condition will subside. After the inflammation is reduced, stretch the affected area before exercising or working to prevent further damage.

Try alternative treatments. Acupuncture can bring quick relief of pain as well as a gradual reduction of inflammation. Deep massage can stimulate circulation in the affected area and loosen tight muscles. Chiropractic sessions can help restore the joints' range of motion.

✳ Diet Recommendations

Eat less meat and more complex carbohydrates. Animal foods are high in arachidonic acid, a precursor to inflammation-causing substances called prostaglandins, which can contribute to inflammation. (For more information, see Basic Guidelines for the Juice Lady's Health and Healing Diet, page 290).

Try vegetable juice fasts. A short juice fast can give your body a chance to remove waste products from inflamed areas. (For more information on the healing power of a fast, see the Juice Fast, page 304.)

✳ Nutrient Recommendations

Bioflavonoids are plant pigments that give fruits and vegetables their bright colors. Two types of flavonoids—quercetin and the anthocyanins—are of particular interest for people with inflammatory conditions. Quercetin inhibits the secretion of histamine and other inflammatory chemicals, thereby limiting the inflammatory response. Anthocyanins concentrate in collagen and help repair this protein-based tissue. In addition, bioflavonoids enhance the actions of vitamin C. *Best juice sources of bioflavonoids:* bell peppers, berries (blueberries, blackberries, and cranberries), broccoli, cabbage, lemons, limes, parsley, and tomatoes.

Essential fatty acids (EFAs), namely the omega-3 fatty acids, are able to inhibit production of inflammatory substances called PG2 prostaglandins, and thereby lessen inflammation severity. Hemp and flaxseed oils are excellent. Krill oil is one of the best sources of EFAs. (For more information on EFAs, see the fats and oils section in Basic Guidelines for the Juice Lady's Health and Healing Diet, page 290.)

Vitamin C deficiency is associated with inadequate bursa formation. This vitamin is also important in the prevention and repair of tissue damage. In addition, it has anti-inflammatory and antihistamine properties, histamine being one of the primary chemicals involved in inflammation. *Best juice sources of vitamin C:* kale, parsley, broccoli, Brussels sprouts, watercress, cauliflower, cabbage, strawberries, papaya, spinach, lemons, limes, turnips, and asparagus.

Zinc is effective in reducing inflammation and contributing to tissue repair. *Best juice sources of zinc:* gingerroot, turnips, parsley, garlic, carrots, spinach, cabbage, lettuce, and cucumbers.

✳ Herb Recommendations

Curcumin, which is the yellow pigment in turmeric, is able to inhibit inflammatory substances. Curcumin is available in supplement form.

✳ Juice Therapy

Gingerroot has been shown in scientific studies to have anti-inflammatory properties. It's also a delicious addition to any juice recipe.

Parsley juice is an excellent source of bioflavonoids and vitamin C. Intake should be limited to a safe, therapeutic dose of one-half to one cup per day. Parsley can be toxic in overdose, and should be especially avoided by pregnant women.

✳ Juice Recipes

Ginger Twist *(pg 332)*   **The Ginger Hopper** *(pg 332)*   **Hot Ginger-Lemon Tea** *(pg 334)*   **Spinach Power** *(pg 341)*   **Morning Energizer** *(pg 337)*   **Orient Express** *(pg 338)*   **Peppy Parsley** *(pg 339)*   **Pure Green Sprout Drink** *(pg 340)* **Wheatgrass Light** *(pg 345)*

Cancer

Cancer is a condition in which cells grow unchecked. Cells have an internal governing code, known as homeostatic control, that directs how they mature and reproduce. When cancer develops, this code goes awry and cells divide faster than they mature, and they reproduce at will, usually producing a tissue mass called a tumor. Cancer cells are malignant, which means they invade surrounding tissue. There are hundreds of types of cancer. Currently, cancer is the second most prevalent cause of death in America.

A multitude of factors, including genes, diet, lifestyle, environment, negative emotions, hormones, and viruses, can contribute to cancer's development. Most cancers develop in a multistep process that can be broken down into two phases—initiation and promotion. During the initiation phase, there is usually a quick, irreversible process that creates a permanent change in a cell's master code, or DNA. Then the promotion phase causes the cell to change into a cancer cell. There is a myriad of promoters—from environmental toxins to poor diet to emotional trauma. Symptoms are as many and varied as the types of cancer that have been identified, but can include weight loss, fatigue, and pain. Researchers estimate that 80 to 90 percent of all cancers are environmentally related. In that broad category, the National Cancer Institute lists diet as the number one contributing factor.

Considering that to be the case, doesn't it make sense that diet should be the number one area to address regarding cancer care? For years, nutrition has been of special interest to me because my mother died of cancer when I was very young. Research confirms that diet will make a tremendous difference in your recovery. Having worked with numerous people who have had cancer, I assure you that juicing can have a major impact on your recovery in addition to whatever treatments you and your doctor choose. Make dietary changes that give your body, and particularly your immune system, the best chance to destroy cancer cells and heal itself at the cellular level. Though the whole subject of nutrition and cancer is far beyond the scope of this chapter, the information presented here will give you an excellent start. For more information, see our book *The Complete Cancer Cleanse* (Thomas Nelson).

✳ Diet Recommendations

Eat a high-complex carbohydrate diet packed with vegetables. Plant-based diets have been shown in hundreds of studies to be effective against agents that promote cancer. All anticancer diets should include lots of vegetables in particular, along with whole grains, such as oats, bran, brown rice, and millet; quinoa (a good source of vegetable protein); raw nuts (except peanuts—they can contain highly carcinogenic aflatoxins); seeds; and legumes (beans, lentils, and split peas). Vegetables and fruit, in particular, help prevent cancer, and vegetables and vegetable juices are an important part of an overall cancer-treatment plan. Eat one serving of cruciferous vegetables such as broccoli, cauliflower, Brussels sprouts, or cabbage several times a week. Also choose fruits and vegetables that are deep yellow, orange, green, or red. They are rich in cancer-fighting compounds. For the best vegetables to prevent and treat cancer, see page 77. (For more information on choosing a healthy diet, see Basic Guidelines for the Juice Lady's Health and Healing Diet, page 290.)

Eat 60 to 75 percent raw food—fruits, vegetables, juices, sprouts, seeds, and nuts. When isolated from their natural fruit or vegetable source, many nutrients that have been tested produced disappointing results. However, when the nutrients are left in their natural combined state, they provide a potent anticancer cocktail.

Eat a high-alkaline diet. Otto Warburg, Ph.D., the 1931 Nobel laureate in medicine, first discovered that cancer cells have a different energy metabolism than healthy cells. He discovered that malignant tumors frequently exhibit an increase in "anaerobic glycolysis"—a process where glucose is used by cancer cells as a fuel, with lactic acid as an anaerobic by-product. The large amount of lactic acid produced by this fermentation of glucose from the cancer cells is then transported to the liver. The conversion of glucose to lactate creates a lower, more-acidic pH in cancerous tissues as well as overall physical fatigue from lactic-acid buildup. Larger tumors tend to exhibit an even higher acidic pH. For this reason, it is very important to eat a high-alkaline diet and avoid sweets, animal proteins, alcohol, coffee, black tea, and refined flour products—all are very acid-producing (see the alkaline diet, page 284).

Avoid all foods and additives that have been linked with cancer. These include processed refined foods (white-flour products) and packaged foods. Eliminate all cooking oils (except virgin olive oil and virgin coconut oil), hydrogenated vegetable oils, hydrogenated peanut butter, margarine, caffeine, and alcohol. Read labels, and avoid all food additives, preservatives, dyes, fillers, and stabilizers. (A good rule: if you can't pronounce it, don't buy it.) Avoid peanuts (actually a legume) as they can contain highly carcinogenic aflatoxins. Buy organically grown food as much as possible because pesticides, fungicides, insecticides, and artificial fertilizers can further weaken your immune system. Use kelp and herbal seasonings instead of salt (with the exception of Celtic sea salt or gray salt, which are rich in minerals). Completely avoid barbecued, fried, and smoked foods. The interaction of fat with high heat creates highly carcinogenic by-products.

Avoid all sugar and refined carbohydrates. Sugars have been shown to feed cancer cells, and possibly to contribute to the formation of the protective coating that envelops these cells. Research from the Karolinska Institute in Sweden showed that people who drink soft drinks or add sugar to their coffee increase their risk of developing pancreatic cancer. And in a case-controlled study of 1,866 women in Mexico, those who derived at least 57 percent of their calories from carbohydrates incurred a risk of breast cancer 2.2 times higher than women with more-balanced diets. These are just two of many studies that link sugar and high-carb foods with increased risk of cancer. If you have cancer, you definitely need to avoid all sweets and refined carbs. Avoid the following: white and brown sugar, dried sugar cane, sugar alcohols such as manitol and sorbitol, honey, maple syrup, and especially all artificial sweeteners, such as aspartame (NutraSweet) and sucralose (Splenda). The only sweeteners recommended in small amounts are stevia, an herbal sweetener sold mainly at health food stores, and agave syrup.

Avoid animal protein. Never eat hot dogs, bacon, luncheon meat, sausage, and smoked or cured meats. Avoid red meat and poultry. Avoid commercially raised animals that are fed hormones to promote fast weight gain; one hormone in particular, diethylstilbestrol (DES), has been implicated in breast cancer and fibroid tumors. As your condition improves, you can add a little poached or broiled cold-water fish, such as salmon, tuna, halibut, trout, mackerel, or sardines to your diet, two or three times per week. Too much protein in general is detrimental to health, but is especially so if you have cancer. Restrict your consumption of dairy products. Instead, use almond or rice milk.

Avoid all soy products. Soy foods contain numerous toxins such as high levels of phytic acid, trypsin inhibitors, toxic lysinoalanine, and nitrosamines along with phytoestrogens, which disrupt endocrine function. Hundreds of epidemiological, clinical, and laboratory studies link soy to cancer, heart disease, digestive distress, thyroid problems, cognitive decline, reproductive disorders, immune system breakdown, infertility, and infantile leukemia. It's also linked to type 1 diabetes and precocious puberty (early maturation, such as breast development and menstruation as early as six years of age) in children who have been fed soy formula. The isoflavones in soy products can depress thyroid function and cause goiters in otherwise healthy children and adults. (Soy is a goitrogen, meaning it blocks iodine absorption.) Watch out for soy oil in salad dressing and as textured vegetable protein in packaged foods. Read all labels.

Drink plenty of vegetable juice. A Japanese study in 2004 found that vegetable juice had a positive effect on the immune system. These findings would come as no surprise to Dr. Max Gerson (the Gerson Clinic), who used carrot-apple juice as the core of his cancer-care program. Famous European health clinics and scores of health practitioners have helped thousands of people successfully make raw juices—preferably made from organic produce—an essential part of an anti-cancer diet.

Raw juices do most of the excellent things that solid raw foods do, but with a minimum strain on the digestive system. The alkalinity of raw vegetables in particular is a powerful ally in your fight against cancer, since this disease develops more easily when the body is too acidic. In addition, raw foods are "alive" with nutrients such as antioxidants that are at the peak of their natural potency. For example, a study published by the American Association for Cancer Research (1999) showed that concentrations of alpha-carotene and lutein (carotenoids) were significantly higher in the vegetable juice group than in the raw or cooked vegetable group, which indicates that they are more concentrated in juice than in raw or cooked veggies. In 2005, investigators found that participants with the highest carotenoid concentrations in their blood—showing that they were eating plenty of vegetables and fruit—had a 43 percent lower risk of either cancer recurrence or a new primary breast cancer, compared with women whose carotenoid levels were lower.

Juices are also rich in phytosterols and sterolins, which can block the development of tumors in colon, breast, and prostate glands by altering cell membrane transfer in tumor growth. Studies indicate that after five days, breast cancer cell cultures supplemented with B-Sitosterol (a phytosterol) had 66 percent fewer breast cancer cells than did controls. Another study showed a 28 percent inhibition of prostate-cancer cell growth after being exposed to B-Sitosterol for five days in vitro. Generally, it is thought that a weak immune system is one of the prerequisites for the development of cancer. By enhancing the function of T cells and the secretion of lymphokines with plenty of freshly made juices, the immune system will stand a better chance of eliminating cancer cells.

Fresh juices are also rich in enzymes, substances that are destroyed by cooking. Enzymes are important for fighting cancer, as they assist pancreatic enzymes in digesting cooked foods. Pancreatic enzymes have the power to destroy the protective mucous barrier that surrounds cancer cells, as do certain enzymes in fruits and vegetables. Dilute all fruit juices by half with water or vegetable juice, and use fruit juice very sparingly to avoid consuming too much fruit sugar—no more than four ounces per day. Juice vegetables instead.

Use juice fasts and cleansing programs. The body eliminates toxins by either directly neutralizing them or excreting them. Toxins the body can't eliminate build up in the tissues, most often in fat cells. It is vitally important that you get rid of stored-up toxins, and that your liver, intestines, and kidneys are all functioning well to assist you in the detoxification process. Studies have shown that people with the poorest detoxification processes are the most susceptible to cancer. Many people have discovered that once they've completed a liver cleanse, the status of their tumors began to change for the better. A complete detoxification program can help rid the body of a host of toxins. (For more information, see the Juice Fast, page 304, and the Cleansing Programs, pages 303–325).

Cleanse your liver. The liver is the key organ of detoxification and hormone metabolism. Your liver is involved in manufacturing hormones from cholesterol, converting thyroid hormones, and manufacturing, breaking down, and regulating sex hormones like estrogen, testosterone, DHEA, and progesterone. When it's not overburdened, the liver will prevent hormones from changing into dangerous metabolites. For example, estrogens break down or are detoxified into estrogen metabolites called 2-hydroxyestrone, 4-hydroxyestrone, and 16-alphahydroxyestrone. These metabolites can have stronger or weaker estrogenic activity—and thus increase or decrease a woman's risk of breast, uterine, and other cancers—depending on how they are metabolized.

Properly metabolizing and excreting hormones is crucial. Research strongly suggests that women who metabolize a larger proportion of their estrogens down the C-16 pathway, as opposed to the C-2 pathway, have elevated breast cancer risk, and that the estrogens metabolized down the C-16 route may be associated with direct toxic effects and carcinogenicity.

Estrogens are metabolized by a series of oxidizing enzymes in the cytochrome P450 family (Phase I of liver detoxification). They are then sent on to Phase II for conjugation. Detoxification enzymes break down all manner of drugs, hormones, and environmental toxins into generally less-harmful metabolites. When Phase II slows down, there is a buildup of toxic intermediates. A healthy, uncongested liver is very important to the detoxification process. However, a healthy, uncongested liver is not the norm; there are too many toxins in our world for most people's livers to detoxify all of them without some assistance. Therefore, a liver cleanse at least twice a year could make a world of difference for you (see the Liver Cleanse, page 310). And a liver support supplement taken daily could be very helpful (see page 348).

✳ Nutrient Recommendations

Antioxidants are found in a number of fruits and vegetables, and have been extensively studied for both their protective and therapeutic actions against cancer. Antioxidants are important because they destroy free radicals, unstable molecules that are always attempting to steal electrons from other molecules. This process sets up a chain reaction that leads to cell damage. Free radicals can cause extensive damage over a period of time, which can lead to cancer. The following antioxidants bind to free radicals, protecting your cells and greatly enhancing your chances of winning the cancer battle:

- **Bioflavonoids** have been shown to have anticancer as well as antiviral and anti-inflammatory properties. They are extremely effective at destroying free radicals. Two flavonoids—nobiletin and tangeretin—boost the activity of a group of enzymes that specialize in ridding the body of such toxins as drugs, heavy metals, and hydrocarbons from auto exhausts. They also enhance the effectiveness of vitamin C. *Best juice sources of bioflavonoids:* bell peppers, berries (blueberries, blackberries, and cranberries), broccoli, cabbage, lemons, limes, parsley, and tomatoes.
- **Carotenes** are plant pigments that have been found to be quite remarkable in their ability to protect the body against free-radical damage. Diets rich in the carotenes are associated with a reduced risk of cancer. Carotenes also have important immune-enhancing capabilities, particularly in stimulating such

immune-system cells as helper T cells that fight cancer. *Best juice sources of carotenes:* carrots, kale, parsley, spinach, Swiss chard, beetroot greens, watercress, broccoli, and romaine lettuce, along with all other orange, yellow, red, and dark green vegetables and fruits.

The best vegetables to prevent and treat cancer include: broccoli (especially broccoli sprouts), Brussels sprouts, Chinese cabbage, celery, turnip greens, spinach, kale, and parsley.

Essential fatty acids (EFAs), and the omega-3s in particular, have powerful anti-cancer properties.

- **Omega-3 fats:** These are fats found in fish and fish oil. The most powerful form of omega-3 oil is its DHA component, which inhibits cancer cell growth. (For more information on omega-3–rich oils, see the fats and oils section in Basic Guidelines for the Juice Lady's Health and Healing Diet, page 290).
- **Conjugated Linoleic Acid (CLA):** This is a special type of fat that reduces inflammation, lowers breast cancer development, and reduces visceral fat.
- **Gamma-Linolenic Acid (GLA):** This potent anti-cancer oil is extracted from evening primrose or borage plants. Studies have shown that it not only prevents breast cancer, it suppresses the growth of existing breast cancers. It can also enhance the effectiveness of tamoxifen against breast cancer.

Iron tablets should be avoided if you have cancer. Excess iron may suppress both the cancer-killing function of the macrophages, immune cells that help in tissue repair, and T- and B-cell activity. Choose a multivitamin without iron.

Selenium works with the enzyme glutathione peroxidase, an antioxidant enzyme that is important in the development of many immune-system cells. *Best juice sources of selenium:* Swiss chard, turnips, garlic, oranges, radishes, carrots, and cabbage.

Vitamin C offers particular immune support for cancer patients. In several studies, it has been shown to increase survival time. It is especially helpful for those going through chemotherapy and radiation, as it appears to enhance the effectiveness of such conventional treatments. *Best juice sources of vitamin C:* kale, parsley, broccoli, Brussels sprouts, watercress, cauliflower, cabbage, strawberries, spinach, lemons, limes, turnips, asparagus.

Vitamin E is an antioxidant that supports the immune system. *Best juice sources of vitamin E:* spinach, watercress, asparagus, carrots, and tomatoes.

Zinc is necessary for enhanced white blood cell functioning, and has been shown to increase production of white cells called T lymphocytes. *Best juice sources of zinc:* gingerroot, turnips, parsley, garlic, carrots, spinach, cabbage, lettuce, and cucumbers.

✳ Herb Recommendations

Astragalus has been shown to restore immune function when the immune system is suppressed as a side effect of chemotherapy. It has also been shown to increase production of antibodies and interferon, two important immune system components, and to increase the activity of helper T cells. Avoid this herb if you have a fever.

Echinacea enhances the immune system. It also acts against viruses, which means it can help you fight off infections if your immune system is not working properly.

✳ Juice Therapy

Beetroot juice has been found to reverse and prevent radiation-induced cancers.

Cabbage juice contains a high concentration of two substances, indole-3-carbinol and oltipaz, that help increase the activity of enzymes that protect against a wide range of cancers.

Carrot juice is one of the richest sources of beta-carotene, and is believed to be able to break down the protective mucous membranes around cancer cells. Cancer expert Dr. Virginia Livingston urged her patients to drink two pints of fresh carrot juice each day. Dr. Max Gerson had his patients drink ten eight-ounce glasses of carrot-apple juice daily, alternating with glasses of green juices.

Garlic juice has been shown in studies to inhibit tumor growth. Onions have similar properties.

Green juices, such as those made from beetroot greens, spinach, parsley, Swiss chard, kale, wheatgrass, and sprouts, are rich in chlorophyll. Research at the University of Texas Systems Cancer Center has found that chlorophyll may block the genetic changes that cancer-causing substances produce in cells.

Parsley juice is rich in bioflavonoids and vitamin C. Intake should be limited to a safe, therapeutic dose of one-half to one cup per day. Parsley can be toxic in overdose, and should be especially avoided by pregnant women.

Pomegranate juice. Studies have shown that pomegranate juice can reverse the development of prostate, lung, and breast cancer. It's rich in polyphenols. High doses of polyphenols prevent and shut down cancerous tumors by cutting off the formation of new blood vessels needed for tumor growth. The amount needed is equivalent to about twenty-five ounces (750 ml) of juice per day. (Polyphenols are commonly found in fruits, vegetables, and green and white tea.) Fresh pomegranate juice is always best because it has not been pasteurized. Commercially prepared juice is required to be pasteurized, which kills vital nutrients.

Tomato juice is rich in lycopene, a very powerful antioxidant that has been shown to be particularly helpful in protecting against prostate cancer. Tomatoes are also rich in p-coumaric and chlorogenic acid, two phytochemicals that block formation of highly carcinogenic nitrosamine compounds within the body.

Wheatgrass juice helps build the immune system. Studies have identified a number of substances in wheatgrass juice that are formidable anticancer agents—one being chlorophyll. Research done on the water-soluble form known as chlorophyllin shows that it prevents assimilation of certain carcinogenic compounds. Chlorophyllin also reduces the oxidative damage caused by radiation and some chemicals. This may explain the effective role that wheatgrass juice plays in an anticancer diet. Wheatgrass juice works best when taken alone (see Sources, page 347, for information on health institutes that use the raw food and juice-fast plans, including wheatgrass juice.)

✳ Juice Recipes

Morning Energizer *(pg 337)* **Triple C** *(pg 344)* **The Ginger Hopper** *(pg 332)*
Sweet Dreams Nightcap *(pg 342)* **Turnip Time** *(pg 344)* **Icy Spicy Tomato**
(pg 335) **Wheatgrass Light** *(pg 345)* **Pure Green Sprout Drink** *(pg 340)* **Salsa
in a Glass** *(pg 340)* **Liver Life Tonic** *(pg 336)* **Calcium-Rich Cocktail** *(pg 329)*
Spinach Power *(pg 341)* **Jack & the Bean** *(pg 335)* **Beet-Cucumber Cleansing
Cocktail** *(pg 330)* **Cabbage Patch Cocktail** *(pg 329)* **Immune Builder** *(pg 335)*
The Revitalizer *(pg 345)*

Candidiasis

CANDIDIASIS is an infection with any species of yeast-like fungus *Candida albicans,* which is naturally present in the intestines; genital tract, mouth, and throat, and on the skin. It normally coexists with friendly bacteria that keep it in check, namely bifidobacteria and acidophilus. When the healthy balance is upset, it overgrows, and can invade other tissues and create a host of problems. This occurs mostly with the use of broad-spectrum antibiotics that destroy healthy microflora, along with a weakened immune system from long-standing illness, stress, lack of sleep, smoking, poor nutrition, overconsumption of sweets and refined carbohydrates, poor digestion, and alcohol. Sugars, refined carbs, and alcohol are the foods of choice for *Candida albicans,* allowing it to proliferate. *Candida albicans* can travel to all parts of the body through the bloodstream. It produces acetaldehyde, a type of alcohol that interferes with normal functioning in various bodily systems. Gastrointestinal symptoms include bloating, gas, cramps, rectal itching, changes in bowel function, and thrush ("white carpet" tongue). Nervous-system reactions include depression, poor memory, irritability, and inability to concentrate. Genitourinary complaints include vaginal yeast infections and recurring bladder infections. Endocrine problems include premenstrual syndrome (PMS) and other menstrual disorders. Immune-system complaints include lowered immunity, allergies, and chemical sensitivities. Overall, candidiasis is characterized by chronic fatigue, loss of sex drive, and malaise.

Although a complete candidiasis-treatment program is beyond the scope of this chapter, the following guidelines will give you an excellent start in getting the infection under control.

On a personal note: I suffered with candidiasis for a number of years. I know firsthand that dietary change is a key to recovery.

❇ Diet Recommendations

Avoid all sugars—natural, refined, and artificial. This also includes all fruit or fruit juice; yeasts love sugars.

Avoid all foods that contain yeast or mold, such as raised breads and other raised flour products, cheese, vinegar, olives, peanuts, alcohol, dried fruit, and melons. Don't eat leftovers; they are much more susceptible to mold growth.

Avoid bottom crawlers such as oysters, clams, and lobster, and deep-sea fish such as tuna, mackerel, and swordfish, which may contain toxic levels of mercury.

Avoid farm-raised fish; they often contain PCBs and not enough omega-3 essential fatty acids, due to their land-based diets. Choose wild-caught fish instead.

Avoid yeast and wheat products (breads, crackers, pasta, etc.) that contain gluten.

Avoid sodium nitrite, found in processed foods such as hot dogs, lunch meats, and bacon.

Avoid monosodium glutamate (MSG), found in many foods as a flavor enhancer.

Avoid hydrogenated or partially hydrogenated oils, and trans fats, found in many processed foods, deep-fried foods, fast food, and junk food.

Choose only grass-fed, organically raised meat and poultry because of the heavy use of antibiotics and hormones in the agriculture industry.

Eat no more than one cup per day of high-carbohydrate vegetables, and **grains.** This category includes potatoes, yams, corn, winter squash, lentils, beans, peas, millet, rice, and barley.

Avoid milk and its products. Milk sugars, like other sugars, promote yeast growth. You can generously eat and juice all vegetables, except those specified above, and sprouts. Wash the vegetables in biodegradable soap and water.

Add ground flax meal to your diet to promote digestive regularity.

Add organic virgin coconut oil; it has antimicrobial properties.

Increase your omega-3 fatty acid intake by selecting ground flax meal, wild-caught salmon, fish oil, avocados, and walnuts.

Eat at least one crushed garlic clove per day.

Drink plenty of water. Increasing your intake of purified water can help your body flush out the toxins released from the yeast. And as the yeast dies off, it needs to be removed or you'll feel worse. Adding a teaspoon of fresh lemon juice to each glass of water will help facilitate the cleansing process.

Increase the use of certain culinary herbs and spices. The following herbs and spices have antifungal and antibacterial properties because of their essential oil content.

Use them often in your cooking: anise, cinnamon, fennel, garlic, gingerroot, lemon balm, licorice, rosemary, and thyme. Garlic has been shown to be more active against *Candida albicans* than the popular drug nystatin, a common antifungal agent. Cooking can destroy garlic's antifungal compound, allicin, so use garlic fresh in salad dressings, on salads, and in juices.

Cleanse the liver. Acetaldehyde, the alcohol produced by *Candida albicans,* can cause a person to feel constantly "hung over." The acetaldehyde puts a strain directly on the liver, which must continually detoxify the alcohol. When the liver becomes overloaded, it cannot filter blood properly. The problem is then magnified as the *Candida albicans* is killed, since this process can release toxins into the bloodstream. Cleansing and supporting the liver is a vital part of candidiasis treatment (see the Liver Cleanse, page 310). Also, short vegetable-juice fasts (no fruit juice!) of one to three days can be quite helpful (see the Juice Fast, page 304).

✳ Nutrient Recommendations

Caprylic acid, derived from coconuts, appears to play an important role in combating *Candida albicans*. This fatty acid apparently coats the gastrointestinal tract and starves the yeast cells. Caprylic acid is easily absorbed in the intestines. Therefore, it is necessary to take a time-released or enterically coated supplement to get a gradual release along the entire gastrointestinal tract. And, you can use virgin coconut oil in cooking, which is rich in caprylic acid.

Cellulase (found in health food stores) is an enzyme that breaks down the outer layer of the *Candida albicans* organism, killing the cell. When the dead cell releases its toxins, the protease enzymes in the product (Candidase) eat them up. This helps prevent die-off symptoms.

Copper helps macrophages, white blood cells that get rid of foreign particles, digest and destroy *Candida albicans*. Studies have shown that when there is a copper deficiency, fewer yeast cells are destroyed, and immune-system functions are impaired. *Best juice sources of copper:* carrots, garlic, gingerroot, and turnips.

Magnesium plays a role in reestablishing a strong immune system in people who have candidiasis. *Best juice sources of magnesium:* beet greens, spinach, parsley, dandelion greens, garlic, beetroot, broccoli, cauliflower, carrots, and celery.

Selenium is essential for a healthy immune system. Tests have shown that a selenium deficiency significantly impairs the ability of white blood cells to kill *Candida albicans*. *Best juice sources of selenium:* Swiss chard, turnips, garlic, radishes, carrots, and cabbage.

Vitamin B₁ (thiamine) has been shown to increase the ability of leukocytes (white blood cells that fight infection and tissue damage) to destroy *Candida albicans*. Also, vitamin B₁ is believed to help combat acetaldehyde production. *Best food sources of vitamin B₁:* seeds, nuts, beans, split peas, millet, buckwheat, whole wheat, oatmeal, wild rice, lobster, and cornmeal. It can also be found, in lesser quantities, in sunflower and buckwheat sprouts, and garlic. It is not found in fruits and vegetables.

Zinc deficiency is thought to play a role in recurring vaginal candidiasis. Zinc is important to a healthy immune system, and helps detoxify metabolic wastes. *Best juice sources of zinc:* gingerroot, turnips, parsley, garlic, carrots, spinach, cabbage, lettuce, and cucumbers.

✳ Herb Recommendations

Barberry, goldenseal, and **Oregon grape** all contain a powerful microbial factor called berberine that is especially effective against *Candida albicans*. Do not use any of these herbs if you are pregnant, and do not use them for more than ten days at a time.

Black walnut can help eliminate both *Candida albicans* and parasites, such as worms, commonly found in people who have candidiasis.

Chamomile contains compounds that kill *Candida albicans*. Traditionally, it is used for diarrhea, indigestion, and colic, all common candidiasis symptoms. Be sure to use German chamomile *(Matricaria recutita)* and not Roman chamomile *(Chamaemelum nobile)*.

Pau d'arco, a Brazilian tree bark, helps eliminate *Candida albicans*.

✳ Juice Therapy

Cranberry juice is commonly used in alleviating bacterial bladder and other urinary tract infections (see Bladder Infections, page 59). Symptoms associated with bladder infection, such as urinary urgency and pain on urination, can be found in people who have candidiasis.

Garlic juice is a potent antifungal agent.

Parsley juice is a good source of zinc. Intake should be limited to a safe, therapeutic dose of one-half to one cup per day. Parsley can be toxic in overdose, and should be especially avoided by pregnant women.

Wheatgrass juice is a potent antifungal agent.

✳ Juice Recipes

Cranberry-Apple Cocktail *(pg 331)*   **Pure Green Sprout Drink** *(pg 340)*   **Ginger Twist** *(pg 332)*   **Magnesium-Rich Cocktail** *(pg 336)*   **Spinach Power** *(pg 341)*   **Sinus Solution** *(pg 341)*   **Triple C** *(pg 344)*   **Afternoon Refresher** *(pg 326)*   **Jack & the Bean** *(pg 335)*   **Garlic Surprise** *(pg 332)*   **Wheatgrass Light** *(pg 345)*

Canker Sores

Mouth sores, known as canker sores, are small ulcers that can appear on the lips, gums, tongue, or insides of the cheeks. They are surrounded by a reddened border and covered with a white or yellowish membrane, and range in size from a pinhead to a quarter. A burning sensation may precede their development. Though quite common, they are very painful. They can be single or clustered, and can persist for a few days to nearly two weeks. Larger sores may cause scarring. Possible causes include stress (see Stress, page 261), candidiasis (see Candidiasis, page 80), food sensitivities or allergies, poor dental hygiene, nutrient deficiencies or trauma caused by vigorous tooth brushing or biting the inside of the cheek.

✳ Diet & Lifestyle Recommendations

Identify food allergies and sensitivities. Reactions to offending foods can cause canker sores. Some of the most common offenders:

- Gluten—the protein found in cereal grains such as buckwheat, wheat, oats, rye, and barley (You may be able to eat these grains sprouted.)
- Fruit and fruit juices: citrus fruit, pineapples, apples, figs, tomatoes, and strawberries
- Dairy: milk and cheese
- Sweets: cakes, pies, cookies, chocolate, candy, soft drinks, muffins, and gum
- Other foods: nuts, shellfish, soy, vinegar, and mustard
- Additives: cinnamonaldehyde (a flavoring agent), benzoic acid (a preservative)
- Other substances: toothpastes, mints, gums, dental materials, metals, medications (Choose toothpastes and mouthwashes that do not contain the foaming agent sodium lauryl sulfate, which can be a causative agent of, or have an aggravating effect upon, canker sores.)

Eat fewer animal products, and drink less coffee. Animal proteins and coffee produce excess acid in the body, which contributes to the development of canker sores.

✳ Nutrient Recommendations

Beta-carotene helps promote faster healing of the mucous membranes. *Best juice sources of carotenes in general:* carrots, kale, parsley, spinach, Swiss chard, beetroot greens, watercress, broccoli, and romaine lettuce.

Folic acid deficiencies can cause canker sores to develop. *Best juice sources of folic acid:* asparagus, spinach, kale, broccoli, cabbage, and blackberries.

Iron deficiencies can cause canker sores. *Best juice sources of nonheme iron, the type found in plants:* parsley, dandelion greens, broccoli, cauliflower, strawberries, asparagus, Swiss chard, blackberries, cabbage, beetroot with greens, and carrots.

Vitamin B$_{12}$ (cobalamin) deficiencies can cause canker sores. This vitamin is not available in fruit or vegetable juices. *Best food sources of vitamin B$_{12}$:* meat, poultry, and fish.

Zinc can be beneficial when there is a zinc deficiency. *Best juice sources of zinc:* gingerroot, turnips, parsley, garlic, carrots, grapes, spinach, cabbage, lettuce, and cucumbers.

✳ Herb Recommendations

Gargle with calendula tea or goldenseal tea to help canker sores heal.

✳ Juice Therapy

Cabbage juice has been shown to heal peptic ulcers. It may also be helpful for mouth ulcers.

✳ Juice Recipes

Triple C *(pg 344)* **The Ginger Hopper** *(pg 332)* . **Spinach Power** *(pg 341)*
Beautiful-Bone Solution *(pg 328)* **Weight-Loss Buddy** *(pg 345)*
Sweet Dreams Nightcap *(pg 342)*

Cardiovascular Disease

CARDIOVASCULAR DISEASE is a general term for diseases that affect the heart and blood vessels. Commonly called atherosclerosis, cardiovascular disease is the leading cause of mortality in the United States and in most industrialized countries. In atherosclerosis, fatty plaques build up in the arterial walls and gradually decrease blood flow to the organs such as the heart. Plaque buildup can weaken the vessel wall, causing a rupture, or plaque can break off from the wall to create a blood-vessel obstruction called an embolism. Symptoms can include angina, which is a squeezing chest pain caused by reduced blood flow to the heart; leg cramps; gradual mental deterioration; weakness; and/or dizziness. Atherosclerosis is also associated with myocardial infarction (heart attack), stroke, and congestive heart failure, which is an inability of the heart to pump blood fast enough to fully meet the body's needs.

The most current theory about how plaque forms is that it follows an injury to the blood-vessel wall. Cholesterol, in the form of low-density lipoproteins (LDLs, the "bad fats"), gathers at the injury site. There, it is oxidized, in a process similar to butter going rancid, which is caused by unstable molecules called free radicals.

The American Heart Association has discovered that people with heart disease all have one thing in common—inflammation. And even though cholesterol-lowering drugs are still a primary treatment of choice, it is interesting to note that scientists are no longer focusing on cholesterol as a factor because more than 60 percent of all heart attacks occur in people with normal cholesterol levels. Currently, researchers are focusing on the following contributors: (1) damaged fats—particularly trans fats (found in margarine, snack foods, and fried foods); (2) the use of oils high in omega-6 fatty acids (polyunsaturated oils), which oxidize easily; (3) inflammation; (4) blood clots; (5) high blood pressure; and (6) high levels of homocysteine, a sulphur-containing amino acid. **Note:** You can get a blood test that measures C-reactive protein (CRP), a marker for blood vessel inflammation. The higher your CRP, the greater your inflammatory activity. And rather than striving to bring down your cholesterol, it appears to be much wiser to bring down inflammation and homocysteine levels.

In 1990, Dean Ornish, M.D., reported from his studies with heart disease patients that comprehensive lifestyle changes such as eating a low-fat vegetarian diet, stopping smoking, practicing stress management, and getting moderate exercise could cause even severe coronary atherosclerosis to regress. Today, many studies support his claims. Maintaining low LDL levels, for example, can reduce the chances of plaque buildup. Recent findings also indicate that it is important to lower levels of homocysteine. If you follow the recommendations noted in this chapter, you should greatly reduce your risk of cardiovascular disease or strengthen a treatment program for an existing problem.

✳ Lifestyle Recommendations

Stop smoking. Smoking not only makes the heart work harder, it also promotes the development of artery-clogging plaque. If you are finding it challenging to stop smoking, increase your vegetable juices and raw foods. One study found that when participants increased their raw foods to just over 60 percent of their diet, 80 percent lost their desire to smoke.

Reduce your stress levels. Stress causes unhealthy changes in hormone balance that can lead to plaque formation. There are many methods you can use to reduce your stress levels, including meditation, prayer, deep breathing, and various kinds of exercises (see Stress, page 261).

Get more exercise. Exercise not only tones your heart, it can also help you maintain a healthy weight (another factor in heart disease) and reduce stress.

✳ Diet Recommendations

Eat a high-complex carbohydrate diet. Fifty percent of your diet should consist of raw fruits, vegetables, sprouts, juices, seeds, and nuts. Studies from all over the world have shown a low incidence of heart disease in places where people eat primarily a high-fiber, low-fat, plant-based diet. This type of diet has been shown to reduce the risk of cardiovascular disease.

Eat six to nine servings of vegetables and fruit each day. A large analysis of almost a quarter of a million people shows that every extra fruit or vegetable serving consumed daily could cut your risk of heart disease by 4 percent. (For more information, see Basic Guidelines for the Juice Lady's Health and Healing Diet, page 290).

Drink a glass of fresh juice daily. Juices are rich in polyphenols (substances found in plants that have antioxidant activity, which has been widely studied regarding heart disease). An equivalent to approximately one glass of wine a day was found to play a beneficial role in combating heart disease, benefiting your circulatory system by facilitating blood-vessel growth. I do not recommend drinking wine because alcohol is a neurotoxin (a substance that destroys nerve tissue). You can get the same effect by drinking fresh vegetable or grape juice. Juices are also rich in soluble fiber, such as the pectins, which have been shown to lower LDL levels. (Oat bran and psyllium seed husk also offer beneficial soluble fiber.) A one- to three-day juice fast can be beneficial as well (see the Juice Fast, page 304).

Eat more fish. Fish has been associated with a reduced cardiovascular risk. The best choices are those taken from cold waters such as salmon, halibut, tuna, cod, trout, and mackerel. These fish contain relatively large amounts of omega-3 fatty acids. Omega-3s have been shown to decrease platelet clumping, thus preventing the formation of vessel-clogging clots and reducing the formation of atherosclerotic plaques. Studies show that when red meat is replaced by fish in the diet, the composition of fatty acids in the blood changes for the better. Omega-3 fatty acids are also found in flaxseed and hemp seeds, which makes them an excellent dietary supplement. For more information, see the fats and oils section in Basic Guidelines for the Juice Lady's Health and Healing Diet (page 290).

Take fish oil (e.g., cod-liver oil, krill oil, EPA, DHA). Omega-3 fatty acids in fish suppress the inflammatory agents that often are unleashed in the body by omega-6 fats such as corn, safflower, sunflower, canola, and soybean oils. Fish oil counters inflammation. Other benefits include:

- Counteracts or prevents cardiac arrhythmia
- Helps prevent thrombosis (a blood clot within a blood vessel)
- Helps prevent fatty deposits and fibrosis of the inner layer forming in the arteries
- Improves endothelial function, a major factor in promoting the growth of new blood vessels
- Lowers blood pressure
- Lowers triglycerides

Avoid unhealthy oils. Polyunsaturated oils (PUFAs)—the omega-6–rich oils—include soybean, safflower, sunflower, corn, and canola. These are *the worst oils* to use in cooking because they are highly susceptible to heat damage due to their large number of double bonds. When heated, toxic chemicals are produced as the oils oxidize. Oxidation causes cross-linking, cyclization, double-bond shifts, fragmentation, and polymerization of the oils, which can cause nearly as much damage as trans fats. Trans fats are found primarily in margarine, hydrogenated vegetable oils, fried foods, and snack foods. Margarine is made through a process called partial hydrogenation, which produces substances called trans-fatty acids. These fatty acids contribute to the development of coronary heart disease and the risk of heart attack. Trans fats in the diet are associated with elevated cholesterol and LDL levels, and with lower HDL (the "good cholesterol") levels.

Choose the best oils. Extra-virgin olive oil is best for cold food preparation, and virgin coconut oil is best for cooking. Coconut oil is very stable and, when heated, won't oxidize easily.

Avoid high-carbohydrate foods. Foods that spike blood sugar spur inflammation. Research at Harvard confirms that women who ate foods with the highest glycemic load had nearly twice as much inflammation. Such foods include white potatoes, white rice, white bread (and other white-flour products like bagels, pasta, and pizza crust), sugar (all sweets) and highly processed cereals. J. Rand Baggesen, M.D., author of *High-Tech Health*, says, "There is no substitute to an active physical lifestyle in combination with a diet that avoids high levels of simple carbohydrates when it comes to health. In 2008, we do not have a medicine as powerful as these simple measures when it comes to avoidance of heart disease and stroke."

Watch your protein. High-protein diets boost inflammation. The Fleming Heart and Health Institute in Omaha found that people on a high-protein diet for a year showed a jump of 62 percent in blood-vessel inflammation, and coronary artery disease worsened.

Don't cook animal protein on high heat, and avoid all fried foods. Researchers at Mount Sinai School of Medicine found that grilling, broiling, and frying meat and poultry has been shown to create damaged proteins called AGEs (advanced glycosylation end products) that trigger inflammation. In diabetics who ate a high AGE-inducing diet, inflammation jumped 35 percent; it dropped 20 percent in those on low AGE-inducing diets. To reduce AGEs, poach or boil chicken, and eat more fish. Broiled fish has about one-quarter the AGEs of broiled steak or chicken. Fruits and vegetables are low in AGEs; cheese is high. In another study, scientists gathered dietary information on more than 9,500 men and women ages forty-five to sixty-four and tracked their health for nine years. Overall, a Western dietary pattern—high intakes of refined grains, fried foods, and red meat—was associated with an 18 percent increased risk for metabolic syndrome, which includes cardiovascular disease. But the one-third who ate the most fried food increased their risk by 25 percent compared with the one-third who ate the least.

Avoid all soda, especially diet. In the study involving 9,500 men and women ages forty-five to sixty-four, researchers tracked their health for nine years and found a correlation between drinking diet soda and metabolic syndrome—the collection of risk factors for cardiovascular disease and diabetes, which include abdominal obesity, high cholesterol and blood-glucose levels, and elevated blood pressure.

Reduce your salt intake. Excessive salt (refined sea salt and common table salt) intake is a common cause of high blood pressure, particularly in salt-sensitive individuals. (The one exception is highly mineralized salt such as Celtic sea salt or gray salt used in moderation. It is best to avoid all other salt.) Though salt restriction is an effective means of decreasing blood pressure, combining salt restriction with a high-potassium diet consisting of plenty of fruits and vegetables will further enhance blood-pressure reduction (see High Blood Pressure, page 175).

Limit coffee consumption. Heavy consumption of coffee—more than three cups per day—increases the risk of heart attack. Drinking green tea is associated with decreased LDL and triglyceride levels, and with increased HDL levels.

Reduce beer consumption. High-alcohol versus low-alcohol beer has been shown to increase LDL levels.

Be aware of the risks of birth control pills. Long-term use of birth control pills may increase artery plaque buildup in your body that may raise your risk of heart disease. In a study of 1,300 healthy women between the ages of thirty-five and fifty-five, Belgian researchers found that there was a 20 to 30 percent increased prevalence of plaque for every ten years of oral contraceptive use.

Get rid of electropollution. Electropollution comes from electric devices such as high-voltage power lines, hair dryers, computers, televisions, cell phones, and radios. Some people are more vulnerable to electropollution and can develop arrhythmias, chest pain, anxiety, and depression. One theory says electropollution has the potential to reduce heart rate variability (HRV)—variations in the heart's beat-to-beat interval. Cardiologist Stephen Sinatra, M.D., has found that a lot of people have poor HRV. He encourages everyone to discharge electropollution from their bodies by grounding themselves by walking barefoot on dirt, sand, or grass. He says it's very important to spend time outside connecting your body (skin) to the earth. This is an excellent way to get rid of electropollution.

✳ Nutrient Recommendations

Antioxidants reduce the oxidation of fats and decrease the ability of platelets to clump together. Increasing intake of the following antioxidant nutrients has been shown to reduce the risk of premature death from coronary artery disease:

- **Beta-carotene** and **vitamin A** are important for good cardiovascular health. Consumption of foods rich in beta-carotene is associated with a lowered risk of nonfatal heart attacks in women, and this nutrient has reduced cardiovascular disease risk among high-risk men. Beta-carotene, also known as provitamin A, is the only form of vitamin A found in fruits and vegetables, and is converted by the body to vitamin A as needed. *Best juice sources of carotenes in general:* carrots, kale, parsley, spinach, Swiss chard, beetroot greens, watercress, broccoli, and romaine lettuce.

- **Coenzyme Q10** is a substance made in the body that inhibits fat oxidation. It also improves the heart's energy production, and has been used with great success in cases of congestive heart failure. *Best food sources of coenzyme Q10:* mackerel, salmon, and sardines; it is not available in fruits and vegetables. Supplement recommendation: 100 mg daily.
- **Folic acid** is responsible for converting homocysteine into the amino acid methionine. A Canadian study showed that low blood levels of folic acid were associated with an increased risk of fatal coronary heart disease. *Best juice sources of folic acid:* kale, spinach and other leafy greens, asparagus, broccoli, cabbage, and blackberries.
- **Magnesium** has been shown to be beneficial for congestive heart failure, arrhythmias, and other heart problems. *Best juice sources of magnesium:* beetroot greens, spinach, parsley, dandelion greens, garlic, blackberries, beetroot, broccoli, cauliflower, carrots, and celery.
- **Selenium** helps prevent the oxidation of LDL. *Best juice sources of selenium:* Swiss chard, turnips, garlic, radishes, carrots, and cabbage.
- **Vitamin C.** Research shows that people with the lowest vitamin C levels had the worst inflammation and peripheral (leg) artery disease. Vitamin C is an important cofactor in the formation of collagen, which strengthens blood-vessel walls. *Best juice sources of vitamin C:* kale, parsley, broccoli, Brussels sprouts, watercress, cauliflower, cabbage, strawberries, spinach, lemons, limes, turnips, and asparagus.
- **Vitamin E.** When diabetic people were given 1,200 IU of vitamin E daily in studies at the University of Texas Southwestern Medical Center, inflammation dropped 30 to 50 percent. Vitamin E is also involved in the growth and repair of the inner lining of arterial walls. *Best juice sources of vitamin E:* spinach, watercress, asparagus, carrots, and tomatoes.

✳ Herb Recommendations

Hawthorn has traditionally been used as a heart tonic. This herb is rich in bioflavonoids, which increase the amount of vitamin C in the fluid that nourishes the body's cells. It also reduces blood pressure and cholesterol levels, and prevents cholesterol from building up in arterial walls. And it helps improve blood supply to the heart by dilating the coronary blood vessels.

✳ Juice Therapy

Apple juice (and apples) have been shown to contain compounds that slow one of the processes that lead to heart disease. These compounds act as antioxidants to delay the breakdown of LDL. When LDL oxidizes, or deteriorates in the blood, plaque accumulates along the walls of the coronary arteries and causes atherosclerosis.

Berry juices, along with cherry juice, are rich in bioflavonoids, which increase the effectiveness of vitamin C.

Cranberry. Based on human studies, researchers have found that drinking three glasses of cranberry juice a day significantly raises levels of HDL in the blood and increases plasma antioxidant levels, reducing the risk of heart disease. Choose 100 percent pure cranberry juice or, better yet, make your own by juicing cranberries and apples. You can also buy cranberry concentrate at health food stores and mix with water and a little stevia.

Garlic juice contains substances that can help delay stiffening of the aorta, the body's main artery. Garlic can also help other arteries to remain elastic, and has been shown to decrease cholesterol and triglyceride levels.

Gingerroot has been shown to reduce inflammation.

Pineapple juice contains bromelain, an enzyme that inhibits platelet clumping.

Pomegranate juice. According to a recent study, antioxidants contained in pomegranate juice may help reduce the formation of fatty deposits on artery walls. Antioxidants are compounds that limit cell damage. Scientists have tested the juice with mice and found that it combats hardening of the arteries (atherogenesis) and related diseases, such as heart attacks and strokes.

✳ Juice Recipes

Sweet & Regular *(pg 343)*   **The Ginger Hopper** *(pg 332)*   **Immune Builder** *(pg 335)*   **Ginger Twist** *(pg 332)*   **Spinach Power** *(pg 341)*   **Peppy Parsley** *(pg 339)*   **Morning Energizer** *(pg 337)*   **Calcium-Rich Cocktail** *(pg 329)*   **Tomato Florentine** *(pg 343)*   **Magnesium-Rich Cocktail** *(pg 336)*   **Beet-Cucumber Cleansing Cocktail** *(pg 328)*   **Cranberry-Apple Cocktail** *(pg 331)*   **Garlic Surprise** *(pg 332)*   **Happy Morning** *(pg 333)*   **Icy Spicy Tomato** *(pg 335)*   **Jack & The Bean** *(pg 335)*   **Memory Mender** *(pg 336)*   **Mood Mender** *(pg 337)*   **Wheatgrass Light** *(pg 345)*

Carpal Tunnel Syndrome

CARPAL TUNNEL SYNDROME (CTS) is a common disorder in the wrist and hand; symptoms include pain, tingling, and weakness in the muscles caused by pressure on the median nerve in the wrist area. The median nerve in the arm passes through the carpal tunnel, a narrow bony passage in the wrist that also contains tendons and ligaments. CTS occurs when this nerve becomes compressed or damaged. Common CTS symptoms include soreness, tenderness, and weakness of the thumb muscles, and/or aching, numbness, tingling, and burning in the fingers. Pain and tingling may extend up the forearm and into the shoulder. Symptoms often worsen with repetitive motion and at night. Women are three to six times more likely to have CTS than men, and most people who develop this disorder are between the ages of forty and sixty.

CTS is often caused by working on the computer for extended amounts of time. With the rise in computer use at work, the incidence of occupationally related CTS (OCTS) is on the rise. Repetitive activities such as those used in typing, massage, carpentry, warehouse work and other jobs that require lifting and carrying, or jackhammer use may result in irritation of the median nerve and/or tendons. CTS can also result from a variety of causes, including wrist injury, hormone imbalances, rheumatoid arthritis (see Rheumatoid Arthritis, page 255), systemic diseases, tumors, blood-vessel changes, nutritional deficiencies, and hyperthyroidism (overactive thyroid). Dietary and lifestyle changes can help ease CTS considerably.

✳ Lifestyle Recommendations

Avoid taking birth control pills. It has been found that the use of birth control pills is associated with an increased risk of developing CTS. They deplete the body's stores of vitamin B_6, a nutrient that is vitally important in fighting CTS (see Nutrient Recommendations, below).

Wear a wrist splint (or splints) at night, at least during the acute phase. These splints, available in any pharmacy, contain a metal insert that keeps the wrists bent, palm out, while you sleep. This position takes stress off the affected tendons, which reduces the chance that you will wake up with numb, painful hands.

Acupuncture can release natural pain-relieving chemicals into the body, which promote circulation and balance the nervous system.

✳ Diet Recommendations

Eat more oats. Oats help nourish nerve tissue. They can be cooked as oatmeal, added to juice, or eaten uncooked as a muesli, a breakfast made with oats soaked in juice, milk, or rice or almond milk along with nuts and dried fruit. Wheat germ can provide extra vitamin B_6.

Avoid eating excess protein. The body needs vitamin B_6 to properly break down proteins. If there is a B_6 deficiency, proteins can break down into toxic substances.

Avoid yellow dyes. Yellow dyes are vitamin B_6–depleting substances.

✳ Nutrient Recommendations

Enzyme supplements may help to reduce tissue swelling associated with carpal tunnel syndrome. It can take several weeks to notice results.

Vitamin B_2 (riboflavin) converts vitamin B_6 into an active form. Take 100mg of vitamin B_2 daily; it's best taken with the other B vitamins as a complex. *Best juice sources of vitamin B_2:* collard greens, kale, parsley, broccoli, and beetroot greens.

Vitamin B_6 (pyridoxine). Researchers have discovered that many people with carpal tunnel syndrome suffer from a B_6 vitamin deficiency, which explains why many sufferers are pregnant women, menopausal women, or women on birth control pills, because these conditions deplete B_6. A study by the Portland (Oregon) Hand Surgery and Rehabilitation Center examined 441 people and found that people with higher levels of vitamin B_6 had fewer CTS symptoms. The environment is full of substances that can deplete the body's B_6 stores. Studies show that supplementing the diet with extra vitamin B_6 increases pain thresholds and reduces swelling associated with CTS. Improvement is usually noted within a few weeks to three months. Fortunately, vitamin B_6 supplementation is simple, inexpensive, and usually very effective. Vitamin B_6 works to strengthen the sheath that surrounds the tendon and thus helps to relieve the pain. Two other B vitamins—B_2 and B_{12}—work in conjunction with B_6 to make the treatment more effective; in addition, folic acid is beneficial. Dosages of 300 mg a day of vitamin B_6 are needed, which far exceeds the Recommended Daily Allowance (RDA) of 2 to 2.5 mg.

You should take high doses of vitamin B_6 in supplement form for no longer than three months and then go to 50 to 100 mg daily as a maintenance dosage. Remember that it can take up to three months for the effects of the supplementation to be felt. It is best to take B vitamins as a complex. Also, drink juices that are B_6-rich and continue these juices for maintenance. *Best juice sources of vitamin B_6:* kale, spinach, turnip greens, bell peppers, and prunes. *Warning:* Vitamin B_6 can be toxic at high levels. Do not take more than the recommended amount. **Vitamin B_{12},** 1,000 mcg daily, and folic acid, 800 mcg daily, are also helpful.

Vitamin C supports connective-tissue health. *Best juice sources of vitamin C:* kale, parsley, broccoli, Brussels sprouts, watercress, cauliflower, cabbage, strawberries, spinach, lemons, limes, turnips, and asparagus.

✳ Herb Recommendations

Yucca's natural steroid properties have been shown to reduce inflammation and obstructions of the joints.

Willow bark oil, applied externally, can help to decrease inflammation and ease pain.

✳ Juice Therapy

Gingerroot juice has anti-inflammatory properties. It is delicious when combined with fruits or vegetables.

Parsley juice is rich in vitamins B_6 and C. Intake should be limited to a safe, therapeutic dose of one-half to one cup per day. Parsley can be toxic in overdose, and should be especially avoided by pregnant women.

✳ Juice Recipes

Calcium-Rich Cocktail *(pg 329)*   Sweet Dreams Nightcap *(pg 342)*   Ginger Twist *pg 332)*   Happy Morning *(pg 333)*   Hot Ginger-Lemon Tea *(pg 334)* Magnesium-Rich Cocktail *(pg 336)*   Mint Refresher *(pg 337)*   Mood Mender *(pg 337)*   Orient Express *(pg 338)*   Wheatgrass Light *(pg 345)*

Chronic Fatigue Syndrome

CHRONIC FATIGUE SYNDROME (CFS) is an illness with a multitude of flu-like symptoms, including extreme fatigue, recurring sore throat, tender lymph nodes, depression, headaches, muscle aches and soreness, loss of concentration and/or memory, and low-grade fever. Unexplained fatigue that lasts at least six months is the principal means of diagnosis, as there is currently no diagnostic test for CFS. Symptoms are often cyclical, lapsing and recurring. Young women are most often affected.

CFS may occur after an illness such as a cold or flu, or it can start during or shortly after a period of high stress. It can also come on slowly without any clear starting point or obvious cause. In some cases, CFS can last for years. Many potential causes for CFS have been investigated, such as Epstein-Barr virus, the yeast *Candida albicans,* parasites, allergies, and various immunological disorders. Another factor thought to be involved is immunologic dysfunction—the inappropriate production of inflammatory cytokines. This results in excessive amounts of nitric oxide and peroxynitrite, which produces fatigue. Some studies have found that people with CFS have lower levels of the hormone cortisol, which is secreted by the adrenal glands. Lowered levels of cortisol may promote inflammation. Thyroid disorders have also been implicated.

Chronic fatigue syndrome does not need to be a lifelong sickness. Many people have recovered well after being sick. Exercise, stress reduction, good nutrition, and detoxification all have amazing benefits and will help with the ups and downs, with the downs becoming less severe and less frequent. A multifaceted approach to healing CFS involves dietary changes (especially those that enhance vitamin and mineral intake), exercise, herbal therapies, nutritional supplements, infection treatment, and counseling on stress management in order to revitalize the immune system and restore biochemical balance. To recover, it takes commitment, persistence, faith that you will get well, and a willingness to do whatever it takes to heal.

On a personal note: I often hear people say that there is no hope for recovery from CFS. There is great hope. I know. Twice I have suffered from such a severe case of CFS that I could not work. Actually, I could barely get out of bed. Now, I am well. (I share my recovery from CFS and my journey to health in the Introduction.)

✳ Lifestyle Recommendations

Control all allergies you may have. Allergies, whether seasonal or food- or drug-related, appear to be a common thread in individuals with CFS. If you have not already done so, have allergy tests performed to pinpoint any problem areas (see Allergies, page 27; see also the Elimination Diet, page 301).

Eliminate yeast and parasitic infections. Much research is currently focused on the role that *Candida albicans* and other yeasts and parasites play in CFS. Though not the cause of this disorder, intestinal pathogens depress the immune system, making the body more susceptible to infections. No fruit or fruit juice is allowed if you have a systemic yeast infection (candidiasis) or parasites (see Candidiasis, page 80, and Parasitic Infections, page 238).

✳ Diet Recommendations

Detoxify your body through cleansing programs. This is a vital first step toward building a healthy immune system. Toxins, both internal and external, must be reduced in order for the body's natural defenses to facilitate the recovery process. Reduce exposure to environmental chemicals from food, air, and water. Eliminate, as much as possible, drugs, dietary toxins, and allergenic foods. Colon cleansing is one of the keys to detoxification; toxins must be eliminated from the bowel, whether in the form of yeasts, parasites, heavy metals, or mucoid waste matter. In addition, the liver must be cleansed along with the gallbladder and kidneys. These must all be detoxified and supported (see the cleansing programs, pages 313–325).

Use massage to encourage draining of the lymphatic system.

Avoid sugar in all forms. Sugar will not give you more energy; rather, it will throw your blood-sugar levels out of balance and inhibit your immune system. Avoid all forms of sugar (white, brown, molasses, corn syrup), either as sweeteners or in processed foods, and avoid honey, sugar alcohols such as mannitol and xylitol, and maple syrup. Fruit, which is high in fruit sugar, should only be a small part of your diet—no more than one piece a day. (Avoid fruit completely if you have candidiasis or parasites.) Avoid drinking fruit juices, with the exception of lemon or lime, because of the concentration of fruit sugars.

Improve your immune function with whole, unprocessed foods. Diet plays a central role in optimum immune function. Eat only whole, natural, unprocessed foods. "Living foods" (raw foods) provide the most potent nutrients to improve your energy level. Strive for a diet in which 50 to 75 percent of your food consists of raw vegetables, vegetable juices, sprouts, nuts, and seeds. (I had to do this in order to get well, and I still do so to maintain my health.) The remainder of your diet should focus on complex carbohydrates, including whole grains such as oats, millet, rye, buckwheat, and brown rice; legumes such as beans, lentils, and split peas; and the herb quinoa. You can have moderate amounts of protein—fish, chicken, eggs, and a small amount of red meat as needed for iron. (Make sure the animal products you choose are from free-range/cage-free animals with no hormones or antibiotics.) Minimize your intake of wheat; it's overconsumed in the Western diet, and much of it is hybrid. As a result, many people are sensitive or allergic to it. As much as possible, your food should be organically grown.

Avoid stimulants and processed foods. Avoid alcohol, caffeine, and tobacco, along with all junk food, fast food, packaged foods, and anything with dyes, preservatives, or additives. These substances can weaken the immune system.

Drink plenty of water. Drink eight to ten eight-ounce glasses of clean, purified water each day. (You can benefit from a water purifier.) Adequate water intake is very beneficial to the immune system.

Use juice fasts to "jump-start" a recovery. Fasting on vegetable juices for one to three days can give your immune system and indeed your entire body a powerful boost. Juice-fasting for short periods of time is probably the single most effective step you can take toward getting well. No one has been able to explain why drinking only fresh vegetable juices for several days works such a miracle, but "miracle" is the right word. Several studies have shown that the nutrients that occur in optimal proportions and quantities in fresh vegetable juices, along with uncooked vegetables and sprouts, boost production of T and B lymphocytes, key components in the immune response, and so increase resistance to illness. In addition, these juices and foods cleanse the spaces between cells. Waste matter can collect in these spaces when cellular metabolism is not functioning well, and become a breeding ground for bacteria and viruses. Poor cellular metabolism also contributes to fatigue (see the Juice Fast, page 304). *On a personal note:* Every year, I take a "health break" for a week of raw foods combined with three days of juice fasting (see Sources, page 347, for a list of health institutes that use this program).

✳ Nutrient Recommendations

B complex vitamins are important to well-functioning nervous and immune systems. They provide energy to people who are stressed or fatigued. The best juice sources of B vitamins overall are green leafy vegetables. *The best food sources, in addition to green vegetables:* whole grains (especially rye, oats, and brown rice), liver, poultry, fish, eggs, nuts, and beans. Folic acid, one of the B vitamins, has been found to be especially helpful to people with CFS. *Best juice sources of folic acid:* asparagus, spinach, kale, broccoli, and cabbage.

Beta-carotene stimulates the immune system and is converted by the body into vitamin A as needed. Both substances help fight infections. *Best juice sources of carotenes in general:* carrots, kale, parsley, spinach, Swiss chard, beetroot greens, watercress, broccoli, and romaine lettuce.

L-carnitine, an amino acid, has been found in low levels in CFS patients. Carnitine plays an essential role in energy production. *Best food sources of carnitine:* avocado, fish, and red meat. It is not found in most fruits and vegetables.

Magnesium affects energy regulation within the body, and it is often found in low amounts in CFS sufferers. *Best juice sources of magnesium:* beetroot greens, spinach, parsley, dandelion greens, garlic, beetroot, broccoli, cauliflower, carrots, and celery.

Vitamin C enhances the ability of immune cells to destroy bacteria and viruses. It also increases production of lymphocytes, the cells that play a key role in cellular immunity. *Best juice sources of vitamin C:* kale, parsley, broccoli, Brussels sprouts, watercress, cauliflower, cabbage, spinach, lemons, limes, turnips, and asparagus.

Zinc offers strong support for the immune system, and helps the body fight viral infections. *Best juice sources of zinc:* gingerroot, turnips, parsley, garlic, carrots, spinach, cabbage, lettuce, and cucumbers.

✳ Herb Recommendations

Astragalus bolsters resistance to disease. Avoid astragalus if you have a fever.

Echinacea fights viral infections.

Goldenseal supports the liver. Avoid this herb if you are pregnant, and do not use it for more than ten days at a time.

Licorice root and **borage** both stimulate the adrenal glands. Avoid licorice if you have high blood pressure, do not use it for prolonged periods of time, and use a medicinal form of the herb, not licorice candy.

Oat straw is useful for nervous exhaustion and low fevers.

Osha root fights viral infections.

✳ Juice Therapy

Beetroot, carrot, and **cucumber** juices (especially beetroot juice) help cleanse the liver and gallbladder. Carrot juice is also helpful in treating fatigue.

Fennel juice helps relieve CFS-associated depression because it contains compounds that help release endorphins, the feel-good chemicals in the brain.

Garlic is a strongly antimicrobial herb effective against bacteria, viruses, and parasites.

Parsley juice is a good source of beta-carotene, magnesium, vitamin C, and zinc. Intake should be limited to a safe, therapeutic dose of one-half to one cup per day. Parsley can be toxic in overdose, and should be especially avoided by pregnant women.

Spinach and **carrot** juices, taken in combination, help with both blood-sugar regulation and liver cleansing.

Wheatgrass juice is a powerful immune builder.

✳ Juice Recipes

Gallbladder-Liver Cleansing Cocktail *(pg 331)*   **Morning Energizer** *(pg 337)*
Spinach Power *(pg 341)*   **Wheatgrass Light** *(pg 347)*   **Allergy Relief** *(pg 326)*
Salsa in a Glass *(pg 340)*   **Memory Mender** *(pg 336)*   **Mood Mender** *(pg 337)*
Magnesium-Rich Cocktail *(pg 336)*   **Sweet Dreams Nightcap** *(pg 342)*

Colds

COLDS are among the most widespread illnesses in the world. The common cold can be caused by a variety of viruses (called rhinovirus) that infect the upper respiratory tract (the nasal passages, sinuses, and throat). Symptoms include general malaise, fever, sneezing, sore throat, headache, and congestion. Most colds last about a week, although a dry cough may linger afterward.

The best thing you can do if you have a cold is to support your immune system—the body's natural defense mechanisms—as opposed to suppressing the symptoms. Actually, the symptoms are a result of the body's attempts to heal. For example, the body releases a potent immune-stimulating compound known as interferon during infections, which is responsible for many of the symptoms. As you assist your body nutritionally, you can help it heal.

While young children can get as many as eight colds a year, that frequency drops off dramatically in adults. By maintaining a healthy immune system, you can protect yourself from getting colds. If you catch more than one or two colds per year, it may be a sign that your immune system needs to be strengthened to prevent future colds. One thing to check is food allergies and sensitivities, which can greatly weaken the immune system.

✳ Diet Recommendations

Drink plenty of fluids. Put a special emphasis on drinking juices (primarily vegetable), herbal teas, and vegetable broths. Increasing fluid intake during an infection will prevent dehydration of the respiratory-tract membranes. When these membranes become dehydrated, virus growth accelerates. Increasing fluids also decreases nasal congestion. If the body is allowed to produce more watery secretions, thicker secretions do not accumulate as easily in the respiratory tract. Inhaling the vapors of spicy soups or simmering herbs, or using a vaporizer can help the nasal tissues. Also, drink lots of hot fluids. Cold viruses multiply fast when the temperature around them is about 90°F. However, they are far less likely to replicate as quickly when their environment heats up. Hot fluids will warm your throat, which should help to impair viral replication. As a bonus, hot fluids have a mild decongestant effect, which helps relieve nasal stuffiness. Hot herbal drinks such as ginger tea are doubly helpful because of their antiviral effect.

Eat light. Foods should be easily digestible, with a strong emphasis on vegetable juices, vegetable soups, broths, salads, and fish.

Make a pot of chicken soup. Also known as "Jewish penicillin," chicken soup has been a mainstay of folk medicine for eight hundred years, ever since the Jewish physician Moses Maimonides recommended it as a cold remedy. Chicken soup really works, as many modern studies have shown. Add lots of garlic to make it the most effective.

Include spicy foods. Any food spicy enough to make your eyes water will have the same effect on your nose, promoting drainage. (Drainage is a good thing, so don't suppress it.)

Avoid mucus-forming foods. This includes dairy products, meat, and wheat products. One study has shown that a compound in milk triggers the release of histamine, a chemical that contributes to runny nose and nasal congestion. This can make your chest, sinus, and nasal congestion worse.

Juice-fast. Go on a short juice fast. Drinking primarily vegetable juices for one to three days can accelerate your recovery. This offers your body a chance to rest from digestive activity and concentrate on fighting the infection. Also, the "aliveness" of raw juices supports the body at the cellular level to speed up the healing process (For more information, see the Juice Fast, page 304.)

Reduce your fat intake. Studies have shown that increased levels of cholesterol, nonessential fatty acids, triglycerides, and bile acids (substances associated with fat intake) inhibit the ability of white blood cells to divide, move to areas of infection, and destroy invading microorganisms.

Avoid sugar. Sugar weakens the immune system. Glucose, the most basic sugar molecule, and vitamin C compete for transport into white blood cells. Sugar competes with vitamin C, impairing the ability of white blood cells to engulf viruses and bacteria. In one study, researchers had volunteers consume 100 grams of sugar, the equivalent of two cans of soda. Then they took blood samples and found that neutrophil (white blood cell) activity had plummeted by 50 percent after consuming the sugar. Five hours later, neutrophil activity still remained substantially below normal. Both refined and natural sugars should be avoided. These include sucrose (table sugar), fructose (fruit sugar), honey, maple syrup, sugar alcohols such as mannitol or sorbitol, and full-strength fruit juice. Fruit juice, if used at all, should be diluted by half with plain water or unsweetened mineral water. Limit fruit juice to no more than four ounces per day (with the exception of lemon, lime, grapefruit, apple, and cranberry), and stay away from all other forms of sugar during an infection.

Avoid alcohol; it's dehydrating. And alcohol acts like sugar in the body in that it competes with vitamin C, which weakens the immune cells' ability to fight infections. It also puts additional strain on the liver, which is already hard at work to detoxify the body during illness.

✳ Nutrient Recommendations

Vitamin A and **carotenes** heal inflamed mucous membranes and strengthen the immune system. Beta-carotene can help increase the number of helper T cells, cells that play a key role in immunity. The body creates vitamin A from beta-carotene. *Best juice sources of carotenes:* carrots, kale, parsley, spinach, Swiss chard, beetroot greens, watercress, broccoli, and romaine lettuce.

Vitamin C and **bioflavonoids** have demonstrated the ability to slow cold and flu infections. Vitamin C has been used extensively to prevent colds and to decrease recovery time and alleviate symptoms. Studies have shown that 2,000 to 5,000 mg of vitamin C a day from the first time symptoms of a cold appear until the cold completely clears up are effective. One of the major problems when you use megadoses of vitamin C, however, is that you may suffer from diarrhea. To avoid this, you can use calcium ascorbate powder, the form of vitamin C that's least irritating to the digestive tract. Take one teaspoon, mixed in vegetable juice or water, four times a day. Bioflavonoids enhance the uptake of vitamin C into immune cells. **Note:** Anyone who suffers from oxalic acid–type kidney stones (rarer than other types of kidney stones) should be extremely cautious in their use of vitamin C. *Best juice sources of vitamin C:* kale, parsley, broccoli, Brussels sprouts, watercress, cauliflower, cabbage, spinach, lemons, limes, turnips, and asparagus. *Best juice sources of bioflavonoids:* bell peppers, broccoli, cabbage, parsley, and tomatoes.

Vitamin E and **selenium** work together to fight infections. Selenium's immune-stimulating effects are enhanced by vitamin E. Studies show these nutrients increase antibody formation. *Best juice sources of vitamin E:* spinach, watercress, asparagus, carrots, and tomatoes. *Best juice sources of selenium:* Swiss chard, turnips, garlic, radishes, carrots, and cabbage.

Zinc shortens the duration and severity of a cold. Zinc blocks the "docking" of the human rhinovirus onto cell membranes, thereby interrupting the infection. If your diet is deficient in zinc, your body could be low in neutrophils and you'll be susceptible to all types of infections. Zinc also reduces inflammation. Zinc lozenges are beneficial when taken at the onset of a cold; the best lozenges are those sweetened with the amino acid glycine. *Best juice sources of zinc:* gingerroot, turnips, parsley, garlic, carrots, spinach, cabbage, lettuce, and cucumbers.

✳ Herb Recommendations

Astragalus strengthens the body's resistance to disease, and reduces the incidence and duration of infection. Do not use it if you have a fever.

Echinacea enhances the activity of the natural killer cells, which may be among the principal mechanisms of immunity against viruses early in the course of an infection. Echinacea has been shown to decrease the frequency of infections, and to reduce the duration and severity of symptoms.

Goldenseal contains the natural antibiotic berberine. Avoid this herb if you are pregnant, and do not use it for more than ten days.

✳ Juice Therapy

Apple juice has antiviral properties. Use tart apples, such as Granny Smiths or pippins, to avoid consuming too much fruit sugar. Drink no more than six ounces daily and dilute by half with purified water.

Beetroot juice (red beet) has been used as a traditional remedy to make cold and flu viruses inactive.

Garlic has antiviral effects. In addition to using garlic juice, consume two to three raw cloves three times a day at the onset of an infection.

Gingerroot juice contains anti-inflammatory compounds. Using fresh gingerroot, in either juice or tea form, at the first sign of a cold may help prevent the cold from progressing, or help to reduce the duration and severity of the symptoms. Gingerroot contains a variety of antiviral compounds. Scientists have isolated several chemicals (sesquiterpenes) in ginger that have specific effects against the most common family of cold viruses, the rhinoviruses. Some of these chemicals are remarkably potent in their antirhinovirus effects. Other constituents in gingerroot, gingerols and shogaols, help relieve cold symptoms because they reduce pain and fever, suppress coughing, and have a mild sedative effect that encourages rest. Besides juicing gingerroot, you can also drink a cup of ginger tea several times a day. To make a tea, add one heaping teaspoon of grated fresh gingerroot to one cup of boiled water, and allow it to steep for ten minutes. If you use dried gingerroot powder, use one-third to one-half teaspoon of powdered gingerroot per cup. Also, see recipe for Hot Ginger-Lemon Tea (page 334).

Grapefruit is great for fighting a cold. It's high in vitamin C and bioflavonoids, and helps detoxify the liver; it's also low in sugar. Add water to dilute sugar concentration. Consult your doctor or pharmacist to make sure that it is OK to consume grapefruit with any prescription medications you're taking.

Jerusalem artichoke juice is rich in inulin, a substance that increases immune-defense mechanisms.

Lemon juice is beneficial because it's rich in vitamin C and bioflavonoids, which helps increase the body's resistance, decreases toxicity, and helps reduce the duration of the illness.

Parsley juice is rich in beta-carotene, bioflavonoids, vitamin C, and zinc, nutrients that support the immune system. Intake should be limited to a safe, therapeutic dose of one-half to one cup per day. Parsley can be toxic in overdose, and should be especially avoided by pregnant women.

Wheatgrass juice is rich in chlorophyll, a powerful blood purifier.

✳ Juice Recipes

The Ginger Hopper *(pg 332)* **Weight-Loss Buddy** *(pg 345)* **Wheatgrass Light** *(pg 345)* **Hot Ginger-Lemon Tea** *(pg 334)* **Magnesium-Rich Cocktail** *(pg 336)* **Sinus Solution** *(pg 341)* **Tomato Florentine** *(pg 343)* **Allergy Relief** *(pg 326)* **Sweet Dreams Nightcap** *(pg 342)* **Turnip Time** *(pg 344)* **Cranberry-Apple Cocktail** *(pg 331)* **Immune Builder** *(pg 335)* **The Revitalizer** *(pg 340)*

Colitis, IBS, and Other Bowel Diseases

THE TERM COLITIS takes in a broad range of intestinal disorders, including two of the most prevalent—irritable bowel syndrome (IBS) and inflammatory bowel disease (IBD). These disorders are more common in women than in men.

In IBS, food moves through the intestines in an uncoordinated, erratic manner, producing alternating bouts of constipation and diarrhea, along with persistent gas, bloating, and abdominal pain. The primary cause is a diet low in fiber and high in refined carbohydrates, often coupled with a sedentary lifestyle, stress, and emotional upsets. It has been noted that symptoms of lactose intolerance, or an inability to digest milk sugar, are similar to those of IBS, and lactose intolerance may be a contributing factor.

IBD is a more severe condition that includes both Crohn's disease and ulcerative colitis. It's associated with inflammation of the joints, eyes, and/or skin, and with an increased risk of colon cancer. Inflammatory bowel disease is thought to be an autoimmune disorder, which is a result of a system that is unbalanced. It's linked to a poor diet and stress, with antibiotics often being a contributing factor.

People suffering with IBD typically eat more refined sugar, butter, margarine, cheese, and meat, and less fruits and vegetables, than healthy individuals. For example, populations in which people eat a traditional, nonprocessed diet have very low rates of Crohn's disease, while the incidence of this disease in the United States has increased by hundreds of percentage points in the last several decades, and rates in Japan have increased markedly with the introduction of Western food.

All autoimmune disorders indicate that the body's immune system has been accidentally triggered to attack specific protein tissues in the body. Often there are underactive T cells (cell-mediated immunity) and overactive, overproduced B cells (humoral immunity). The original cause can be leaky gut syndrome; therefore, autoimmune diseases have a very close connection with inflammatory bowel diseases. It's thought that this results from the constant irritation of infection(s) such as viral, bacterial, fungal, parasitic, protozoan, and yeasts such as *Candida albicans* that are not successfully treated. In IBD, the overactive B cells can attack a particular part(s) of the body, such as the bowel. Vaccinations can also trigger an imbalance in T and B cells.

Crohn's disease, or regional enteritis, is an inflammation that can affect any part of the digestive tract, while ulcerative colitis only affects the large intestine. Symptoms include bloody diarrhea, cramps in the lower abdomen, abdominal tenderness, loss of appetite and weight, flatulence, malaise, low-grade fever, and anal irritation. Anal fissures, hemorrhoids, fistulas (abnormal channels), and abscesses may form. In Crohn's disease, chronic inflammation causes the intestinal walls to become thick and rigid, and the bowels may become narrow and obstructed.

✳ Lifestyle Recommendations

Eliminate yeast, bacterial, and parasitic infections. Parasitic or bacterial infections may be a contributing factor in bowel diseases. There is circumstantial evidence that first attacks and occasional relapses of ulcerative colitis are related to infection with bacteria such as Salmonella, and bacterial infection has been reported in about 13 percent of Crohn's disease patients. You should be tested to find out if you are harboring disease-causing organisms.

Pathogenic bacteria in the colon are commonly found in most bowel diseases. They produce toxins, which further irritate the digestive system. The intestinal tract can take on the characteristics of a waste dump. The healthy gut bacteria can become overpowered and destroyed by bad bacteria and/or yeast infections such as *Candida albicans*. Treatment of the bacteria by drugs is only a temporary solution because the opportunity exists for their reestablishment. Proper diet together with the reestablishment of good bacterial flora is essential. The bad bacteria must be starved to death by removing their primary food source, which is carbohydrates, from the diet; otherwise treatment will not be successful. The pathogens will simply return after treatment ends because they are opportunistic. If you have a systemic yeast infection (candidiasis) or parasites, no fruit or fruit juice is allowed (see Candidiasis, page 80, for a complete list of what to avoid).

✳ Diet Recommendations

Eat a high-fiber, low-fat (except good fats), low-sugar diet to treat IBS and prevent IBD. Fiber can help regulate intestinal function. Include high-fiber foods, such as vegetables, fruit, whole grains (except wheat), oat bran, guar gum, and psyllium, in your diet. These high-fiber foods have a positive effect on intestinal flora; the beneficial microbes are essential to proper digestion. Avoid wheat bran, which may be too irritating, and avoid all insoluble fiber if you have active IBD. These foods are too harsh and must be eliminated until the intestines heal. In this case, vegetable juice is very beneficial because it offers nonirritating soluble fiber and antioxidants that are healing for the intestinal tract.

Avoid animal proteins as much as possible except for fish, which contains the healing omega-3 fatty acids. It's also easier to digest than meat.

Reduce simple and refined carbohydrate consumption. The consumption of refined and high-sugar carbohydrates generally shows disease effects in the following manner:

- Body fat accumulation, which leads to obesity, diabetes, heart disease, cancer, gallbladder disease, and degenerative bone diseases.
- Damage to the intestinal tract, which leads to leaky gut syndrome, IBD, and a medical textbook listing of autoimmune diseases.

The primary high-carbohydrate foods to avoid are sugars, including table sugar, fructose, corn syrup, honey, pure maple syrup, brown rice syrup, and agave, along with flour products. (The only sweetener recommended is stevia, found at health food stores.) Greatly reduce consumption of whole grains, fruit, milk products, sweets, and starchy vegetables.

Avoid mucus-forming foods. Eliminate sugar in all forms (cakes, cookies, muffins, pies, pastries, ice cream). Avoid butter, margarine, other dairy products, fried foods, spicy foods, wheat products, and all junk food such as chips and soft drinks, along with coffee. These foods encourage the secretion of intestinal mucus, and prevent the uptake of nutrients. (For more information on a healthy diet plan, see Basic Guidelines for the Juice Lady's Health and Healing Diet, page 290.)

Drink plenty of fresh vegetable juice and water. Anyone with IBS, and especially IBD, is at increased risk for malnourishment. Fresh juices are nutrient-rich and very helpful in keeping people with any form of bowel disease well nourished. Juices are easily digested and contain high concentrations of vitamins, minerals, and enzymes. They also contain phytonutrients that may help protect against colon cancer. Carotene-rich juices, such as carrot, kale, parsley, and spinach, help heal the intestinal mucosa. Also, juice is rich in plant sterols and sterolins, which are plant fats present in fruits vegetables, and all plants. They are biologically active molecules that significantly enhance the immune system. Sterols/sterolins help the immune system from becoming too stressed and overproducing B cells while underproducing T-cells, an action responsible for the autoimmune response.

Drink plenty of water. Include at least two quarts of purified water per day. Herbal teas can make up part of your water intake. Avoid caffeine and alcohol. If you have a weak digestive system, be sure to drink all fluids at room temperature.

Avoid soda. One study found an increase in Crohn's disease among people who consumed large amounts of soft drinks. Also, iced and carbonated beverages stimulate peristalsis, or the movement that propels food through the intestines. Drink beverages that are closer to room temperature.

Identify food allergies and intolerances. Allergies and intolerances to dairy products, corn, wheat, and foods that contain carageenan, a stabilizer used in processed foods, can contribute to IBD and IBS. If you are allergic to wheat and have IBS, switch to oat or rice bran cereals, flours, and breads (see Allergies, page 27; see also the Elimination Diet, page 301).

Colon-cleanse and juice-fast. There have been several case reports of people who have experienced considerable relief from colitis after a short juice fast (see the Juice Fast, page 304, and the Intestinal Cleanse, page 307).

✳ Nutrient Recommendations

Beta-carotene and **chlorophyll** help heal the intestinal tract. *Best juice sources of carotenes:* carrots, kale, parsley, spinach, Swiss chard, beetroot greens, watercress, broccoli, and romaine lettuce. *Best juice sources of chlorophyll:* all dark green vegetables.

Enzymes. Even before we develop a chronic health problem, eating predominantly cooked food begins to burden our colon and tissues with undigested protein and mucus. This contributes to inflammation and an autoimmune response. With every cooked meal you eat, it is wise to take digestive enzymes to stop further deterioration and improve digestion and assimilation. Years of accumulation of partially digested proteins, and the buildup of mucus in the intestinal tract, requires a good colon cleanse (see the Intestinal Cleanse, page 307).

Glutamine, an amino acid, is needed for the production of rapidly dividing cells such as those lining the intestines. It has been shown to prevent atrophy of the intestines' mucosal lining. Glutamine is available in most fruit and vegetable juices.

Omega-3 fatty acids, especially EPA and DHA, have been shown to reduce inflammation. In bowel disorders there is usually an increased level of chemicals derived from inflammatory fatty acids in the colon, serum, and stools. Omega-3s fight this effect. One double-blind study showed a reduced rate in relapse in Crohn's disease when nine enterically coated fish-oil capsules were taken every day. Cod-liver oil is very beneficial; you may take one tablespoon daily, which also provides vitamin D, essential for calcium integration. (Boron is also helpful.) Once the calcium status of the body is improved, the immune system tends to function better. Hemp oil is rich in omega-3 and omega-9 fatty acids; take one teaspoon hemp oil daily. (For more information on omega-3 oils, see the fats and oils section in Basic Guidelines for the Juice Lady's Health and Healing Diet, page 290.)

Vitamin C is particularly important in preventing fistula formation, such as fistulas between the colon and bladder. Also, vitamin C is an important antistress nutrient, and is helpful for IBS. *Best juice sources of vitamin C:* kale, parsley, broccoli, Brussels sprouts, watercress, cauliflower, cabbage, spinach, lemons, limes, turnips, and asparagus.

✳ Herb Recommendations for Crohn's Disease

Boswellia serrata is an herb used in Ayurvedic, or traditional Indian, medicine for its anti-inflammatory effects.

✳ Herb Recommendations for IBS

Chamomile, lemon balm, rosemary, and **valerian** aid the gastrointestinal tract.

Peppermint oil, in enterically coated capsules, relieves IBS symptoms by inhibiting gastrointestinal contractions; it also relieves gas. The enteric capsule coating is important, as it allows the oil to pass undigested through the stomach and reach the colon.

✳ Herb Recommendations for Ulcerative Colitis

Goldenseal is an anti-inflammatory for the gut; it's helpful in resolving bacteria and mucus problems that contribute to bowel and digestive disorders.

Irish moss and **marshmallow root** are traditional remedies that soothe irritated intestinal mucous membranes. Avoid Irish moss if you are allergic to carageenan.

Licorice, an anti-inflammatory that helps the adrenal glands make extra cortisone, reduces excess stomach acidity and heals ulcerations.

Slippery elm soothes inflammation.

Note: Food intolerances and *Candida albicans* overgrowth are very common with bowel diseases and must be eliminated for the herbal formulas to do their work. *Candida albicans* overgrowth is often due to killing the good bacteria in the bowel with antibiotics and steroids (see Candidiasis, page 80).

✳ Juice Therapy

Beetroot juice is thought to contain enzymes that restore healthy cellular respiration and cellular energy.

Cabbage juice has been scientifically documented to heal ulcers. It also contains phytonutrients that inhibit tumor growth and strengthen the immune system.

Daikon radish juice is used in traditional Oriental medicine to help dissolve hardened accumulations in the intestines.

Pear and **carrot** juices combine to form a traditional remedy for a weak digestive system.

Sprouts can be juiced and they are an excellent source of sterols and sterolins.

Tomato juice is packed with lycopene, a powerful antioxidant that helps protect against digestive tract cancers.

✳ Juice Recipes for Crohn's Disease

Triple C *(pg 344)*   **Antiulcer Cabbage Cocktail** *(pg 327)*   **Orient Express** *(pg 338)*
Salsa in a Glass *(pg 340)*   **Morning Energizer** *(pg 337)*   **Ginger Twist** *(pg 332)*

✳ Juice Ingredient Recommendations for IBS

Carrot juice is rich in beta-carotene.

Fennel and **mint** juices promote digestion and relieve gas, and can help to ease the intestinal spasms common in IBS.

Gingerroot juice aids in the absorption of nutrients, and is excellent for easing indigestion, colic, and flatulence. It is an anti-inflammatory agent.

✳ Juice Recipes for IBS

Mood Mender *(pg 337)*   **Morning Energizer** *(pg 337)*   **Beet-Cucumber**
Cleansing Cocktal *(pg 328)*   **Colon Cleanser** *(pg 330)* **Happy Morning** *(pg 333)*
Wheatgrass Light *(pg 345)*   **Mint Refresher** *(pg 337)*   **The Ginger Hopper** *(pg 332)*

✳ Juice Ingredient Recommendations for Ulcerative Colitis

Beetroot greens juice is rich in chlorophyll, a blood purifier.

Cabbage juice has been shown to be effective in healing ulcers.

Carrot juice is rich in beta-carotene, which helps heal the digestive tract.

Mango, papaya, and **pineapple** juices are all rich in enzymes that help digestion. Studies have shown that bromelain, an enzyme in pineapple, and papain, an enzyme in papaya, aid digestion, reduce inflammation, and enhance wound healing.

Wheatgrass juice is loaded with chlorophyll and beta-carotene. Both compounds have healing properties that are especially beneficial for the intestinal mucosa.

✳ Juice Recipes for Ulcerative Colitis

Spinach Power *(pg 341)*   **Triple C** *(pg 344)*   **Wheatgrass Light** *(pg 345)*
Mood Mender *(pg 337)*   **Sweet Dreams Nightcap** *(pg 342)*

Constipation

Constipation is the infrequent passage of small, hard, dry bowel movements that are usually difficult and painful to pass. If you have dark stools that fall quickly in the water, that usually indicates insufficient dietary fiber or too little water consumption. On the other hand, an ideal bowel movement is medium brown, the color of plain cardboard or a walnut shell. It leaves the body easily with no straining or discomfort, and has the consistency of toothpaste. It should be large, soft, and fluffy, and approximately four to eight inches long. There should be little gas or odor. It should enter the water smoothly and fall slowly. Food should take no longer than twenty-four hours to move through the system, and since we usually eat two or three times a day, we should have two to three bowel movements daily.

When constipated, a person may feel sluggish, bloated, and uncomfortable. Waste material that lingers in the intestines can cause problems. It can block the absorption of valuable nutrients from the food you eat and the nutritional supplements you take. The waste material can also putrefy, becoming toxic. These toxins can then pass through the intestinal wall into your bloodstream. Chronic constipation can lead to everything from bad breath, fatigue, malnutrition, indigestion, hemorrhoids, headaches, and varicose veins to diverticulosis, depression, and diseases like cancer, especially colon cancer.

The most common causes of constipation are eating a low-fiber diet, drinking too little water, and not getting enough exercise.

Highly refined, low-fiber foods, such as those which most Americans eat, in conjunction with inadequate fluid intake and exercise, is the main reason so many Americans suffer from this condition. Surveys indicate that constipation affects more than four million Americans, who spend $725 million on laxatives yearly. And it's one of the most common digestive complaints, accounting for 2.5 million visits to the doctor each year.

✳ Lifestyle Recommendations

Get regular exercise. To prevent or reverse constipation, you need to exercise at least thirty minutes a day, three days a week. Aerobic exercise, such as walking, swimming, or step aerobics, helps keep the bowels regular.

Get treatment for parasites and *Candida albicans*. Parasites and *Candida albicans* can cause constipation. If you don't know if you have either, your doctor can send your stool specimen to Genova Diagnostics or Great Plains Laboratory for testing for the presence of pathogens (for more information on testing, see www.gdx.net or www.greatplainslaboratory.com).

✳ Diet Recommendations

Eat a high-fiber, complex-carbohydrate diet. A diet rich in whole grains, fruits, vegetables, and legumes (beans, lentils, split peas) helps prevent and treat constipation. A high-fiber diet aids in cleansing and toning the intestinal tract. (Be aware that vitamin B deficiency and insufficient potassium may result in loss of bowel tone.) You can sprinkle ground flaxseed on your cereal or morning smoothie and over salads and soups to get more fiber. Or, soak a tablespoon of flaxseed (golden is best) overnight in a glass of water and eat them in the morning. (For more information, see Basic Guidelines for the Juice Lady's Health and Healing Diet, page 290).

Eat fewer foods high in fat and refined foods. Fatty foods include red meat and dark-meat poultry, eggs, and dairy products. Especially reduce intake of cheese, margarine, fried foods, and fast foods. Omit sugar products, including table sugar, powdered sugar, brown sugar, and corn syrup, as well as desserts and prepared foods that contain these sugars. Refined flour products include all items made with white flour, such as bread, crackers, pasta, and pizza dough. These foods do not contain enough fiber to keep food moving through the intestines. They are considered colon-clogging foods.

Drink plenty of water. That means at least two quarts per day.

Use juicing, juice fasting, and colon cleansing. Many people have reported that once they started drinking any combination of fresh juices, they became very regular (see the Juice Fast, page 304, and the Intestinal Cleanse, page 307). A couple of juices are especially helpful in treating constipation. Prune juice is a well-known laxative. You can juice the plums that are used to make prunes, if you can find them. Boysenberry juice is another gentle laxative. (If you have a weak digestive system, drink juices only at room temperature.) Juice fasts and intestinal cleansing can be very helpful in correcting constipation.

✳ Nutrient Recommendations

Calcium and **magnesium.** Calcium combines with excess bile and fat in the colon to form a harmless substance, which is excreted with your stool. It's recommended that you take 1,000 to 1,500 mg daily of calcium citrate. Because calcium can cause constipation, it's recommended that you take 500 to 750 mg of magnesium citrate at the same time, which helps prevent constipation. It's best to divide the doses and take half in the morning and half in the evening. Magnesium is needed for normal muscle function, including intestinal muscles. One study examined the intake of magnesium with constipation in 3,835 women and found that low magnesium intake was associated with constipation. *Best juice sources of magnesium:* beetroot and beetroot greens, spinach, Swiss chard, collard greens, parsley, broccoli, and carrots.

Fiber supplements. Psyllium seed, a bulking agent, is a common remedy for constipation. Make sure you take it with water; see the package directions. Be aware however, that psyllium can be drying to the colon. You may achieve better results with ground flaxseed or pectin. Or, you can combine these fibers.

Probiotics. There is some evidence that probiotic supplements may relieve constipation. For example, one study looked at the effect of a probiotic beverage containing a strain of beneficial bacteria called *Lactobacillus casei Shirota* (65 milliliters a day) or a placebo in people with chronic constipation. The probiotic drink resulted in significant improvement in severity of constipation and stool consistency.

Vitamin C is helpful in preventing constipation. It's also particularly helpful in preventing fistula formation (abnormal openings), such as fistulas between the colon and bladder. Start by taking 500 mg of vitamin C daily. You can increase in 500-mg increments to bowel tolerance and then cut back 500 mg. This will help you determine the dose best for you. *Best juice sources of vitamin C:* kale, parsley, broccoli, Brussels sprouts, watercress, cauliflower, cabbage, strawberries, spinach, lemons, limes, turnips, and asparagus.

✳ Juice Therapy

Apple, parsley, pear, and **radish** juices stimulate intestinal motion. Parsley juice intake should be limited to a safe, therapeutic dose of one-half to one cup per day. Parsley can be toxic in overdose, and should be especially avoided by pregnant women.

Boysenberry juice is a gentle laxative.

Prune juice is a well-known laxative. You can juice the plums that are used to make prunes, if you can find them.

✳ Juice Recipes

Sinus Solution *(pg 341)*   **Colon Cleanser** *(pg 330)*   **Spinach Power** *(pg 341)*
Beet-Cucumber Cleansing Cocktail *(pg 328)*   **Gallbladder Cleansing
Cocktail** *(pg 331)*

Cravings

OVER TIME, human beings have learned that certain tastes, especially salty and sweet, signal the presence of important nutrients. Salt is essential for the body's water balance, while sweet foods are rich in the calories needed for energy. This attraction to salt and sweet was vital for our ancient ancestors, who lived in a hunter-gatherer environment, worked hard in warmer weather, and usually found food scarce in the winter. They often lived off stored-up body fat in the winter months. Because these tastes were so important to early humankind's survival, they involve more than just the taste buds, and are associated with changes in brain chemistry and hormone balance as well.

Times have changed. Now, most people have experienced frustrating urges for things like potato chips, chocolate, ice cream, or peanut butter on a steady basis, and know firsthand Webster's definition of crave, which is to "want greatly." Getting rid of food urges means getting to the root of the cause. Even though you think you're hungry for a quart of strawberry cheesecake ice cream or a bag of honey-mustard pretzels, that isn't what your body needs.

Cravings for such strange items as dirt, starch, or paint are referred to as pica. Recorded for centuries, this phenomenon has been explained as a need for minerals. And that's the current explanation for most familiar cravings—a deficiency of specific nutrients. Cravings can also be due to food allergies (see Allergies, page 27), blood-sugar imbalances (see Hypoglycemia, page 180), candidiasis (see Candidiasis, page 80), or hormonal changes during the premenstrual phase of the menstrual cycle (see Menstrual Disorders, page 211). Or, of course, pregnancy.

In this section, you can find what you crave most often, and put into practice the recommendations for modifying your diet to curb your cravings. And the next time an uncontrollable urge to munch strikes, make a big glass of one of the recommended juices and start getting to the root of your cravings.

✳ Juicing for all Cravings

Because fresh juices have been broken down and are so easy to digest, the body can readily utilize them. They are power-packed with nutrients the body can use right away. Most people who juice on a regular basis find they aren't as hungry. Cravings for many things lessen and often disappear over time.

✳ Alcohol and Cigarette Cravings (Addictions)

Nutrition is the main focus to beat alcohol cravings. When alcohol is consumed over a period of time, it affects the body's chemistry. Once you get in the habit of drinking alcohol on a regular basis, your body gets used to the alcohol in the bloodstream and reacts with withdrawal symptoms when you stop drinking. Then it releases a trigger to crave more alcohol. Your lifestyle, and especially nutrition, can dramatically influence these triggers, so changing the way you eat and your attitudes will help reduce those cravings. Here's what you can do:

Make 60 to 65 percent of your diet raw food. Alcohol cravings appear to lessen, and even disappear, when a diet high in raw foods is introduced. A 1985 study put thirty-two people with high blood pressure on a six-month diet, which included 62 percent uncooked foods. This diet succeeded in lowering the participants' blood pressure and balancing blood cholesterol and fats, and it promoted weight loss. But the interesting part is that 80 percent of those who regularly drank alcohol abstained without suggestion or encouragement. A similar percentage of smokers quit smoking.

Dr. John Douglas, who worked with addiction patients at the Kaiser Permanente Medical Center in Los Angeles, also discovered that such a diet eaten over a span of several weeks caused his patients not to want as many cigarettes or alcoholic drinks as before. He concluded that a diet rich in such raw foods as vegetables, fruits, juices, sprouts, seeds, and nuts must sensitize the body to what is good for it and what is not. He noted that raw sunflower seeds were particularly effective in depressing the cravings associated with addiction. Sunflower sprouts should have a similar effect, and can be juiced. Fresh vegetable juice can significantly help you reach a daily goal of 60 to 65 percent raw food.

Reduce sugar and caffeine intake. Studies with humans have shown that greatly reducing one's intake of sugar and caffeine can directly lower alcohol cravings. In the case of sugar, this means avoidance of processed desserts and treats; sodas; dried fruits; and fruit juices, except in limited amounts (like four ounces of juice diluted with water). In the case of caffeine, the benefits would come from elimination of caffeinated sodas; coffee and tea, unless decaffeinated; and chocolate, except raw cacao, which is unsweetened and high in antioxidants (found at health food stores). Both sugar and caffeine can have an impact on your blood-sugar regulation. There has been evidence in the research that stabilizing blood sugar can help reduce alcohol cravings. A second step is to make sure that your diet is filled with nutrient-rich foods so that you can get all the nourishment your body needs, including help in supporting your liver and other detoxification processes.

Increase amino acids and nutrients that support serotonin, a neurotransmitter that affects alcohol and tobacco cravings. Low serotonin may excite these cravings (for more information on serotonin and the amino acids and a diet that facilitates improvement, see causes of Carb Cravings, page 121). Also, dopamine is the neurotransmitter that is most likely out of balance when heavy caffeine or stimulant drugs are desired (see page 122 for more information on amino acids and how to balance them in the body).

Vitamin B$_1$, also known as thiamine, cannot be held in the body and is crucial to level blood sugar. You could benefit by taking a B complex vitamin. *Best juice sources of thiamine:* sunflower and buckwheat sprouts.

L-glutamine, an amino acid, has also been used to help reduce cravings for alcohol and sugar.

✴ Juice Recipes

Pure Green Sprout Drink *(pg 340)*   **The Ginger Hopper** *(pg 332)*   **Spinach Power** *(pg 341)*   **Wheatgrass Light** *(pg 345)*

Sugar and high-carbohydrate cravings. If you consistently desire sweets, refined grains (breads, crackers, pasta), and such starchy vegetables as potatoes, winter squash, and corn, you have a carbohydrate craving. This can contribute to a condition known as insulin resistance. Being insulin resistant means your body stops responding to insulin, and instead grabs every calorie it can and deposits it as fat. So no matter how little you eat, you will gradually gain weight. Your cells cannot absorb the glucose they need, so they signal your brain that you need more carbohydrates, and in particular, sugars, and the more you eat, the more you want. The result is persistent food cravings and weight gain. This can lead to obesity and sabotage attempts at dieting and hunger control. If you have typically eaten a low-fat, high-carbohydrate diet for a number of years, the chances are strong that you have become at least partially insulin resistant. (Carbohydrate craving is fairly common during the premenstrual phase due to hormone imbalances.)

✳ Causes of Carb Cravings

Low blood sugar and/or low serotonin signals the brain that it needs a pick-me-up. This signal causes a sugar craving, or what is often referred to as a carbohydrate craving. Serotonin is our basic feel-good hormone. If serotonin is low, we can feel sad or depressed, or experience anxiety, headaches, and poor sleep. Hormonal imbalances, low protein intake, and/or weak digestion can lead to low serotonin. Unfortunately, sugars and simple carbohydrates release a short burst of serotonin, which makes us want them often when serotonin is low. We usually feel good for a moment but soon return to our low-serotonin state, and then crave more sugar and simple carbohydrates. It's a downward spiral, and sugar and other refined carbs make the situation worse.

Carbohydrates have a molecule that looks very much like that of the neurotransmitter serotonin. People often crave carbohydrates when serotonin is insufficient. When the amino acids that help to create serotonin are consumed along with a healthy diet of a wide variety of proteins, these cravings typically subside (see page 122 for the amino acid protocol). When serotonin is low, other cravings occur as well, such as cravings for alcohol. Extreme carbohydrate cravings are also caused when the blood-glucose level of the brain is too low. The brain realizes that a quick boost is needed. Keeping proteins consistently infused into the diet and complex carbohydrates is one of the most effective ways to improve this issue. Proteins break down into amino acids to create neurotransmitters. A variety of proteins is important to offer the brain an array of neurotransmitter precursor nutrients.

Adrenal fatigue can cause carb cravings. If you are under a lot of stress, or suffer from insomnia or sleep deprivation, you are probably exhausted much of the time. This leads to adrenal fatigue or adrenal exhaustion, which signals the body that it needs a pick-me-up. You may resort to sugar, high-carbohydrate snacks, or coffee during the day and carbohydrates or alcohol at night, all of which exacerbate the problem. You may benefit from getting an adrenal test and supporting your adrenal glands nutritionally.

✳ Lifestyle Recommendations

Stress reduction and emotional healing. An extended period of physical or psychological stress produces stress hormones such as cortisol and adrenaline, which can interfere with the synthesis of the brain neurotransmitter serotonin. Serotonin conveys the positive sensations of satiety, satisfaction, happiness, and relaxation. It's known to unlock at least fourteen different receptor types, each thought to have a distinct role in influencing our moods, impulses, appetites, and motivation. It regulates cravings, and when converted to melatonin, helps us sleep well. Therefore, reducing stress and dealing with emotional issues can greatly improve serotonin levels.

✳ Diet Recommendations

Recognize protein deficiency, which can cause a craving for sweets, and may contribute to low serotonin levels. Serotonin is produced from the essential amino acid (protein unit), L-tryptophan, which is obtained from food. (Turkey and eggs are among the best sources of L-tryptophan.) L-tryptophan is converted to serotonin with the assistance of vitamin B_6 (pyridoxine) and magnesium. Aim for three to four servings of protein per day, and vary your protein sources; include nuts, seeds, legumes (beans, lentils, split peas), eggs, and muscle meats such as beef, chicken, turkey, and fish. Choose organically fed, free-range or cage-free, and no antibiotics or hormones. Strict vegans can become protein-deficient fairly easily. If you're vegan, make sure each day you eat at least two to three cups of legumes (beans, lentils, or split peas) complemented by whole grains, nuts, seeds, and sprouts.

Follow the hypoglycemia diet. See the chapter on Hypoglycemia, page 180.

✳ Nutrient Recommendations

Amino acid support. There is a relationship between insulin resistance and absorption of amino acids. It is believed that insulin resistance may interfere with the absorption of essential amino acids such as phenylalanine and tyrosine, which are forerunners of brain neurotransmitters such as dopamine and norepinephrine. Insulin resistance is also believed to result in a dysfunction of dopamine metabolism. Dopamine conveys the sensation of pleasure.

Also, serotonin is converted from the amino acid L-tryptophan. L-tryptophan breaks down into 5-hydroxytryptophan (5-HTP) for the creation of serotonin. The body often needs larger amounts of this amino acid than we get from food. Additionally, other cofactors such as B vitamins and enzymes must be present for this to occur. Since L-tryptophan breaks down into 5-HTP at a very low percentage, 5-HTP is often taken as a supplement. Dosages should be based on testing, however. B vitamins are among the necessary nutrients for the creation and transport of L-tryptophan and 5-HTP into serotonin, and should also be taken as part of the complete brain wellness plan. Also, varied protein consumption is imperative with this program. You may greatly benefit from an amino acid supplement program tailored to your body's specific needs.

Chromium helps to regulate blood sugar, and improves glucose tolerance by increasing insulin's efficiency. Eat more foods rich in chromium, such as chicken, eggs, broccoli, and whole grains (barley in particular). *Best juice sources of chromium:* apples, parsnips, spinach, carrots, lettuce, string beans, and cabbage. If after increasing your intake of these foods and juices you still crave sweets, try a chromium supplement of 50 to 200 mcg. (Liquid, trivalent organic chromium is best.) Vitamin E, vanadium (a trace mineral), and evening primrose oil may also be helpful. *Best juice sources of vitamin E:* spinach, watercress, asparagus, carrots, and tomatoes. *Best juice sources of vanadium:* parsley, green beans, carrots, cabbage, garlic, tomatoes, and radishes. Evening primrose oil can be taken in supplement form.

Folic acid is involved in serotonin production, so a deficiency could affect serotonin levels. *Best juice sources of folic acid:* asparagus, spinach, kale, beetroot with greens, broccoli, cabbage, and blackberries.

Probiotics, enzymes, and **betaine HCL.** Taking probiotics such as kombucha, kefir, or supplemental probiotics (found at health food stores) will help improve weak digestion, plus enzymes and betaine HCL will help you digest cooked foods and protein more effectively.

✳ Juice Recipes

The Ginger Hopper *(pg 332)* **Beautiful-Skin Cocktail** *(pg 328)* **Triple C** *(pg 344)* **Sinus Solution** *(pg 341)* **Tomato Florentine** *(pg 343)* **Spring Tonic** *(pg 342)* **Weight-Loss Buddy** *(pg 345)* **Wheatgrass Light** *(pg 345)*

Ice cravings (pogophagia). If you continually reach for ice cubes to crunch, you may have what is known as pogophagia. A craving for ice is often a sign of anemia. Anemia can be the result of iron, vitamin B_{12} (cobalamin), and/or folic acid deficiency (see Anemia, page 39). *Best juice sources of nonheme iron, the type found* *in plants:* parsley, dandelion greens, broccoli, cauliflower, strawberries, asparagus, Swiss chard, blackberries, cabbage, beetroot with greens, and carrots. *Best juice sources of folic acid:* asparagus, spinach, kale, broccoli, cabbage, and blackberries.

✳ Juice Recipes

Spinach Power *(pg 341)*   **Morning Energizer** *(pg 337)*   **Triple C** *(pg 344)*
Calcium-Rich Cocktail *(pg 329)*

Peanut butter cravings. Do you ever find yourself scooping out spoonfuls of peanut butter, never even bothering to spread it on crackers or bread before you eat it? Unless you buy the natural brands that contain only peanuts and salt, it may be the corn syrup or other sugars you're actually craving. Or it may be that you are copper deficient; peanuts are rich in copper. There are better sources of copper, however, that are lower in fat and without the carcinogenic aflatoxins found on peanuts. *Best juice sources of copper:* carrots, garlic, gingerroot, and turnips.

✳ Juice Recipes

The Ginger Hopper *(pg 332)*   **Garlic Surprise** *(pg 332)*   **Beet-Cucumber**
Cleansing Cocktail *(pg 328)*   **Ginger Twist** *(pg 332)*   **Immune Builder** *(pg 335)*

Salty-food cravings. If potato chips, pretzels, bacon, or salted popcorn is your desire, it may be the salt you're after. Salt cravings can be a symptom of sickle-cell anemia, Addison's disease, adrenal fatigue, various muscular disorders, high blood pressure (see High Blood Pressure, page 175), or diabetes (see Diabetes Mellitus, page 131). A common cause of occasional salt cravings is adrenal stress. Caffeine consumption and other lifestyle stressors can weaken the adrenal glands, allowing blood-pressure levels to drop and bringing on fatigue. Increasing salt intake can temporarily help the symptoms, but can have negative long-term effects. Also, magnesium deficiency has been shown to cause salt cravings in animals. If you crave salt, reduce your consumption of table salt (sodium chloride), and increase your consumption of natural sodium from vegetables such as celery, along with Celtic sea salt or gray salt, which is rich in minerals, magnesium, pantothenic acid, potassium, vitamin B$_6$ (pyridoxine), vitamin C, and zinc, all of which help to support your adrenal glands. *Best juice sources of magnesium:* beetroot greens, spinach, parsley, dandelion greens, garlic, blackberries, beetroot, broccoli, cauliflower, carrots, and celery. *Best juice* *sources of pantothenic acid:* broccoli, cauliflower, and kale. *Best juice sources of potassium:* parsley, Swiss chard, garlic, spinach, broccoli, carrots, celery, radishes, cauliflower, watercress, asparagus, and cabbage. *Best juice sources of Vitamin B_6:* kale, spinach, turnip greens, bell peppers, and prunes. *Best juice sources of Vitamin C:* kale, parsley, broccoli, Brussels sprouts, watercress, cauliflower, cabbage, strawberries, spinach, lemons, limes, turnips, and asparagus. *Best juice sources of zinc:* gingerroot, turnips, parsley, garlic, carrots, spinach, cabbage, lettuce, and cucumbers.

✳ Juice Recipes

Magnesium-Rich Cocktail *(pg 336)*   **Liver Life Tonic** *(pg 336)*   **Spinach Power** *(pg 341)*   **Beautiful-Skin Cocktail** *(pg 328)*   **Peppy Parsley** *(pg 339)*

Sour-food cravings. If you crave lemons, limes, or other sour foods, you may need acetic acid to help detoxify toxins released from undigested proteins. Toxins build up in the body when foods putrefy in the intestinal tract (see Constipation, page 114; also see the Intestinal Cleanse, page 307). Drink a teaspoon of lemon juice in a glass of water to provide acetic acid. Vitamin B_2 (riboflavin) may also be helpful. *Best juice sources of vitamin B_2:* collard greens, kale, parsley, broccoli, and beetroot greens.

Chlorophyll, found abundantly in green juices, is another nutrient that can help detoxify the system and reduce cravings for sour foods.

✳ Juice Recipes

Magnesium-Rich Cocktail *(pg 336)*   **Pure Green Sprout Drink** *(pg 340)*   **Allergy Relief** *(pg 326)*   **Peppy Parsley** *(pg 339)*   **Wheatgrass Light** *(pg 345)*

Depression

DEPRESSION is a feeling of unhappiness, sadness, hopelessness, worthlessness, gloom, and self-reproach that lasts longer than the passing blue mood. Often, depressed people hide from society and lose interest or pleasure in usual activities. Their sex drive may decrease, and they may be irritable. They may tend to sleep a lot or hardly be able to sleep at all, feel jittery, lack concentration, lose appetite, or be constantly hungry. They may have headaches, backaches, or digestive problems, and may get sick more often, since depression saps the immune system. If severely depressed, a person may become suicidal. For most people, though, depression is not severe; they can still function, but do so with more effort and struggle.

Depression is often linked to a lack of the main neurotransmitter serotonin, but also involves the stimulating brain chemicals dopamine and norepinephrine. Serotonin is created from the amino acid L-tryptophan, which is fairly hard to derive in large quantities from diet. This is why so many Americans have depression, sleep disorders, anxiety, and problems with stress, since serotonin plays a role in all of these. Stress causes us to use up our inhibitory or calming neurotransmitters such as serotonin more quickly than we can create them from our diet. But when we give our body the amino acids it needs, and establish balance between the stimulating and calming neurotransmitters (brain chemicals), symptoms such as depression may abate.

Stimulants of any kind cause a depletion of neurotransmitters. The most likely offenders are caffeine and many medications used for focus and energy. Factors that can exacerbate the situation include: alcohol, high-sugar or low-protein intake, blood-sugar imbalance, candidiasis, poor thyroid or adrenal function, nutrient deficiencies, smoking, food allergies, stress, hormone imbalances, prescription drugs, and environmental toxins.

Many medications are used to help redistribute neurotransmitters, but they cannot make "fresh" or "new" neurotransmitters. Some of these medications work on one neurotransmitter (the SSRIs such as Paxil, Prozac, Celexa, Strattera, Wellbutrin) and some, such as Effexor and Cymbalta, work on more than one. Treating depression with a wide variety of prescription drugs can have side effects, some quite severe. Various amino acids, nutritional supplements, and dietary changes have been shown to be very effective in not only alleviating symptoms, but also addressing the root of the problem. And they have few, if any, side effects. However, they usually take longer to bring relief. If you are already taking a prescription antidepressant, be sure to see a doctor before switching to another plan. In most cases, you may need to decrease your prescription medication gradually. And remember, nutritional therapy will work best if you follow an overall treatment plan that includes a whole-foods diet with varied protein sources and plenty of vegetables and vegetable juices.

✳ Lifestyle Recommendations

Get enough sleep. This helps prevent depression. Serotonin affects sleep, and sleep affects serotonin. If you suffer from insomnia, see Insomnia and Jet Lag, page 202.

Make time for regular exercise. Movement boosts serotonin. Indulge in a brisk walk for a healthy dose of serotonin and dopamine. Both serotonin and dopamine are released while you walk. Exercise tones not only your body, making you feel better physically, but also your mind by releasing endorphins, the feel-good brain chemicals. That is why you feel happy, euphoric, yet very clear-minded after working out for at least thirty minutes.

Stop smoking. Smoking leads to depression by decreasing tryptophan levels. It also decreases vitamin C, which can lead to depression. Depression may, in turn, make it more difficult to quit smoking. Thus, by addressing your depression, you may find it easier to kick the smoking habit and by stopping smoking, you may help your depression (see Cravings, page 118).

Get fifteen minutes of sunshine every day. Sunshine stimulates serotonin production. When it's cold outside, sit next to a window.

Schedule joyful moments into each day. Any activity or person that brings you joy actually raises serotonin. Engaging in a kind act raises serotonin. Speak encouraging words to yourself and others; your thoughts and words affect your body. Each day, do something you love. Feelings of love get serotonin pumping.

✳ Diet Recommendations

Avoid sugar and refined carbohydrates. Depression can be caused by low blood-sugar levels (hypoglycemia). This disorder develops when there is not enough of the right fuel to keep blood-sugar levels steady. Eliminate all refined carbohydrates; this includes sweets such as cakes, candy, cookies, and ice cream, and white-flour products such as bread, pasta, pizza, and rolls, plus all junk food. This may be challenging if emotional stress leads to a craving for sweets, since they provide quick bursts of emotional and physical energy. But they leave you feeling burned out and depressed in the end. During times of stress, it is important to maintain even blood-sugar levels by eating complex carbohydrates, like vegetables, whole grains, and legumes, along with varied sources of protein, which help increase brain serotonin. Also, eat high-energy snacks, such as raw vegetables, fruit, fresh vegetable juices, raw nuts, and seeds to keep blood-sugar levels even and ward off depression (see Hypoglycemia, page 180; Cravings, page 118; see also Basic Guidelines for the Juice Lady's Health and Healing Diet, page 290).

Reduce coffee consumption. Stimulants cause a depletion of neurotransmitters, which can cause depression. Several studies have looked at caffeine intake and depression. In a study of healthy college students, moderate and high coffee drinkers scored higher on a depression scale than did low users. Other studies have shown that depressed patients tend to consume fairly high amounts of caffeine. In addition, the intake of caffeine has been linked with the degree of depression in psychiatric patients—the higher the intake of caffeine, the more severe the depression. It is recommended that you drink no more than three cups of coffee per day, and make them on the weaker side. Studies indicate that a combination of caffeine and sugar is even worse for depression, hence sugar or syrup in your coffee, or coffee and doughnuts, are definitely on the "omit list."

Avoid food additives. These substances are linked with depression. Read food labels, and avoid anything that has chemicals and other additives. Particularly avoid MSG, which can cause a stimulatory effect in the brain that causes a depletion of serotonin. Be aware that MSG is not always labeled as such, but sometimes as hydrolyzed vegetable protein, Accent, Ajinomoto, and natural meat tenderizer. A good rule is not to buy what you can't pronounce.

Eliminate foods that can cause allergies. Food allergies can cause you to feel more defensive and depressed (see Allergies, page 27; see also the Elimination Diet, page 301).

Eat more raw foods—fresh fruit, vegetables, and vegetable juices. People who consume a diet high in raw foods and juice have found that these lift their spirits. Juice fasting for one to three days can be very helpful; many people have reported a great sense of well-being following a juice fast (see the Juice Fast, page 304).

✳ Nutrient Recommendations

Amino acids can help balance neurotransmitters, which are the natural chemicals that facilitate communication between brain cells. These chemicals direct our emotions, memory, mood, behavior, sleep, and learning abilities. The neurotransmitters are manufactured in the body from amino acids—our protein building blocks in food. The major neurotransmitter involved in preventing and reversing depression is serotonin, along with the stimulating brain chemicals dopamine and norepinephrine. When serotonin is low, you feel anxious, aggravated, moody, or depressed. Serotonin is converted from the amino acid L-tryptophan, which breaks down into 5-hydroxytryptophan (5-HTP) for the creation of serotonin. Other cofactors such as B vitamins and enzymes must be present for this to occur. Since L-tryptophan breaks down into 5-HTP at a very low percentage, 5-HTP is often taken as a supplement. Dosages should be based on testing, however. B vitamins are among the necessary nutrients for the creation and transport of L-tryptophan and the breakdown of L-tryptophan into 5-HTP to make serotonin, and should also be taken as part of the complete brain wellness plan. Also, varied protein consumption is imperative with this program; include nuts, seeds, beans, eggs, and muscle meats such as fish, chicken, turkey, and beef. (Choose organically fed, free-range/cage-free, and no hormones or antibiotics.) For more information on amino acid testing, see page 350.

Folic acid and **vitamin B$_{12}$** (cobalamin) are important depression fighters; deficiencies of either or both are associated with depression. Alcohol and aspirin usage contribute to folic-acid deficiencies. *Best juice sources of folic acid:* asparagus, spinach, kale, broccoli, cabbage, and blackberries. Vitamin B$_{12}$ is not available in fruits and vegetables. *Best food sources of B$_{12}$:* meat, poultry, and fish.

Magnesium deficiency can cause numerous psychological changes, including depression. The symptoms of magnesium deficiency include poor attention, memory loss, depression, fear, restlessness, insomnia, tics, cramps, and dizziness. Magnesium levels have been found to be significantly lower in depressed patients than in controls. A supplement of 200 to 400 mg of magnesium glycinate may improve your mood. Also, this form of magnesium is very calming. *Best juice sources of magnesium:* beetroot with greens, spinach, Swiss chard, collards, parsley, and sunflower sprouts.

Omega-3 fatty acids are essential fatty acids (EFAs) that play an important role in fighting depression. Low levels of omega-3 fatty acids in the diet have been associated with increased rates of depression. Omega-3s are crucial to brain function and health. They make up the insulation for neurons. This insulation is necessary since neurotransmitters conduct on the outside of this fatty-acid coating. They're available from fish, fish oil, grass-fed animals (not grain-fed), and some nuts and seeds like walnuts, flax, and hemp. Lower levels of omega-3 consumption have been linked to increased rates of depression and possibly suicide. This can be attributed to omega-3 deficiencies affecting serotonin and dopamine transmission in the frontal cortex and hippocampus. Another biochemical cause of depression is a genetic inability to manufacture enough prostaglandin E1 (PGE 1) which is an important brain metabolite derived from EFAs. You may benefit from increasing your omega-3s by taking flaxseeds and hemp seeds, along with fish oil such as krill and cod-liver oil, and by eating more cold-water fish such as salmon, trout, mackerel, and halibut, along with grass-fed beef. (For more information, see the fats and oils section in Basic Guidelines for the Juice Lady's Health and Healing Diet, page 290.)

S-adenosylmethionine (SAM or SAMe)

SAMe is a synthetic form of a compound formed naturally in the body from the essential amino acid methionine and adenosine triphosphate (ATP), the energy-producing compound found in all cells in the body. There have been several studies on the use of SAMe for depression. It has been hypothesized that SAMe increases the availability of the neurotransmitters serotonin and dopamine. SAMe has been shown to be comparable to prescription antidepressants in action. Two meta-analyses have examined the available evidence and concluded that SAMe was superior to placebo in treating depressive disorders and approximately as effective as standard tricyclic antidepressants. A 2002 Italian study found SAMe to be as effective as imipramine, one of the original tricyclic antidepressants, and SAMe subjects reported fewer side effects than subjects who took imipramine. Recommended dosage: 400 to 1,600 mg daily.

Vitamin C and **bioflavonoids,** especially rutin, have been shown to help people with depression. *Best juice sources of vitamin C:* kale, parsley, broccoli, Brussels sprouts, watercress, cauliflower, cabbage, spinach, lemons, limes, turnips, and asparagus. *Best juice sources of bioflavonoids:* bell peppers, berries (blueberries, blackberries, and cranberries), broccoli, cabbage, lemons, limes, parsley, and tomatoes.

Vitamin D. We get it from the sun, but in the winter and on dark, dreary days, we should supplement our diet with vitamin D. One study found that depression during winter months was significantly reduced among study subjects who took high daily doses of vitamin D for a period of one year. Cod-liver oil is a good source of vitamin D along with omega-3 fatty acids.

✳ Juice Therapy

Celery juice. According to European folklore, celery helps you forget your troubles from a broken heart and soothes your nerves at the same time. It's probably the butyl phthalide (a phytochemical) in celery, which is known to have sedative properties.

Dark green juices are rich in chlorophyll and many other nutrients that have been shown to be very helpful for depression.

Fennel juice has long been used as a tonic to help release endorphins into the bloodstream. Endorphins create a mood of euphoria and help dampen anxiety and fear.

✳ Juice Recipes

Pure Green Sprout Drink *(pg 340)*   **Mood Mender** *(pg 337)*   **Happy Morning** *(pg 333)*   **Morning Energizer** *(pg 337)*   **Peppy Parsley** *(pg 339)*   **Wheatgrass Light** *(pg 345)*   **Mint Refresher** *(pg 337)*   **Spinach Power** *(pg 341)*   **Beautiful-Skin Cocktail** *(pg 328)*   **Salsa in a Glass** *(pg 340)*

Diabetes Mellitus

DIABETES MELLITUS is a condition in which the body cannot properly regulate blood-sugar levels. This gives rise to symptoms that include fatigue and increased thirst. Diabetes mellitus includes several conditions. In type 1 diabetes, also known as insulin-dependent or juvenile-onset diabetes, the body's own immune system destroys cells in the pancreas called beta cells. Beta cells secrete insulin, the hormone that helps most of the body's cells take in glucose (the cells' main fuel source) from the blood. Because there is little or no insulin in the blood, the person must take insulin in order to survive. Type 1 diabetes generally develops sometime in childhood but can occur in adults.

In type 2 diabetes, also known as adult-onset or noninsulin-dependent diabetes, the pancreas may not make insulin well, or it may secrete insulin, but there may be a problem with the insulin receptors on the body's cells; there may not be enough receptors, or the receptors may be insensitive to insulin. Without enough insulin, or proper utilization of it, glucose stays in the blood. It appears that the hormone leptin is largely responsible for the accuracy of insulin-signaling and whether or not one becomes insulin resistant (see next page for explanation). This condition usually develops after a person reaches age forty. It can be controlled by diet and, in some cases, by medication. But if type 2 diabetes is not controlled, it can progress to the point that additional insulin is required. Symptoms of type 2 diabetes may include fatigue, thirst, weight loss, blurred vision, and frequent urination. Some people have no symptoms. A blood test can show if you have diabetes.

A third type of diabetes is known as gestational diabetes mellitus (GDM). It occurs for the first time during pregnancy, and usually disappears after a woman gives birth. GDM is usually controlled well with dietary changes. These changes must continue after delivery, though, because women who develop GDM have a much higher chance of developing type 2 diabetes later in life.

Diabetes can have a number of long-term complications, including atherosclerosis, susceptibility to infection, and damage to the eyes, nerves, and kidneys. Therefore, it is very important to control your blood-sugar levels with diet even if you are not experiencing any symptoms.

✳ Diet Recommendations

Treatments that concentrate merely on lowering diabetics' blood sugar while raising their insulin levels can actually worsen rather than remedy the problem of metabolic miscommunication. They just trade one problem for another. Science is telling us that we must eat a diet that maximizes the accuracy of insulin- and leptin-signaling, allowing our cells to better listen to the body's life-giving messages. This is where the true remedy lies. That means emphasizing good fats, eliminating all sugar and refined-flour products, and reducing nonfiber carbohydrates, including starches. Following are specific recommendations that have proven effective for many diabetics.

Avoid sugar, sweets, and all other simple carbohydrates, and limit high-starch foods. This includes cookies, candies, cakes, pies, ice cream, and items made with processed white flour, including bread, rolls, pasta, and pizza. Limit starchy vegetables such as potatoes, winter squash, corn, and peas. Be aware that many breads, muffins, bagels, and pasta say they are whole grain, but they are not. Very few of these products are actually all whole grain. They are mostly white flour with a few whole grains thrown in. There are only a few breads that are actually all whole grain: Ezekiel and other sprouted-grain breads. Fruit also contains simple carbohydrates, so don't eat more than one piece per day. Limit your intake of fruit juice to no more than four ounces daily, and dilute it by half with water or vegetable juice. Avoid alcohol, as it is a simple carbohydrate that acts like sugar in the body.

Consuming simple carbohydrates and high-starch foods can contribute to a condition known as insulin resistance, in which there is too much insulin in the bloodstream. Being insulin resistant means that your body stops responding to insulin, and instead grabs every calorie it can and deposits it as fat. Your cells cannot absorb the glucose they need, so they signal your brain that you need more carbohydrates. This is part of what is termed the "metabolic syndrome," which is a cluster of common pathologies—abdominal obesity linked to an excess of visceral fat, insulin resistance, dyslipidemia (an unhealthy fat profile), and hypertension. This syndrome is occurring at epidemic rates, with dramatic consequences for human health worldwide, and appears to have emerged largely from changes in our diet in recent decades, along with reduced physical activity. An important but not well-appreciated dietary change has been the substantial increase in fructose intake, which appears to be an important causative factor in this syndrome. The best sweetener for diabetics (and the only one I recommend) is stevia, available at health food stores in powder or liquid drops.

Avoid all soda. Researchers have found a correlation between drinking soda, including diet soda, and metabolic syndrome. Scientists gathered dietary information on more than 9,500 men and women ages forty-five to sixty-four and tracked their health for nine years. The risk of developing metabolic syndrome was 34 percent higher among those who drank just one can of diet soda a day compared with those who drank none.

Fruit. Some fruits and berries are acceptable for diabetics, but many are not. For example, avocados, strawberries, raspberries, cranberries, mountain ash, blackberries, pomegranates, pears, lemons, limes, grapefruit, and dog rose hips are good choices. All other fruit, such as cherries, plums, grapes, pineapple, oranges, bananas, and chestnuts, are not. They contain too much sugar.

Eat complex carbohydrates and whole, unprocessed foods. Vegetables, whole grains, and legumes (beans, lentils, split peas) are made up of complex carbohydrates. These carbohydrates require more time for your digestive system to break them down into fuel. Since digestion takes more time, glucose is released into the bloodstream more slowly and evenly than with simple carbohydrates, which tend to dump glucose into your bloodstream all at once. Whole foods are good sources of fiber, which also helps regulate blood sugar. Limit consumption to no more than three to four cups per week of starchy vegetables such as potatoes, yams, winter squash, peas, and corn; they are processed into fuel more quickly than other vegetables.

Eat more of your vegetables raw, and drink fresh vegetable juices. Dr. John Douglas of the Kaiser Permanente Medical Center in Los Angeles found that raw vegetables are better tolerated by diabetics than cooked vegetables, and that raw foods help stabilize blood-sugar levels. Dr. Max Bircher-Benner of the European Bircher-Benner clinic successfully used raw vegetable juices in treating diabetics. When juicing, make sure you juice primarily vegetables rather than fruit. Focus on vegetables that are low in sugar content. As a general rule, vegetables that are grown aboveground are low in sugar, while those grown belowground are higher in sugar—this includes beetroot, carrots, white potatoes, sweet potatoes, and yams. You can add a small amount of carrot, beetroot, or green apple to the juice to make it more delicious. But the key is only a small amount diluted with lots of greens. (For more information, see Principle 1 in Basic Guidelines for the Juice Lady's Health and Healing Diet, page 290.)

Eat smaller, more frequent meals, and include a little protein at each meal or snack. Diabetics do best eating several small meals throughout the day, rather than two or three large meals. Eating more frequently, and eating a little protein at each meal or snack, helps keep blood sugar at a relatively constant level, which is far better than inducing big surges in blood sugar by eating a large meal. One way to accomplish this goal is to save a portion of each meal and eat it later as a snack.

Reduce your consumption of animal products. Research shows that reducing animal proteins in your diet lowers the risk of developing severe diabetes complications. You do not need to eat a strictly vegetarian diet. You can choose fish over other animal proteins more often, and eat only small quantities of meat and poultry. Cold-water fish such as salmon, tuna, halibut, cod, trout, and sardines contain oils called essential fatty acids that can help make your cells more receptive to insulin.

❋ Nutrient Recommendations

Blackberry leaf. Steep two tablespoons of dried, crushed blackberry leaves for thirty minutes in one cup of boiling water, filter, and drink one-third cup three times a day. This remedy helps to normalize blood-sugar levels in diabetics.

Chromium makes insulin more effective at the cellular level. It is a component of glucose tolerance factor (GTF), which helps the cells take up glucose and helps regulate blood-sugar levels. Studies have found low levels of chromium in people with diabetes. There are many promising studies suggesting that chromium supplementation may be effective in preventing and treating diabetes. *Best juice sources of chromium:* green peppers, parsnips, spinach, carrots, lettuce, string beans, and cabbage.

Copper deficiency may impair glucose tolerance. *Best juice sources of copper:* carrots, garlic, gingerroot, and turnips.

Magnesium deficiency is the most common mineral deficiency seen in diabetics. There is experimental and clinical evidence that the amount of magnesium in the Western diet is insufficient to meet individual needs and that magnesium deficiency may contribute to insulin resistance. Some studies suggest that low magnesium levels may worsen blood-glucose control in type 2 diabetes and that supplementation may help with insulin resistance. For example, a study examined the effect of magnesium in sixty-three people with type 2 diabetes and low magnesium levels who were taking the medication glibenclamide. After sixteen weeks, people who took magnesium had improved insulin sensitivity and lower fasting glucose levels. Animal studies indicate a pivotal role of magnesium in glucose homeostasis and insulin secretion and action. Experimental and clinical studies suggest that magnesium intake may lower the risk of hypertension and type 2 diabetes, may decrease blood triglycerides, and may increase HDL cholesterol levels. *Best juice sources of magnesium:* leafy green vegetables such as beetroot greens, spinach, parsley, and dandelion greens, along with garlic, beetroot, broccoli, cauliflower, carrots, and celery.

Vitamin B₃ (niacin), like chromium, is a component of GTF. *Best food sources of vitamin B₃:* brewer's yeast, rice and wheat bran, peanuts, turkey, chicken, and fish. It is not available in vegetables and fruits.

Vitamin C metabolism can be disrupted by diabetes, and a deficiency can lead to problems with glucose regulation. Vitamin C levels are typically lower in people with diabetes, even when they take supplemental C. *Best juice sources of vitamin C:* kale, parsley, broccoli, Brussels sprouts, watercress, cauliflower, cabbage, spinach, lemons, limes, turnips, and asparagus.

Vitamin E needs increase with diabetes, and this vitamin can help to decrease the amount of insulin required. *Best juice sources of vitamin E:* spinach, watercress, asparagus, carrots, and tomatoes.

Zinc plays an important role in the production and storage of insulin. There is some research showing that people with type 2 diabetes have suboptimal zinc levels due to decreased absorption and increased excretion of zinc. *Best juice sources of zinc:* gingerroot, parsley, garlic, carrots, and spinach.

✳ Herb Recommendations

Gymnema sylvestre is an herb used in Ayurvedic (traditional Indian) medicine. In animal studies, it has been shown to reduce blood-sugar levels in individuals with high sugar levels, while not affecting those individuals with normal levels.

Cinnamon. A couple of studies have found that cinnamon improves blood-glucose control in people with type 2 diabetes.

Cinnamon Tea

Although many people like to simply sprinkle cinnamon on oatmeal, having cinnamon in tea is another option. You can find cinnamon in chai tea, but that is often sweetened, which is not good for diabetics. It is best is to make your own cinnamon tea using a recipe like this.

    1 cinnamon stick
    1 cup boiling water

1 decaffeinated black tea bag

Pinch or drop of stevia

1. Place the cinnamon stick in a cup.
2. Add the boiling water and steep, covered, for 10 minutes.
3. Add the tea bag. Steep for 1 to 3 minutes.
4. Sweeten to taste, if desired.

✳ Juice Therapy

Bitter melon is a green melon that can be found in Asian markets. It has been used for centuries by Chinese and East Indians to treat diabetes; it enhances glucose metabolism and lowers blood-sugar levels. Bitter melon is prepared by juicing the fruit and the seeds and mixing them with other desired juices and water.

Brussels sprouts juice is good for diabetics and hypoglycemics; it also promotes healthy skin and increases male potency.

Cabbage juice was found in one study to help diabetics; it is suspected of having an insulin-like activity.

Celery juice is good for diabetics and for people who have sweet cravings and obesity.

Garlic juice lowers blood-sugar levels. It also helps the body fight off infections, which tend to occur more frequently when diabetes is present.

Jerusalem artichoke juice possesses unique properties for treating types 1 and 2 diabetes. Eat two to three raw Jerusalem artichokes or drink their juice (from one-third to one full glass) three times a day twenty minutes before a meal to help stabilize blood-sugar levels.

String bean juice has been used to support the pancreas. It is recommended that five cups of string bean juice be consumed throughout the day; one cup with breakfast, lunch, and dinner, and two juice snacks. Green bean juice is very strong-tasting and is better tolerated when mixed with milder-tasting juices, such as carrot and celery.

✳ Juice Recipes

Note: Most of the juice recipes should be modified for diabetes. Use only one or two carrots per juice, one-half small beetroot, and one-half green apple. Concentrate on low-sugar vegetables and leafy greens.

Beautiful-Skin Cocktail *(pg 328)* **Triple C** *(pg 344)* **Weight-Loss Buddy** *(pg 345)* **Jack & the Bean** *(pg 335)* **Morning Energizer** *(pg 337)* **Tomato Florentine** *(pg 343)* **Cabbage Patch Cocktail** *(pg 329)* **Garlic Surprise** *(pg 332)* **Immune Builder** *(pg 335)* **Orient Express** *(pg 338)* **Pancreas Helper** *(pg 338)* **Peppy Parsley** *(pg 339)* **Pure Green Sprout Drink** *(pg 340)* **Spring Tonic** *(pg 342)* **Super Green Sprout Drink** *(pg 342)* **The Revitalizer** *(pg 340)* **Wheatgrass Light** *(pg 345)*

Diverticulosis and Diverticulitis

DIVERTICULOSIS is a condition in which little pouches called diverticula develop along the intestinal walls, generally the large intestine wall. Diverticula are created when pressure is exerted against the intestinal wall. This pressure is strongest in the sigmoid area, the place where the large intestine is narrowest. Not surprisingly, the sigmoid area is also the place where most diverticula are found. These intestinal pouches occur at weak points, such as between fibers in the intestinal muscles or where arteries enter the bowel wall. Diverticulosis is usually symptomless, although there may be rectal bleeding and vague feelings of intestinal distress. It's often a consequence of chronic constipation (see Constipation, page 114), as dry, hard stools require more force to pass.

Diverticulitis is a condition in which a diverticulum (pouch or sac in the lining) of the colon ruptures. The rupture results in infection in the tissues that surround the colon. Diverticulitis symptoms include abdominal pain, abdominal cramps, diarrhea, constipation, fever, and bloating. Abscesses can form, as can fistulas—abnormal connections between the bowel and other organs. Both conditions tend to develop after middle age.

Chronic gastrointestinal diseases, such as diverticulitis, may result in malnutrition, which impairs both digestion and absorption of nutrients. Nutrient insufficiency leads to a decrease in digestive enzyme production and decreased cell growth. A whole-foods diet and the recommendations that follow can ease both malnutrition and the underlying diverticulitis.

✳ Diet Recommendations

During an attack (acute) you should choose a very-low-fiber diet (insoluble fiber). The very best choice is to juice vegetables such as carrots, celery, watercress, lettuce, cucumbers, and green apples for two to three days (see the Juice Fast, page 304). During an attack, stick with liquids such as purified water, peppermint herbal tea, and freshly made vegetable juices to help your colon heal. Then progress to a semisolid diet of steamed vegetables, mashed sweet potatoes or yams, and grated vegetables. You may add oatmeal or quinoa.

To prevent further attacks, once your symptoms improve, gradually add high-fiber foods back into your diet. While you're healing, avoid nuts, seeds, and popcorn (see page 140). Start with 5 to 15 grams of fiber per day and work up to 25 to 35 grams per day. Continue to eat a high-fiber diet. Diverticular disease was rare in the United States prior to the twentieth century, since people used to eat a diet that contained a lot more fiber. Roughage is vital for digestive-tract health. Both soluble and insoluble fiber holds water and increases fecal bulk, and soluble fiber combines with water to form a gel that lubricates the stool. Juice contains soluble fiber. Fiber makes stools softer and easier to pass. Insoluble fiber generally decreases transit time, the time it takes food to travel from one end of the digestive tract to the other, and soluble fiber normalizes transit time. In a long-term follow-up study among male health professionals, eating dietary fiber, particularly insoluble fiber, was associated with about a 40 percent lower risk of diverticular disease. The importance of eating a high-fiber diet rich in vegetables, fruits, sprouts, whole grains, and legumes (beans, lentils, split peas) cannot be overemphasized. (For more information on dietary goals, see Basic Guidelines for the Juice Lady's Health and Healing Diet, page 290.)

Take supplemental fiber. Use pectin, flax fiber, psyllium husk, guar gum, or oat bran, along with acidophilus, the friendly bacteria that aid digestion. Together, they help prevent constipation. Avoid supplemental fiber, though, during a period of active inflammation, as it can aggravate the problem.

Juice-fast during an acute phase. A vegetable juice diet gives the bowel a rest, and provides soluble fiber. Carrots, cabbage, and green juices are especially healing for the intestinal tract (see the Juice Fast, page 304). If you have a weak digestive system, drink the juices at room temperature. (Do not chill, since this is taxing on the digestive tract). The Intestinal Cleanse can also be quite beneficial (see page 307).

Avoid irritating foods. Nuts, seeds, and popcorn can become trapped in the diverticula, causing inflammation. Dairy products, especially cheese (small amounts of plain yogurt are acceptable), red meat, fried foods, fatty foods, hot sauces, spices, sugar, refined flour products, alcohol, coffee and caffeine-containing colas and teas, soda, and processed foods can cause intestinal irritation and/or constipation.

✳ Nutrient Recommendations

Beta-carotene helps heal the mucous membranes that line the intestinal tract. *Best juice sources of carotenes in general:* carrots, kale, parsley, spinach, Swiss chard, beetroot greens, watercress, broccoli, and romaine lettuce.

Digestive enzymes are present in raw food but are destroyed by cooking. For the body to digest and absorb food, it needs ample amounts of enzymes. Often, by the time we reach our forties our glands and organs are beginning to fall short in producing enough enzymes to maintain optimum health. Taking supplemental enzymes will help improve digestion and thus improve colon health.

Probiotics help maintain the natural balance of microflora in the intestines. Studies have shown that probiotics are effective in treating colon diseases.

Vitamin K deficiency has been linked to intestinal disorders. *Best juice sources of vitamin K:* turnip greens, broccoli, lettuce, cabbage, spinach, watercress, asparagus, and string beans.

✳ Herb Recommendations

Fenugreek seed, flaxseed, licorice, marshmallow root, and psyllium seed soothe and protect the mucosa that lines the intestines. Avoid licorice if you have high blood pressure, do not use for prolonged periods of time, and use a medicinal form of the herb, not licorice candy.

✳ Juice Therapy

Pear juice has traditionally been used for weak digestive systems; pear and apple juices provide pectins (soluble fiber), which help improve elimination.

Wheatgrass juice is especially healing for the digestive tract. It can also be used as an implant into the colon during a colonic or placed in the water for an enema.

✳ Juice Recipes

Antiulcer Cabbage Cocktail *(pg 327)* **Morning Energizer** *(pg 337)* **Natural Diuretic Cocktail** *(pg 338)* **Colon Cleanser** *(pg 330)* **Immune Builder** *(pg 335)* **Peppy Parsley** *(pg 339)* **Pure Green Sprout Drink** *(pg 340)* **Triple C** *(pg 344)* **Wheatgrass Light** *(pg 345)*

Eczema (Atopic Dermatitis)

ECZEMA is an intensely itchy, inflammatory skin disorder that is commonly found on the hands, face, wrists, elbows, and knees. It can occur at any age but is most common in infants and often disappears by eighteen months of age (although it can recur later in life). It is characterized by patches of red, itchy, dry, thickened skin. There are various types of lesions, scratches, papules, red patches, weeping areas, and scaly areas with small blisters. Eczema leaves the skin vulnerable to bacterial and/or viral infection.

Eczema can be caused by a host of factors, including heredity, diet, stress, candidiasis (see Candidiasis, page 80), and environmental pollutants and irritants. (Another type of eczema, contact dermatitis, is most often caused by exposure to poison ivy or oak.) Many eczema sufferers have a personal or family history of such allergic conditions as hay fever or hives. Although it is known that certain genetic factors may be involved in eczema, some experts say that heredity may be more related to familial environment, such as similar diet and lifestyle. Since World

War II, the numbers of new cases of eczema have continued to rise steadily. This suggests that environmental pollution, along with consumption of refined and fast foods, and a deficiency of essential fatty acids, may be strong factors in its development.

Breast milk is the best food for an infant who has eczema (or any infant, for that matter). The mother should eat a diet rich in the nutrients and juices covered in this chapter. If you or an older child are prone to this condition, the following suggestions can help.

✳ Lifestyle Recommendations

Reduce exposure to irritating metals. Several studies have found a correlation between eczema and allergy to gold or nickel. Not wearing gold and nickel jewelry is an obvious start, but it is also important to avoid gold or nickel fillings and gold and nickel in cosmetics. Common sources of nickel also include stainless-steel cookware.

✳ Diet Recommendations

Eat a high-fiber, whole-foods diet that includes plenty of raw fruits, vegetables, and vegetable juices. A high-fiber diet greatly facilitates elimination, and good elimination is vital in easing eczema. Drinking plenty of fresh vegetable juices and water is also important for proper elimination (see Constipation, page 114).

Drink only purified water. Tap water contains toxic compounds that have been known to make eczema symptoms worse. Drink only pure, clean water, and make sure that you drink at least eight eight-ounce glasses per day.

Liver/gallbadder detox. When the liver and gallbladder are congested, the body suffers the effects of poor assimilation of fat-soluble nutrients, which can play a role in the development of eczema, psoriasis, and dry skin. If you complete liver and gallbladder cleanses, your symptoms could clear up quickly (see pages 310–320 for the Liver Cleanse and the Gallbladder Cleanse).

Avoid sugar and refined flour products, which quickly turn to sugar. Avoid all sugar (such as table sugar, fructose, honey, and maple syrup) and refined-flour products (such as bread, rolls, pizza, and pasta). These substances can contribute to a weakening of the immune system, which is where abnormalities associated with eczema originate.

Eliminate animal products, with the exception of fish. Meat and dairy products contain arachidonic acid, a fatty acid that contributes to the inflammation experienced in eczema and psoriasis. Animal fats can aggravate itching and irritation. Many people experience an improvement in their symptoms after adopting a vegetarian or vegan diet, with the addition of fish.

Eliminate food allergens. Many studies have demonstrated a strong correlation between the onset of eczema and consumption of such foods as milk and other dairy products, wheat, corn, soy, peanuts, and eggs. There are many accounts in which a skin rash has been alleviated when allergenic foods were eliminated from the diet. Several studies have shown that a gluten-free diet can have remarkable effects on the skin lesions of eczema and psoriasis sufferers. Gluten is a protein found in wheat, rye, barley, and oats. (Rice and corn are gluten-free.)

Use juice-fasting and cleansing diets to rid your body of toxins. Eczema can be a sign that the body isn't eliminating toxins efficiently. One to three days of juice fasting will help cleanse the lymphatic system, which is an important part of treating eczema. The skin, also known as the "third lung," is partially responsible for clearing toxins from the body, but cannot perform this vital function if the lymphatic system is sluggish. The liver is another important elimination organ. When it is overtaxed, it becomes incapable of doing its job correctly, and waste products build up in the bloodstream and lymph. Excess waste contributes to inflammation and thus to outbreaks of eczema (for more information, see the Juice Fast, page 304, and the Liver Cleanse, page 310).

Eat more raw foods. One very large survey study found that people who ate a lot of raw food experienced significant improvement in skin disorders. Increase your intake of raw foods to 60 to 75 percent of your diet.

✳ Nutrient Recommendations

Bioflavonoids help control factors involved in inflammation and allergic reactions. *Best juice sources of bioflavonoids:* bell peppers, berries (blueberries, blackberries, and cranberries), broccoli, cabbage, parsley, and tomatoes.

Digestive enzymes improve digestion and may help decrease eczema's severity. Ness Formula enzymes are the best supplemental enzymes I've found; they are available through some doctors' offices or you can order them (see Sources, page 347). Bitter leafy green vegetables, such as kale, mustard greens, and dandelion greens, also help promote the flow of digestive juices. They can be juiced, mixed with milder-tasting juices (such as carrot and green apple, or lemon). Drink prior to eating.

Essential fatty acids (EFAs) are vital to your skin's health. Researchers stress the importance of eating a diet that is rich in EFAs, which exist in two forms, omega-3 and omega-6 fatty acids, in the treatment of eczema, with omega-3s being the most important. Studies have shown that the breast milk of mothers whose children have eczema is low in EFAs. Cold-water fish such as salmon, trout, tuna, herring, mackerel, halibut, and sardines are rich in omega-3s. They are also plentiful in flaxseeds and hemp seeds, cod-liver oil, and krill oil. (For more information, see the fats and oils section in Basic Guidelines for the Juice Lady's Health and Healing Diet, page 290.)

Folic acid is at a low level in eczema and psoriasis sufferers. *Best juice sources of folic acid:* spinach, kale, beetroot and mustard greens, broccoli, and cabbage.

Probiotics, or "good" bacteria, are live microbial organisms naturally found in the digestive tract. They are thought to suppress the growth of potentially harmful bacteria, improve immune function, and strengthen the digestive tract's protective barrier. A long-term study showed that probiotics were very effective in preventing eczema in infants.

Vitamin A deficiency can cause a thickening of the skin, a condition typically found in eczema. Carotenes, found in fruits and vegetables, are converted in the body to vitamin A as needed. *Best juice sources of carotenes:* carrots, kale, parsley, spinach, Swiss chard, beetroot greens, watercress, broccoli, and romaine lettuce.

Zinc is necessary for the conversion of EFAs into anti-inflammatory substances called prostaglandins. *Best juice sources of zinc:* gingerroot, turnips, parsley, garlic, carrots, spinach, cabbage, lettuce, and cucumbers.

✳ Herb Recommendations

Burdock root, dandelion root, garlic, goldenseal, and **red clover** are all lymph-cleansing herbs. Avoid goldenseal if you are pregnant, and do not use it for more than ten days at a time.

✳ Juice Therapy

Beetroot, cabbage, carrot, celery, cucumber, parsley, and **spinach** juices all help cleanse the lymphatic system and the liver. Cucumber juice can also relieve itching when applied directly to the skin. A combination of carrot juice (ten ounces) and spinach juice (sixteen ounces) has been shown to be beneficial for eczema.

Green juices, such as **wheatgrass, parsley, kale,** and **spinach,** are rich in chlorophyll, which is a blood purifier. These are very helpful in healing eczema.

Parsley juice is rich in beta-carotene and zinc. Intake should be limited to a safe, therapeutic dose of one-half to one cup per day. Parsley can be toxic in overdose, and should be especially avoided by pregnant women.

✳ Juice Recipes

Magnesium-Rich Cocktail *(pg 336)* **Spinach Power** *(pg 341)* **Pure Green Sprout Drink** *(pg 340)* **Wheatgrass Light** *(pg 345)* **Allergy Relief** *(pg 326)* **Afternoon Refresher** *(pg 326)* **Morning Energizer** *(pg 337)* **The Ginger Hopper** *(pg 332)* **Ginger Twist** *(pg 332)* **Triple C** *(pg 344)* **Immune Builder** *(pg 335)* **Jack & the Bean** *(pg 335)* **Liver Life Tonic** *(pg 336)* **Peppy Parsley** *(pg 339)* **Super Green Sprout Drink** *(pg 342)*

Epilepsy and Seizures

SEIZURES involve uncontrolled electrical discharges from nerve cells, called neurons, in the brain, resulting in abnormal synchronization of electrical activity. They can cause loss of consciousness and uncontrolled muscle movements called convulsions, as well as tingling, temporary loss of speech, staring, and inattentiveness. A seizure can also be as subtle as numbness in part of the body, a brief loss of memory, sparkling or flashes, sensing an unpleasant odor, a strange epigastric sensation, or a sensation of fear. The medical syndrome of recurrent, unprovoked seizures is termed epilepsy, but seizures may occur in people who do not have epilepsy. Epilepsy is a disease characterized by recurring seizures in which the brain produces sudden bursts of electrical energy that disrupt other brain functions. Some people have daily attacks, while others have long periods of time, up to a year or two, between episodes. Many children diagnosed with epilepsy outgrow their seizures.

If a seizure affects many different areas of the brain at once, a generalized seizure occurs. This can cause a loss of consciousness and convulsions. If only one small part of the brain is affected, a partial seizure occurs. A partial seizure causes less-dramatic symptoms, the exact nature of which depends on the location of the misfiring neurons. Within both basic categories are many forms of epileptic seizures, each characterized by a specific pattern of symptoms.

Seizures can be triggered by factors such as lack of sleep; alcohol consumption; stress; hormonal changes associated with the menstrual cycle; food sensitivities such as gluten, soy, or dairy; heavy metal toxicity; cell damage by toxins known as free radicals; pesticide poisoning; head injury; drug toxicity; aspartame (NutraSweet); infection such as encephalitis or meningitis; fever leading to convulsions; metabolic disturbances, such as hypoglycemia, hyponatremia or hypoxia; or lesions in the brain (abscesses, tumors) in both epileptics and nonepileptics.

✳ Diet Recommendations

Eat a high-fat, low-carbohydrate diet. Clinical trials have confirmed that a high-fat diet works "better than any other regimen," according to Dr. John Freeman, director of the Pediatric Epilepsy Clinic at the Children's Center in Baltimore, who created the ketogenic diet (KD). One study of 150 children whose seizures were poorly controlled by medication found that about one-quarter of the children had a 90 percent or better decrease in seizures with the KD, and another half of the group experienced a 50 percent or better decrease in their seizures. The MCT diet (medium-chain triglycerides) is currently most recommended, which is a modified ketogenic diet in which more carbohydrates and proteins are used to reduce the problems associated with a high fat intake without sacrificing the benefits of the high-fat diet. Virgin coconut oil is one of the best sources of MCTs available. (For more than seventy delicious recipes using coconut oil, see my book *The Coconut Diet;* also, see Sources for information on virgin organic coconut oil.)

The Low Glycemic Index Treatment (LGIT). It is best to combine the KD (MCT diet) with the LGIT, which was developed in 2002 as an alternative nutritional therapy to the ketogenic diet. (The LGIT focuses on carbohydrates that have a low glycemic index, which means they're low in sugar.) High fiber is important because fiber (unlike processed foods) must be broken down. This slows sugar absorption, thereby avoiding drastic fluctuations in blood sugar. Less-processed foods such as beans, brown rice, and rolled oats are examples of foods that help slow sugar absorption. Multivitamin and mineral supplementation with additional calcium supplementation is required while on the LGIT/KD to reduce the risk of deficiencies.

Choose a gluten-free diet. A significant percentage of epileptic patients are sensitive to a protein called gluten, and avoiding foods that contain it has been beneficial for many people. A 1948 *American Journal of Physiology* article documents seizures in dogs fed wheat gluten, along with blindness, ataxic neurological symptoms, and death. (If you have a pet that's experiencing seizures, buy only gluten-free pet food and doggie treats. Or, better yet, make your own pet food with ground meat, a little brown rice, and vegetables.) Eliminate all gluten-containing foods (including wheat, buckwheat, oats, rye, and barley) from your diet. Instead, you can use rice, rice flour, potatoes, potato flour, corn, cornmeal, and other gluten-free breads and flour products.

Choose organic food. Eating organic food means fewer heavy metals and pesticides, which have been implicated in epilepsy.

Avoid the artificial sweetener aspartame (NutraSweet). The National Cancer Institute shows a significant increase in aspartame-related seizures and malignant brain tumors since 1985, about two years after aspartame was introduced on the market. Critics have been looking at early studies and have come away puzzled as to how the FDA could deduce human "safety" concerning aspartame. One of the studies conducted in 1972, titled *52 Week Oral Toxicity Infant Monkey Study* (SC-18862), gave aspartame to seven infant rhesus monkeys for fifty-two weeks. All medium- and high-dose monkeys showed increased phenylalanine levels in their blood and exhibited brain seizures, starting at about seven months into the experiment. The seizures were of the grand mal type. One monkey, of the high-dose group, died after three hundred days. The cause of death was not determined because the data were lost. Once the aspartame was omitted from the monkeys' diets, the brain seizures ceased. GARD originally stood for the "glutamate/aspartate restricted diet," named after its limitation of these two nonessential amino acids that are the parent compounds of MSG and aspartame (NutraSweet). They are termed "excito-toxins" and are known to be triggers of seizures. Many pilots appear to be particularly susceptible to the effects of aspartame ingestion. They have reported numerous serious toxicity effects, including grand mal seizures in the cockpit. Nearly one thousand cases of pilot reactions have been reported to the Aspartame Consumer Safety Network Pilot Hotline. Foods containing aspartame include diet soft drinks, gum, ice cream, sweetened yogurt, frozen yogurt, cookies, candy, and other dessert items that are labeled "sugar free."

Eliminate vitamin D–fortified milk and milk products. According to Lewis B. Barnett, M.D., head of the Hereford Clinic and Deaf Smith Research Foundation in Hereford, Texas, calciferol (synthetic vitamin D_2), like fluorine, tends to bind magnesium. This substance is added to pasteurized milk, and enhances the likelihood of seizures, because low magnesium levels can contribute to seizures. This synthetic form of vitamin D is ten times more active than the natural form in binding magnesium. For this reason the natural vitamin, as found in fish-liver oils, will not cause magnesium depletion, whereas calciferol does.

Avoid caffeine. Studies show that caffeine may affect seizure frequency, making epilepsy more difficult to control. Foods containing caffeine include coffee and green, white, and black tea, soft drinks, and chocolate. Some medications also contain caffeine.

Juice vegetables. Although the specific underlying cause of epilepsy and seizures is often unknown, research has found that damage caused by free radicals can predispose the brain to seizures. Oxidative stress has been identified as a major factor in epileptic seizures. It appears that the brains of people with epilepsy are under considerable oxidative stress from free radicals. Studies have shown that epileptics are low in many antioxidants, including glutathione, superoxide dismutase, and vitamins E, C, and A. Studies have found that the combination of vitamins E and C protect nerve cell membranes from oxidation in people with post-traumatic seizures. Freshly made vegetable juices are loaded with antioxidants.

✳ Nutrient Recommendations

Amino acids. Epilepsy and seizures can often be improved with magnesium, omega-3 fatty acids (fatty cold-water fish and fish oils), and balancing neurotransmitters with amino acid therapy. A seizure of any kind causes a spilling of a large quantity of neurotransmitters. This can lead to neurotransmitter depletion, ultimately causing a great imbalance in brain chemicals. This is often one of the contributing factors to seizures becoming worse over time—the imbalance becomes greater. Many patients with seizure activity have elevated excitatory or stimulating neurotransmitters and quite low levels of inhibitory or calming neurotransmitters. This imbalance is more likely to allow for seizure activity. Balancing the neurotransmitters can help tremendously in alleviating seizures. B vitamins and varied protein consumption are imperative with this program; include nuts, seeds, beans, eggs, and muscle meats such as fish, chicken, turkey, and beef. (Choose organically fed, free-range/cage-free, and no hormones or antibiotics.) For information on neurotransmitter testing, see Sources, pages 350–352.

Magnesium. According to Dr. Lewis B. Barnett, M.D., head of the Hereford Clinic and Deaf Smith Research Foundation in Hereford, Texas, stunning improvements in epileptic seizures have been observed in his work when patients have been placed on high doses of magnesium gluconate. When magnesium deficiencies occur, epilepsy can be one of the results. Magnesium deficiency can also manifest in hyperirritability. Deficiencies may occur because of a malfunctioning pituitary gland. Also, ingesting fluoride can cause deficiencies because it bonds with magnesium in the blood, forming the insoluble magnesium fluoride. This means that the magnesium cannot be assimilated by the pituitary gland, with the consequent failure of the pituitary gland to function properly, which leads to symptoms of magnesium deficiency. (Fluoride is prevalent in water, toothpaste, and dental treatments.) To get the best results, you should supplement your wellness program with magnesium gluconate. Drink only purified water and use only fluoride-free toothpaste. Avoid all fluoride dental treatments. And include plenty of magnesium-rich juices. *Best juice sources of magnesium:* beetroot greens, spinach, Swiss chard, collard greens, parsley, dandelion greens, garlic, beetroot, and broccoli. Also, include plenty of avocados and raw sunflower seeds.

Manganese is a mineral that has been found in low levels in the blood and hair of epileptics. Those with the lowest levels of manganese typically have the highest number of seizures. *Best juice sources of manganese:* spinach, beetroot greens, Brussels sprouts, carrots, broccoli, cabbage, and beetroot.

Selenium is important in certain enzyme reactions that may play a role in protecting nerve cells from free-radical damage. Selenium deficiency may be an important triggering factor for seizures, and subsequent nerve damage, in people with epilepsy. *Best juice sources of selenium:* Swiss chard, turnips, garlic, radishes, carrots, and cabbage.

Sodium, known to many people as a substance to avoid, can help people who are prone to seizures. Studies have shown that epileptics with the lowest sodium concentrations in their bloodstreams have the highest number of seizures. It's not recommended that you increase your use of table salt (sodium chloride), but rather that you consume more fresh sodium-rich vegetables and juices. (The best salt to use is mineral-rich Celtic sea salt or gray salt.) *Best juice sources of sodium:* Swiss chard, beetroots with greens, celery, spinach, watercress, turnips, carrots, parsley, sunflower sprouts, cabbage, garlic, and broccoli.

The B vitamins are essential for many functions in the central nervous system. Vitamin B_6 and folate are critical cofactors in the production of many neurotransmitters. Of particular relevance in epilepsy, B_6 (pyridoxine) is required to convert the principal excitatory neurotransmitter, glutamate, into the primary inhibitor neurotransmitter, gamma-aminobutyric acid (GABA) in the brain. A reduction in GABA levels increases the chance of seizures. Some doctors have used an intravenous form of this vitamin for a week, followed by supplemental use, to completely control seizures in their patients. *Best juice sources of vitamin B_6:* kale, spinach, turnip greens, and bell peppers. Vitamins B_1, B_3, B_{12}, and carnitine are required for the maintenance of the myelin sheath that surrounds neurons and affects their ability to conduct coherent impulses.

Vitamin E. Researchers at the University of Toronto found that the frequency of seizures was reduced by more than 60 percent in ten of the twelve children taking 400 IU of vitamin E daily for three months. Six of them had a 90 to 100 percent reduction in seizures. By comparison, none of the twelve children who took placebos (inactive substances) along with their medication improved significantly. But when the children who were taking placebos were switched to vitamin E, seizure frequency was reduced by 70 to 100 percent in all of them and there were no adverse side effects. *Best juice sources of vitamin E:* sunflower sprouts, spinach, asparagus, and carrots.

Zinc levels have been shown in studies to be lower in epileptics than in other people. *Best juice sources of zinc:* gingerroot, turnips, parsley, garlic, carrots, spinach, cabbage, lettuce, and cucumbers.

✳ Juice Therapy

Carrot, beetroot, and **cucumber** juice in combination have been found helpful for epilepsy.

✳ Juice Recipes

Allergy Relief *(pg 326)* **Morning Energizer** *(pg 337)* **Spinach Power** *(pg 341)*
The Ginger Hopper *(pg 332)* **Orient Express** *(pg 338)* **Pure Green Sprout Drink** *(pg 340)* **Turnip Time** *(pg 344)* **Wheatgrass Light** *(pg 345)*

Eye Disorders

THE eyes are subject to a number of disorders such as floaters, cataracts, macular degeneration, and other eye diseases like glaucoma and detached retina or myopia. They are caused by weakness and inflammation in the tissues that compose and surround the eyes. Many eye disorders are caused by toxins known as free radicals.

Floaters are small clumps of gel that form in the vitreous and appear as spots, threads, or fragments of cobwebs, which float slowly before the eyes. Although they appear to be in front of the eyes, they are actually floating in the vitreous and are seen as shadows by the retina.

A cataract is a loss of transparency or a clouding of the eye's lens. This clouding is often caused by free-radical damage to some of the proteins and fats in the lens, damage that causes white spots to develop. When this happens, the lens cannot transmit light to the retina at the back of the eyeball, a situation that causes progressively blurred vision. Cataracts can result from eye diseases, surgery, or injury; systemic diseases; or exposure to ultraviolet light, radiation, or toxins, and, along with macular degeneration, are the primary causes of blindness and visual impairment in people over fifty-five. Diabetics run an increased risk of cataract development. Cataracts affect about 50 percent of all Americans over age seventy-five.

Like cataracts, age-related macular degeneration (AMD) occurs more often in older people. This disorder is marked by damage to a spot called the macula, which lies at the center of the retina. In dry macular degeneration, damage is caused by pigment deposits. In wet macular degeneration, the leakage of blood or other fluid causes scarring in the macula. Symptoms include dim or distorted vision, especially while reading, with a gradual loss of precise central vision and blank spots in the field of central vision. Systemic disease and toxin exposure contribute to macular degeneration.

✳ Lifestyle Recommendations

Stop smoking. Tobacco contains significant amounts of cadmium, and high amounts of cadmium in the eye lens have been linked with both cataracts and macular degeneration. Cigarette smoke is also loaded with free radicals and aldehydes, which attack proteins and fats in the eyes.

Detox your body. Pectin (soluble fiber, high in apples) may help remove unwanted metals and toxins from the eyes, and L-methionine has the ability to chelate toxic metals, all of which may be important in the treatment of floaters, as well as cataracts and AMD.

On a personal note: I had floaters for what seems to have been most of my life. Today, they are gone. I noticed that they had disappeared after a series of detoxes, an increase in drinking fresh vegetable juices, and incorporating the amino acid program. (For more information on the amino acid program, see Sources, page 350).

✳ Diet Recommendations

Eat more fruits and vegetables, especially spinach and other dark leafy greens, and drink fresh vegetable juices. Studies show that people who ate spinach and other dark greens five or more times per week reduced their risk of developing cataracts by between 47 and 65 percent (see the recipe for Awesome Green Smoothie, page 327). Dark greens are rich in carotenoids, specifically lutein and zeaxanthin, substances that are important antioxidants. In addition, tomatoes are associated with lower risk of cataracts; they're also rich in carotenes (see "Antioxidants," below).

Avoid sweets and refined carbohydrates. Sugars promote osmotic pressure (swelling of the lens), and increase the risk of free-radical damage. In a fourteen-year study of women sponsored by the USDA Human Nutrition Research Center it was found that those women who consumed the highest amount of simple carbohydrates were 2.5 times more likely to develop cataracts than those whose intakes were the lowest.

✳ Nutrient Recommendations

Antioxidants. Research indicates that a diet rich in antioxidants can help prevent and, in some cases, partially reverse (or correct) eye disorders. Antioxidants protect the eyes from oxidative damage. Research shows that vitamins C and E, lutein and zeaxanthin (carotenoids), beta-carotene, and zinc are all vital for eye health. Carotenes, in particular, destroy free radicals, which helps prevent and treat retinal disorders. One study showed that supplementation with vitamin A and carotenes can halt or reverse blindness in children with vitamin A deficiency. Another study found that the subjects who consumed the most vitamin C, vitamin E, beta-carotene, lutein, zeaxanthin (all antioxidants), and folate had the lowest incidence of cataracts. Curcumins are phytonutrients that help protect the eye lens from degeneration. They are available in supplement form, and are present in both gingerroot and turmeric. There's a definite link between these nutrients and proper vision. *Best juice sources of carotenes:* carrots, kale, parsley, spinach, Swiss chard, beetroot greens, watercress, broccoli, and romaine lettuce.

On a personal note: I received a letter several years ago from a lady who said she had been declared legally blind. When she started juicing and following the dietary program from my juice book, her vision was restored to normal.

Glutathione is a protein that plays an important role in protecting cells against free-radical damage. It has been shown to help prevent cataract formation. *Best juice sources of glutathione:* asparagus, broccoli, and tomatoes.

Omega-3 fatty acids. Omega-3 fatty acids may protect our eyes from the development and progression of retinopathy, a deterioration of the retina. A mice study published in the journal *Nature Medicine* supports increasing the ratio of omega-3 to omega-6 fatty acids with the finding that omega-6 fatty acid over-consumption is associated with an increased risk of retinopathy. *Best sources of omega-3s:* fish oil, flaxseeds, hemp seeds, and fatty cold-water fish.

Quercetin, a bioflavonoid, can help prevent diabetic cataracts by decreasing the accumulation of sorbitol (a sugar alcohol formed from glucose), which is toxic in the lens. *Best juice sources of quercetin:* berries and parsley.

Selenium can, when taken in supplement form, restore the cellular activity of glutathione. Studies have shown that a large number of people with cataracts have low levels of selenium. *Best juice sources of selenium:* Swiss chard, turnips, garlic, radishes, carrots, and cabbage.

Vitamin C can slow the development of both cataracts and macular degeneration. The Nurses Health Study, conducted through Tufts University, found that those nurses who supplemented their diet with vitamin C for at least ten years had the lowest prevalence of cataracts. *Best juice sources of vitamin C:* kale, parsley, broccoli, Brussels sprouts, watercress, cauliflower, cabbage, spinach, turnips, and asparagus.

Vitamin E helps prevent both cataracts and macular degeneration. It is also helpful in halting and reversing the progress of these conditions. *Best juice sources of vitamin E:* spinach, watercress, asparagus, carrots, and tomatoes.

✳ Juice Therapy

Apple juice may help remove unwanted metals and toxins from the eyes.

Blueberry juice helps improve eyesight.

Carrot juice is very helpful for strengthening the eyes and improving vision.

✳ Juice Recipes

Beet-Cucumber Cleansing Cocktail *(pg 328)*   **Happy Morning** *(pg 333)*
Icy Spicy Tomato *(pg 335)*   **Orient Express** *(pg 338)*   **Tomato Florentine** *(pg 343)*
Morning Energizer *(pg 337)*   **The Ginger Hopper** *(pg 332)*   **Turnip Time** *(pg 344)*

Fibrocystic Breast Disease

Fibrocystic breast disease (FBD) is a benign cystic condition of the breasts that is fairly common, affecting at least 20 percent of women of reproductive age. FBD is thought to be associated with hormonal activity, primarily estrogen, and is thought to be caused by poor hormonal metabolism.

The lumps that characterize FBD can be either firm or soft, and move freely beneath the skin. These lumps form when fibrous tissue surrounds cysts and thickens like scar tissue, which causes pain. There is rapid fluctuation in the size of the masses at different times in a woman's hormonal cycle, with tenderness and lumpiness often increasing during the premenstrual phase. Symptoms vary in severity, ranging from mild discomfort to severe pain.

FBD is usually caused by a hormonal imbalance. High estrogen levels can cause excess breast tissue growth, especially if the body doesn't produce enough progesterone, a hormone that limits estrogen's activity. Excess dietary estrogens have been implicated in FBD. Women who eat meat have estrogen levels that are 50 percent higher than those found in vegetarian women. While all animal protein contains some estrogen, this problem is intensified when cows, pigs, sheep, chickens, and turkeys are fed hormone growth stimulants, as this causes estrogens to be passed on to people when the meat and dairy are ingested. A diet that reduces estrogen levels can help ease the pain and discomfort of FBD. Iodine deficiency and abnormal breast milk production have also been linked to FBD. You should note that while most breast lumps are benign, all such lumps should be brought to a doctor's attention.

✳ Lifestyle Recommendations

Progesterone. Women who have low progesterone may benefit from natural progesterone. However, if FBD is due to too much estrogen, it is not corrected by adding progesterone. This is a common therapeutic mistake. When estrogen is too high, supplementing progesterone does not lower estrogen. It may temporarily mask the problem and help only minimally, or do nothing but increase the hormonal load on the body. It will not restore hormonal balance in this case. Pathologies and liver burden will progress. An alternative approach would be to forgo the progesterone and reduce the estrogen, improve hormonal metabolism by improving liver function, improve lymphatic drainage, and optimize local circulation by massaging the breast. (An excellent way to improve lymphatic action is the Lymphasizer, a gentle-motion exercise machine that you use by lying on the floor with your feet in grooves. The machine moves your body like a fish swims in water. It improves the lymphatics as well as organ function [see Sources, page 348]). Improve liver function with the Liver Cleanse, page 310.

What about taking prescription medication? Some medical doctors say that taking a drug (usually a testosterone analog) to suppress excess estrogen may offer worse side effects than the disease. Besides being expensive, there are unwanted side effects, and many of them are masculinizing: hair growth on the face and body, male pattern baldness, and lower pitch to the voice, along with acne, seborrhea, vaginal dryness, and sagging smaller breasts. You can read more on this subject at www.fibrocystic.com.

✳ Diet Recommendations

Reduce meat consumption. In the United States and Canada, ranchers routinely give synthetic estrogen to their cattle and farmers give it to their chickens. As a result, the cattle and chickens bloat and retain water, and the estrogen-laden meat is heavier and especially tender, while fat builds up and marbles through the meat. This means the ranchers and farmers can get more money for their cattle and chickens because the meat weighs more and is extra tender. The European Union has banned Canadian and United States beef from being imported, citing worries about increasing the rate of breast cancer in Europe. Purchase only organically grown, without antibiotics or hormones, free-range or cage-free meat, chicken, and turkey, and eat only small portions of these foods occasionally until the FBD is controlled. The idea is to exclude dietary animal estrogens from your diet.

Eat mainly vegetables and legumes (beans, lentils, split peas). A high-complex-carbohydrate, whole-foods diet is the best choice. This diet should be mostly vegetarian, except for fish and occasional free-range/cage-free meat or poultry dishes. In addition, a diet that consists of whole grains, vegetables, fruit, and legumes has been shown to decrease symptoms of premenstrual breast tenderness and swelling (see Menstrual Disorders, page 211). Studies have shown that women who maintain a vegetarian diet are actually able to excrete two to three times more estrogen than omnivorous women. This could, in part, explain why studies show that vegetarian women have a lower incidence of breast cancer. The fiber in such a diet is beneficial because fiber decreases the time it takes food to move through the colon. The longer waste stays in the intestinal tract, the more estrogen is reabsorbed into the bloodstream. You can obtain plenty of fiber from legumes (beans, peas, and lentils); vegetables such as Brussels sprouts, broccoli, and carrots; raw fruits such as apples, oranges, and pears; and grains, particularly bran and oats. Fresh vegetable juice has soluble fiber. Additional fiber may be obtained from dietary supplements in the form of powders such as apple pectin powder or fiber capsules. (For more information, see Basic Guidelines for the Juice Lady's Health and Healing Diet, page 290.)

Drink freshly made juice. A diet rich in fruits and vegetables benefits women with FBD. Phytochemicals present in fruits and vegetables assist enzymes in the body in detoxifying harmful compounds. Freshly made vegetable juice helps you easily increase your intake of vegetables.

Detox the body. Scientists now believe that intake of too many xenoestrogens ("xeno" means foreign) that come from the myriad of synthetic estrogens or chemicals that mimic estrogen in our environment can cause fibrocystic breast disease, breast cancer, and endometrial cancer. These chemicals that affect the hormonal systems of the human body occur at one hundred to one thousand times greater concentration than that of normal human hormones. Research has demonstrated that two weak xenoestrogens may act synergistically to give a strong "estrogen" response. Some xenoestrogens like DDE (a metabolite of DDT) may persist in the body fat for decades. Many of these mimicking hormones were once thought to occur only in pesticides. Now, however, many of the newly discovered xenoestrogens are found in everyday materials once thought to be inert substances. This means that periodic detoxes are of the utmost importance in the care and treatment of FBD (see the cleanse programs on pages 303–325).

Cleanse the liver. Liver congestion can lead to the development of fibrocystic breasts. It's the liver's job to metabolize hormones. The liver removes active estrogens from circulation, conjugating them and releasing them to the gastrointestinal tract for elimination. When the liver is inundated with too much work, such as processing numerous hormones; emulsifying fats and cholesterol; and removing toxins, pesticides, drugs, alcohol, and other substances from the blood, it may have a difficult job metabolizing estrogens. When the bowels are constipated or when there are undesirable bacterial flora present such as an overgrowth of *Candida albicans,* estrogens that have been conjugated (joined with other substances) in the liver for elimination are unconjugated (broken apart) in the intestine, reabsorbed, and returned to the liver a second and even third time, adding to the liver's workload.

Avoid methylxanthines, which occur in coffee (both caffeinated and decaffeinated), cola, root beer, chocolate, and black tea. They will aggravate fibrocystic disease. Caffeine is known to stimulate overproduction of fibrous tissue and cyst fluid.

✳ Nutrient Recommendations

Iodine is required for production of thyroid hormones. There is an association between low thyroid function and FBD. Iodine is especially abundant in seafood, including fish, and sea vegetables such as nori and hijiki. *Best juice sources of iodine:* lettuce, spinach, and green bell peppers.

Vitamin A has helped reduce breast pain and decrease breast cysts in some women. The body can convert beta-carotene, found in fruits and vegetables, to vitamin A. *Best juice sources of beta-carotene:* carrots, kale, parsley, spinach, Swiss chard, beetroot greens, watercress, broccoli, and romaine lettuce.

Vitamin B complex. In 1942, a researcher found that B vitamin deficiency hindered the liver's ability to metabolize estrogen levels in both animal and human test subjects. Adding B vitamin supplementation can help to decrease the severity of PMS, heavy menstrual bleeding, and fibrocystic breast disease.

Vitamin E can ease inflammation, neutralize free radicals, and stabilize hormone levels. *Best juice sources of vitamin E:* spinach, watercress, asparagus, carrots, and tomatoes.

✳ Herb Recommendations

Gotu kola has been used naturopathically to treat FBD. **Vitex agnus castus,** also known as chaste tree fruit, has been shown to normalize hormone levels.

✳ Juice Therapy

Asparagus, cantaloupe (with seeds), **cucumber, lemon, parsley,** and **watermelon** juices are natural diuretics, or substances that remove excess water from the body.

Beetroot juice is a good liver cleanser, as is the juice of **artichoke leaf.**

Parsley juice is a rich source of beta-carotene. Intake should be limited to a safe, therapeutic dose of one-half to one cup per day. Parsley can be toxic in overdose, and should be especially avoided by pregnant women.

✳ Juice Recipes

Morning Energizer *(pg 337)*   **Afternoon Refresher** *(pg 326)*   **Natural Diuretic Cocktail** *(pg 338)*   **Magnesium-Rich Cocktail** *(pg 336)*   **Calcium-Rich Cocktail** *(pg 329)*   **Spinach Power** *(pg 341)*   **Beet-Cucumber Cleansing Cocktail** *(pg 328)* **Colon Cleanser** *(pg 330)*   **Gallbladder-Liver Cleansing Cocktail** *(pg 331)*   **Liver Life Tonic** *(pg 336)*   **Peppy Parsley** *(pg 339)*   **The Revitalizer** *(pg 340)*

Fibromyalgia Syndrome

FIBROMYALGIA Syndrome (FMS) is an autoimmune disorder that affects 10 to 20 million people in the United States and Canada. FMS patients have eleven out of the sixteen tender or trigger points in four quadrants, which results in widespread pain. FMS is a chronic neurotransmitter disorder of the central nervous system. Other common symptoms include fatigue, morning stiffness, sleep disturbances, anxiety, depression, and cognitive dysfunction (fibro-fog!), to name a few. There are distinct changes in brain chemistry, such as decreased amounts of serotonin and increased levels of P-substance.

Symptoms of FMS can be triggered or aggravated by a number of conditions, including overwork, depression, or anxiety, and fluctuations in temperature or humidity levels.

The cause of fibromyalgia is unknown, and there are no simple answers to conditions such as FMS. Causes lie in a mix of factors, including nutritional deficiencies; toxicities; bowel dysbiosis (unbalanced microbial colony in the gut);

inadequate stress-coping abilities; sensitivities and allergies; inappropriate or excessive medication; inadequate blood-sugar control; hormonal imbalances; poor posture; breathing dysfunction; current or past viral, parasitic, yeast, or bacterial infections; impaired organs of digestion and elimination; and emotional distress. There are certainly no magic bullets that can remedy the situation, which may have taken many years to evolve. It's imperative to address the underlying causes; otherwise treatments will succeed only in masking or moderating symptoms. Good nutrition is imperative in fighting any disease, but especially if you are dealing with a condition as difficult to treat as FMS.

Making the dietary changes suggested below can help you recover. The health care required to restore immunity and reverse FMS begins at home with diet and lifestyle changes; not with a magic pill, but by eliminating factors that impair health and by giving the body the best chance possible to heal.

✳ Diet Recommendations

Eliminate sugar and white-flour products. Correction of this condition may lie as much in what you avoid eating as in what you consume. Completely avoid simple carbohydrates (sugar and white flour). It has been found that a significant percentage of FMS patients have hypoglycemia, or low blood sugar (see Hypoglycemia, page 180), and do not tolerate carbohydrates well. You should eliminate all sweets, such as cakes, pies, frozen yogurt, candy, cookies, and ice cream; all fruit juice (it's too high in fruit sugars) with the exception of lemon, lime, grapefruit, cranberry, and green apple; and all refined-flour (white-flour) products, such as bread, rolls, pizza, and pasta. Limit fruit intake to no more than one or two servings per day because of the sugar.

Avoid alcohol and caffeine; alcohol blocks proper glucose (blood-sugar) usage, and caffeine alters glucose levels.

Eat a whole-foods diet. Increase vegetable and protein servings, and choose only whole-grain products. (For more information on healthy eating, see Basic Guidelines for the Juice Lady's Health and Healing Diet, page 290.)

Detox the body. There appears to be a complex role of toxic exposures in chronic illnesses such as FMS, chronic fatigue syndrome (CFS), and Gulf War Illnesses (GWI). They are characterized by similar symptoms, suggesting that there may be some overlap in the underlying causes, with toxicity being the focus. Autoimmune diseases such as FMS have been linked to vaccines as one source of toxicity along with a host of environmental toxins, additives, and contaminants in our food, air, and water; pesticides; and industrial chemicals. The organs of elimination get overwhelmed trying to deal with all this toxicity, and it builds up throughout the body, causing pain and making us sick. It is interesting to note that in Chinese medicine, shoulder and neck pain are connected to gallbladder congestion. (see the Gallbladder Cleanse, page 318). Detoxification of the organs of elimination is quite helpful for FMS recovery (see pages 303–325).

Juice plenty of vegetables. Juicing vegetables, short juice fasts, and detoxing the body, especially the colon, liver, and gallbladder, will help you make huge strides toward recovery. Vegetable juices can help tremendously in healing aching muscles and sore joints. I suggest two to three glasses of vegetable juice per day. Omit fruit from all juice recipes, except for lemon, lime, and green apple (unless citrus causes joint pain for you; then omit lemon and lime). Also, a short vegetable-juice fast of one to three days can be very healing (see the Juice Fast, page 304). You could benefit by spending a week at a raw foods and juicing detox center to kick off your cleansing, rejuvenating lifestyle (see Sources, page 347, for recommendations).

Make 60 to 75 percent of your diet raw food. Several studies have shown that a diet consisting primarily of raw fruits, vegetables, green salads, carrot and other vegetable juices (two to three glasses per day), nuts, seeds, and dehydrated foods over a two- to three-month period with some cooked food at dinner produced significant improvements in pain, flexibility, joint stiffness, and quality of sleep. Those who were overweight experienced a significant reduction in weight.

✳ Nutrient Recommendations

Amino acids can help balance neurotransmitters, which are the natural chemicals that facilitate communication between brain cells. Pain is a very significant part of fibromyalgia, and it uses up the neurotransmitters serotonin and dopamine. Dopamine, the feel-good neurotransmitter, is made from dl-phenylalanine. Dl-phenylalanine will make dopamine at a little slower rate than l-tyrosine, but the benefit is that it reduces the breakdown of endorphins—those natural pain relievers. Anxiety is also often a problem in fibromyalgia since serotonin levels have been utilized quickly due to pain. In many studies 5-HTP has been used successfully to balance serotonin and has helped people with FMS and CFS.

When neurotransmitters are balanced, you'll be able to sleep well again. Getting a good night's sleep, which means seven to nine hours of deep, restful sleep for most people, is a key to your recovery (see Insomnia, page 202, for more information).

Glutamate is often a causal factor in excessive pain as well as migraine headaches. This is a good reason to avoid monosodium glutamate (MSG) and to read labels because it's added to many packaged foods (see Migraine Headaches, page 216, for a list of products containing MSG). The drug Topamax reduces excessive glutamate excretion. Taurine, however, does the same thing; it will reduce glutamate and norepinephrine in cases where it is elevated.

B vitamins are among the necessary nutrients for the creation and transport of L-tryptophan and 5-HTP into serotonin. They should be taken as part of the complete brain-wellness plan. Also, omega-3 fatty acids and varied protein consumption are imperative as well. For information on neurotransmitter testing and the amino acid program, see Sources, page 350.

Magnesium levels in fibromyalgia patients have been found to be significantly lower than in other people. Also, enzymes that depend on vitamin B require an adequate supply of magnesium. *Best source of supplemental magnesium:* magnesium glycinate. *Best juice sources of magnesium:* beetroot greens, spinach, parsley, dandelion greens, garlic, beetroot, broccoli, cauliflower, carrots, and celery.

Malic acid is a fruit acid extracted from apples. In recent years, evidence has suggested that fibromyalgia pain is the result of local hypoxia (oxygen deficiency) to the muscles. For instance, patients with fibromyalgia have low muscle-tissue oxygen pressure in affected muscles. Malic acid appears to reverse hypoxia's inhibition of glycolysis (carbohydrate breakdown) and energy production, possibly improving energy production and reversing the negative effect of the hypoxia. While studies also used magnesium supplements, due to the fact that magnesium is often low in fibromyalgia patients, the rapid improvement following malic acid treatment, as well as the rapid deterioration after discontinuation, suggests that malic acid is the most important component. Recommended dosage is 1,200 mg twice a day.

SAMe (S-adenosylmethionine) is an amino acid that has been studied regarding treatment of fibromyalgia. A couple of preliminary studies suggest that SAMe may help. A small double-blind study evaluated the effect of SAMe or placebo in seventeen people with fibromyalgia, eleven of whom also had depression. The number of tender points decreased after taking SAMe but not placebo, and depression, as assessed by two rating scales, improved.

In another double-blind study, forty-four people with fibromyalgia took 800 mg of SAMe a day or placebo. After six weeks, there were statistically significant improvements in pain, fatigue, morning stiffness, mood, and activity. However, tender point score, muscle strength, and mood (evaluated by the Beck Depression Inventory) were not significantly better with SAMe than placebo.

Vitamin B$_1$ (thiamine) has helped a number of fibromyalgia sufferers, according to investigative reports. *Best food sources of vitamin B$_1$:* seeds, nuts, beans, split peas, millet, buckwheat, whole wheat, oatmeal, wild rice, lobster, and cornmeal. It can also be found, in lesser quantities, in sunflower and buckwheat sprouts, and garlic. It is not found in fruits and vegetables.

✴ Juice Therapy

Apple and **cranberry** juice are excellent sources of malic acid.

Fennel juice has been used as a traditional tonic to help release endorphins into the bloodstream. Endorphins create a mood of euphoria, and help dampen anxiety and fear.

Garlic juice offers a healthy amount of vitamin B$_1$, and has antibiotic properties.

Parsley juice is rich in magnesium. Intake should be limited to a safe, therapeutic dose of one-half to one cup per day. Parsley can be toxic in overdose, and should be especially avoided by pregnant women.

Sprout juice provides the most concentrated natural source of vitamins, minerals, enzymes, and amino acids. Sprouts are considered by many to be one of nature's most perfect healing foods.

Wheatgrass juice has been proven over many years to benefit people by cleansing the lymph system, building the blood, restoring balance in the body, removing toxic metals from the cells, nourishing the liver and kidneys, and restoring vitality.

✳ Juice Recipes

Mood Mender *(pg 337)* **Turnip Time** *(pg 344)* **Pure Green Sprout Drink** *(pg 340)* **Magnesium-Rich Cocktail** *(pg 336)* **Peppy Parsley** *(pg 342)* **Morning Energizer** *(pg 337)* **Afternoon Refresher** *(pg 326)* **Tomato Florentine** *(pg 343)* **Icy Spicy Tomato** *(pg 335)* **Thyroid Tonic** *(pg 343)* **Wheatgrass Light** *(pg 345)*

Gallstones and Liver–Gallbladder Congestion

LOCATED DIRECTLY UNDER THE LIVER, the gallbladder is a small, pear-shaped sac that functions as a reservoir for bile (created by the liver), which the body uses to digest fats. The gallbladder is connected to the liver and intestines by tiny ducts, called bile ducts. Hard accumulations called gallstones can form in the gallbladder, liver, and bile ducts.

Because of the introduction of chemicals and preservatives into our food, pesticide spraying, large amounts of caffeine, phosphoric acid, refined and artificial sweeteners in desserts, snack foods, soft drinks, drugs (legal and illegal) and alcohol, the demand on the liver to detoxify the body has greatly increased. This contributes to liver and gallbladder congestion. When the liver is constantly stagnant, sediment often settles out of the bile and forms accumulations that resemble stones, sand, or mud.

Generally stones form when cholesterol combines with bile salts and bilirubin (a reddish yellow pigment). If the bile contains too much of any one of these substances, under certain conditions it can harden into stones and accumulate in the gallbladder and liver. Over time, the number of stones, sand, or mud increases, taking up significant space in the gallbladder and liver. When this happens, there is very little space to store new bile in the gallbladder. Since the body needs bile to help it digest fat and absorb nutrients like vitamins and minerals, gallbladder congestion results in malabsorption (poor absorption of nutrients) and poor digestion, along with a host of other symptoms. Obesity is associated with gallstones, as is rapid weight loss caused by a very-low-calorie diet.

If a stone blocks a bile duct, it usually produces nausea, vomiting, and severe pain that may last for several hours. These symptoms often appear after a high-fat meal. If the gallbladder becomes inflamed, there is severe pain in the upper right

Symptoms of gallstone congestion

- Neck and back pain
- Pain or tenderness under the rib cage on the right side
- Pain between the shoulder blades
- Light or chalky-colored stools
- Indigestion after eating (heartburn), especially fatty or greasy foods
- Bitter fluid reflux after eating
- Nausea
- Dizziness
- Bloating
- Gas
- Burping or belching
- Feeling of fullness or poor food digestion
- Diarrhea (or alternating from soft to watery stools)
- Loss of libido
- Constipation—frequent need for laxatives
- Headache over eyes, especially the right eye

abdomen, accompanied by nausea, vomiting, and fever. (This condition must be treated immediately, or it can become life-threatening. Call your doctor or go to the emergency room at the nearest hospital.)

✳ Diet Recommendations

Follow the gallbladder cleansing diet. A considerable amount of research suggests that a fiber-depleted, refined-foods diet contributes to gallstone development. Make 50 to 75 percent of your diet raw food, such as fruits, vegetables, sprouts, juices, nuts, and seeds. Include plenty of dark leafy green salads, beetroot, apples, whole grains, and extra-virgin olive oil. You can have fish and a moderate number of organic eggs, but omit other animal products.

At least one week before a liver/gallbladder flush, the diet should be vegan (no animal foods) with emphasis on raw and lightly cooked vegetables, seeds, nuts, sprouts, vegetable juices, and a moderate amount of fresh fruit. Eat more pears since they have a specific healing effect on the gallbladder. A tablespoon of extra-virgin olive oil should be taken twice a day. Olive oil serves as a stimulant for the production of bile and lipase, a fat-digesting enzyme. High-quality extra-virgin olive oil also helps prevent gallstone formation.

Avoid high-fat foods: red meat; fried foods; butter; commercial oils including soy, corn, safflower, sunflower, and canola; margarine; and spicy foods. Use only extra-virgin olive oil or virgin coconut oil. Gallbladder-cleansing foods include pears, parsnips, seaweed, lemons, limes, and turmeric. Radishes are known to remove stones. For twenty-one days eat one to two radishes a day between meals, and drink three cups of cleavers tea or five cups of chamomile tea a day.

Drink fresh juices. Drink plenty of fresh juice: apple, pear, beetroot, carrot, purple cabbage, dark leafy greens, gingerroot, and lemon juices are all very good. These juices help cleanse the liver and colon, which improves gallbladder function.

Detox the gallbladder and liver. We all need to maintain our gallbladder and liver (along with all other organs) just as we maintain our car. And just as we can't drive our cars continually without maintenance and not expect a breakdown, so we can't push our bodies year after year without maintenance of our organs of elimination without experiencing problems. You can develop gallstones in the liver as well as the gallbladder. Gallstones in the liver are a major impediment to maintaining good health, youthfulness, and vitality and a big reason why people become ill and have difficulty getting well. In Chinese medicine it is well known that neck, shoulder, and back problems are often the direct result of inadequate bile flow and liver congestion. Low bile flow is also a contributor to joint pain because the synovial fluid around the joints will decrease, sometimes causing terrible pain. Liver congestion and stagnation are contributors to many of the most common health problems, yet conventional medicine has no way to diagnose them. Blood tests are not helpful because liver enzyme levels are elevated only when there is advanced liver cell destruction, as in hepatitis.

The gallbladder flush can help dissolve and purge stones, sand, or mud from the gallbladder and liver. A detoxification plan for the liver and colon will also support the gallbladder, and the Kidney Cleanse helps support the liver. Follow the Gallbladder, Liver, Kidney, and Intestinal Cleanses (pages 307–325).

Avoid all sweets and refined-flour products. Studies show that sugar consumption is higher among people with gallstones. Sugar may influence gallstone composition. Eliminate all sweets, including chocolate, cake, candy, cookies, pie, ice cream, frozen yogurt, and soft drinks. Also avoid refined-flour products, including bread, rolls, pizza, and pasta. Choose only whole-grain products, including whole-grain pasta (available at health food stores).

Avoid alcohol—its connection to liver damage and congestion is well known. "Drink even one beer and take a look at a slice of your liver under a microscope; you'll see death to liver cells," says Sandra McClanahan, M.D. Alcohol is absorbed into the bloodstream from the stomach and intestines, and must first go through the liver before circulating around the whole body. So, the highest concentration of alcohol is in the blood flowing through the liver. As little as one ounce of alcohol can damage the liver, resulting in fatty deposits. As the liver breaks down alcohol, by-products are formed, such as acetaldehyde and free radicals (toxic molecules that damage cells), and some of them are more toxic and injurious to the body than alcohol itself, even when nutrition is adequate. The damage caused by free radicals can include the destruction of essential components of cell membranes. Alcohol also depletes a store of liver peptides called GHS, which helps us detoxify chemicals.

Prevent constipation. Studies show that transit time (the time it takes food to move through the intestinal tract) is much slower among women with gallstones, and could be a contributing factor to gallstone formation (see Constipation, page 114). Consider the Intestinal Cleanse (see page 307).

✳ Nutrient Recommendations

Vitamin C can help prevent gallstone formation. It's needed to convert cholesterol to bile acids. Women who have higher blood levels of vitamin C have a reduced risk of gallstones. Studies show that ascorbic acid–deficient guinea pigs frequently develop gallstones, and ascorbic acid may also reduce the risk of gallbladder disease in humans. Among women, increase in serum ascorbic-acid level has been independently associated with a 13 percent lower prevalence of gallbladder disease and gallstones. Some in the medical profession believe that vitamin C can cause gallstones, but there does not appear to be any evidence to support this; rather, it's the opposite. *Best juice sources of vitamin C:* kale, parsley, broccoli, Brussels sprouts, watercress, cauliflower, cabbage, strawberries, spinach, lemons, limes, turnips, and asparagus.

✳ Herb Recommendations

Milk thistle (silymarin) has been used in traditional medicine to cleanse and support the liver. (see Sources for recommendations.)

✳ Juice Therapy

Apple and **spinach** juices are helpful in preventing constipation, and are good for the colon and gallbladder.

Beetroot, celery, dandelion, and **lemon** juices have been used to cleanse and support the liver.

Carrot, beetroot, and **cucumber** juices are traditional remedies to cleanse the gallbladder.

Daikon radish juice is used in Chinese medicine to help eliminate excess fat from the body.

Jerusalem artichoke juice helps support the liver and pancreas, and helps normalize blood-sugar levels.

Purple cabbage, carrot, beetroot with leaves, lemon, apple, and **gingerroot** juice is a helpful combination for the liver and gallbladder.

Pear juice helps prevent constipation, and is good for the gallbladder.

Tomato juice, with a pinch of cayenne or a dash of hot sauce, can provide energy and help revitalize the liver and adrenal glands.

✳ Juice Recipes

Colon Cleanser *(pg 330)*   **Beet-Cucumber Cleansing Cocktail** *(pg 328)*   **Natural Diuretic Cocktail** *(pg 338)*   **Peppy Parsley** *(pg 339)*   **Morning Energizer** *(pg 337)*   **Liver Life Tonic** *(pg 336)*   **Gallbladder-Liver Cleansing Cocktail** *(pg 331)*   **The Revitalizer** *(pg 340)*   **Orient Express** *(pg 338)*   **The Ginger Hopper** *(pg 332)*   **Magnesium-Rich Cocktail** *(pg 336)*   **Pure Green Sprout Drink** *(pg 340)*   **Salsa in a Glass** *(pg 340)*   **Icy Spicy Tomato** *(pg 335)*

Gout

Gout is one of the most painful forms of arthritis. It occurs when too much uric acid builds up in the body. The body produces excess uric acid and/or is unable to eliminate it. Excess uric acid crystallizes in the joints and other tissues and can lead to:

- Sharp uric acid crystal deposits in joints, often in the big toe
- Deposits of uric acid (called tophi) that look like lumps under the skin
- Kidney stones from uric acid crystals

For many people, the first attack of gout occurs in the big toe (also the ankle or heel). Attacks often occur during the night after a person overeats and drinks such purine-rich foods as meat, poultry, fish, alcohol, fried foods, and rich desserts. (Because this type of diet was beyond the means of most people until the middle of the twentieth century, gout is sometimes called "the rich man's disease.") Often, the attack wakes a person from sleep; the toe is very sore, red, warm, and swollen. As the disease progresses, more joints can be affected, attacks can last for longer periods of time, and deformities can develop. There is also a higher risk of kidney dysfunction and kidney stones.

✴ Diet Recommendations

Increase vegetables, fruit, and vegetable juice. Eat plenty of raw fruits and vegetables. Raw fruits, vegetables, and juices should make up at least 50 percent of your diet. A large portion of your diet should consist of vegetables and whole grains, such as brown rice, millet, barley, and buckwheat. Popcorn lightly salted (without added butter or oil) makes a good snack.

Avoid foods rich in purines. Purines are components of alcohol and certain foods such as animal products that metabolize into uric acid in the body. A study published in *The New England Journal of Medicine* (2004) found that people who ate the most meat were 40 percent more likely to have gout and those who ate the most purine-rich fish and seafood were 50 percent more likely to have gout than those who ate the least.

Foods high in purines include:

- hearts
- herring
- mussels
- yeast
- smelt
- sardines
- sweetbreads
- anchovies

- grouse
- mutton
- veal
- bacon
- liver
- salmon
- turkey
- kidneys

- partridge
- trout
- goose
- haddock
- pheasant
- scallops

Note: Some vegetables, though high in purines, have not been found to cause gout. They include peas, beans, mushrooms, cauliflower, and spinach.

Avoid rich foods such as gravy, consommé, concentrated sweets, pastries, cakes, and pies. And avoid all white-flour products and sugar. Restrict animal fat consumption; it's believed to reduce the normal excretion of uric acid.

Avoid all alcohol, especially beer. Ethanol increases the production of uric acid. Studies of gout sufferers show that many patients consume above-average amounts of alcohol.

Eat cherries. One-half pound of cherries (fresh or frozen) each day for two weeks has been shown to prevent attacks. Or drink fresh cherry juice—eight to sixteen ounces per day. You may prefer to use black cherry juice concentrate and mix it with water or take cherry fruit extract as a pill (1,000 mg three times per day during an attack; 1,000 mg per day to prevent attacks). Cherries and other dark red berries (hawthorn berries) contain anthocyanins that increase collagen integrity and decrease inflammation. Studies show that people with gout who consumed the cherry diet daily had no attacks of gout, and their blood levels of uric acid were reduced to normal. A number of patients reported greater freedom of movement in finger and toe joints. Dark purple-red, yellow, red, sweet, and sour—all varieties appear to be equally effective. The effective ingredient in cherries is not known, but keracyanin, the coloring pigment, is suspected to be the beneficial agent. Strawberry and celery juices have also been found to be beneficial.

✳ Nutrient Recommendations

Potassium causes uric acid crystals to go into solution so they can be eliminated. Eat plenty of fruits and vegetables and drink freshly made vegetable juices and you should not need to take a potassium supplement. *Best juice sources of potassium:* parsley, Swiss chard, spinach, broccoli, celery, radishes, watercress, red cabbage, beetroot, raspberries, cherries, strawberries, and lemons.

Vitamin C may help lower serum uric acid by increasing its excretion. Clinical studies have shown that by taking vitamin C supplements, you can increase urinary excretion of uric acid and reduce blood levels of uric acid. According to the University of Maryland Medical Center, vitamin C taken in high doses can help decrease blood uric-acid levels, but should not be taken without a health-care professional's supervision. There's a small subset of people with gout that will actually get worse with high levels of vitamin C. Also, a single high dose can free up too much uric acid and cause kidney stones. For this reason, it is probably best to start with a dose of 500 mg per day and slowly increase the dosage daily until your uric-acid levels start to fall. For gout sufferers, it's best to take vitamin C supplements in a buffered form, as this is nonacidic. *Best juice sources of vitamin C:* kale, parsley, broccoli, Brussels sprouts, watercress, cauliflower, cabbage, strawberries, lemons, limes, and turnips.

✳ Herb Recommendations

Devil's claw reduces pain and inflammation. Dose is 750 mg three times per day in capsule, or 1 teaspoon three times per day of tincture between meals during attacks. Do not take devil's claw if you have diabetes or take blood-thinning medication.

Stinging nettle can be used to help support kidney function, which is often compromised as the body tries to rid itself of excess uric acid. Take 250 mg three times per day or make a tea by steeping three to four teaspoons of dried leaves or root in two-thirds cup boiling water for five minutes. Strain and cool. Drink three to four cups a day. Do not take stinging nettle if you have diabetes or high blood pressure, are taking blood-thinning medication, or are pregnant.

✳ Juice Therapy

Cherry juice contains gout-fighting compounds; **strawberry** and **celery** juices have also been found to be beneficial.

Gingerroot juice is an anti-inflammatory agent.

Lemon juice helps prevents gout attacks by stimulating the formation of calcium carbonate in the body. Calcium carbonate neutralizes acids in the body, including the uric acid that triggers gout attacks. After each meal drink the juice of one freshly squeezed lemon in a glass of lukewarm water.

Parsley juice is effective in combating and flushing uric acid from the tissues, which eases painful limbs and joints. Take one teaspoon of parsley juice three times daily for six weeks. Wait three weeks before taking again. Intake should be limited to a safe, therapeutic dose of one-half to one cup per day. Parsley can be toxic in overdose, and should be especially avoided by pregnant women.

✳ Juice Recipes

Water can be added to any of the recipes below in order to reduce concentrations of fruit sugar.

Gout-Fighting Tonic *(pg 333)*   **Waldorf Twist** *(pg 345)*   **The Ginger Hopper** *(pg 332)*   **Ginger Twist** *(pg 332)*   **Allergy Relief** *(pg 326)*   **Natural Diuretic Cocktail** *(pg 338)*   **Peppy Parsley** *(pg 339)*   **Pure Green Sprout Drink** *(pg 340)* **Afternoon Refresher** *(pg 326)*

Herpes

THERE ARE SEVERAL TYPES of herpesviruses, but the most common are herpes simplex 1 and 2. Type 1 (HSV-1) is most commonly seen as cold sores on the lips, while type 2 (HSV-2) is most commonly found in the genital area, and is also known as genital herpes. Both types cause painful, highly contagious blisters that occur either singly or in multiple clusters. The development of the blisters is often preceded by a burning or itching sensation, and the initial infection may be accompanied by mild fever. Those who have suppressed immune systems, either through stress, disease, or medications, have more frequent and longer-lasting outbreaks.

After entering the body, the herpesvirus never leaves, although it may be dormant for long periods of time. Recurrences of HSV-1 may be triggered by certain foods, fever, colds, allergies, sunburn, and menstruation. Recurrences of HSV-2 may be triggered by illness, stress, certain foods, sunburn, sexual intercourse, and menstruation.

Since the herpesvirus cannot be eliminated from the body, it is important to keep the virus in a dormant state. The best way to do this is to control, as much as possible, factors that activate it and to build your body's immune defenses.

✳ Lifestyle Recommendations

Practice stress management. Emotional stress has been cited as the number-one cause of frequent or repeated herpes outbreaks..While stress is a fact of life, with practice we can control our response to it. It might help to remember that what drives the stress response is often fear. Most often fear starts with our thoughts, so when stressful, fearful thoughts enter your mind, reject them right away, before they take hold in your body.

✳ Diet Recommendations

Choose foods high in lysine, an amino acid that retards the growth of the herpesvirus. High-lysine foods include fish, chicken, turkey, eggs, and vegetables. Especially increase your consumption of lysine-rich foods during outbreaks.

Eat high-alkaline foods. Promoting an alkaline state discourages the growth of herpes. Broccoli has been shown in lab studies using monkey and human cells to interfere with herpes reproduction. This action is attributed to indole-3-carbinol (I3C), a compound found in broccoli and other cruciferous vegetables such as cabbage, kale, cauliflower, and Brussels sprouts. *High-alkaline foods:* green and yellow vegetables, especially yams and leafy greens; fruits and whole grains, especially millet.

Avoid foods high in arginine, an amino acid necessary for the herpesvirus to grow. Eat the following high-arginine foods sparingly, and avoid them completely during an outbreak: all nuts, but especially almonds, cashews, and peanuts; sunflower seeds; soy; and chocolate.

Eliminate or significantly reduce acidic foods. Keeping the body pH level in balance is crucial since the herpesvirus grows much faster in an acidic environment.

Foods and beverages that foster acidity include processed foods, coffee (including decaf), soft drinks, sugar, dairy, alcohol, white vinegar, muscle meats, fried foods, and white-flour products. If you have a tendency toward frequent outbreaks, you may want to reduce or eliminate these foods from your diet.

✳ Nutrient Recommendations

Beta-carotene increases the action of interferon, an immune system–enhancing protein that inhibits virus development. In addition, beta-carotene stimulates white blood cells to kill more viruses. *Best juice sources of carotenes in general:* carrots, kale, parsley, spinach, Swiss chard, beetroot greens, watercress, broccoli, and romaine lettuce.

Lysine is an amino acid that retards the growth of the herpesvirus. The recommended supplemental dosage is 500 to 1,000 mg per day.

Polyphenols have inactivated viruses in test tubes, and they have the potential to do the same thing in the body. *Best juice sources of polyphenols:* apples, blueberries, and purple grapes.

Vitamin C and **bioflavonoids** offer powerful immune-system support, and studies show that vitamin C helps reduce blister formation. *Best juice sources of vitamin C:* kale, parsley, broccoli, Brussels sprouts, watercress, cauliflower, cabbage, strawberries, papaya, spinach, lemons, limes, turnips, and asparagus. *Best juice sources of bioflavonoids:* bell peppers, berries (blueberries, blackberries, and cranberries), broccoli, cabbage, lemons, limes, and parsley.

Vitamin E strengthens the immune system. *Best juice sources of vitamin E:* spinach, watercress, asparagus, and carrots.

Zinc stops viruses from reproducing, and supports and strengthens the immune system. *Best juice sources of zinc:* gingerroot, turnips, parsley, garlic, carrots, spinach, cabbage, lettuce, and cucumbers.

✳ Herb Recommendations

Echinacea and **goldenseal** support the immune system. Avoid goldenseal if you are pregnant, and do not use it for more than ten days at a time.

Garlic is known to kill herpes simplex and influenza virus in test tubes. It also stimulates the immune system. It contains several helpful compounds, including allicin, which is one of the plant kingdom's most potent antibiotics. Take several cloves of raw garlic per day during an outbreak. If you don't want garlic breath, try chopping it up into very small pieces and divide them into doses of a size you can swallow. Place them one dose at a time on a spoon, and swallow, with water. Don't chew it. This should help spare your breath. You can also add a clove or two to your vegetable juice drinks.

✳ Juice Therapy

Carrot, blueberry, parsley, and **spinach** juices contain concentrated amounts of the nutrients that are most helpful in controlling herpes infections. Parsley juice intake should be limited to a safe, therapeutic dose of one-half to one cup per day. Parsley can be toxic in overdose, and should be especially avoided by pregnant women.

✳ Juice Recipes

Morning Energizer *(pg 337)* **Spinach Power** *(pg 341)* **Ginger Twist** *(pg 332)* **Triple C** *(pg 338)* **Tomato Florentine** *(pg 343)* **Colon Cleanser** *(pg 330)* **The Ginger Hopper** *(pg 332)* **Antiviral Cocktail** *(pg 327)* **Cabbage Patch Cocktail** *(pg 329)* **Cranberry-Apple Cocktail** *(pg 331)* **Garlic Surprise** *(pg 332)* **Happy Morning** *(pg 333)* **Immune Builder** *(pg 335)* **Peppy Parsley** *(pg 339)* **Pure Green Sprout Drink** *(pg 340)* **Super Green Sprout Drink** *(pg 342)* **Wheatgrass Light** *(pg 345)*

High Blood Pressure (Hypertension)

HIGH BLOOD PRESSURE is a blood pressure reading of 140/90 mmHg or higher, and both numbers are important. Pre-hypertension is blood pressure between 120 and 139 for the top number, and between 80 and 89 for the bottom number. (Unless treated, people with pre–high blood pressure could end up with high blood pressure.) Below 120/80 is normal.

Nearly one in three Americans has high blood pressure. Once it develops, it usually lasts a lifetime. The good news is that it can be lowered and controlled by natural methods. High blood pressure is called the silent killer because it usually has no symptoms. Some people may not find out they have it until they have trouble with their heart, brain, or kidneys. When high blood pressure is not found and treated, it can cause the heart to enlarge, aneurysms (small bulges) to form in blood vessels, arteries to harden, blood vessels in the kidneys to narrow, and blood vessels in the eyes to burst. It can lead to stroke.

Everyday lifestyle choices can contribute to the development of high blood pressure; they include high caffeine consumption (more than three cups daily); alcohol, sugar, fat, and salt; and a diet that contains too few fruits and vegetables. Additionally, high stress; lack of exercise; deficiencies of vitamins, minerals, and essential fats; and some drugs can contribute to hypertension.

✳ Lifestyle Recommendations

Stop smoking. Smoking can contribute to high blood pressure.

Get regular exercise. Aerobic exercise—generally, any type that doesn't involve lifting weights—can help lower blood pressure. Exercise for at least thirty minutes three times a week; walking, swimming, and aerobic dance or step aerobics are all good choices.

Practice relaxation techniques. Activities such as deep-breathing exercises, biofeedback, and progressive muscle relaxation can all help lower blood pressure.

✳ Diet Recommendations

Eat your vegetables! Studies show that making 60 percent or more of your diet vegetables, fruit, juices, sprouts, seeds, and nuts can lower your blood pressure. Juicing can help you reach this goal with ease. Eat more fatty cold-water fish such as salmon, tuna, herring, mackerel and halibut for their beneficial omega-3 fatty acids. Include more onions, garlic, celery, olive oil, and organically grown fruits and vegetables, especially leafy greens and cruciferous vegetables such as broccoli, cauliflower, Brussels sprouts, and cabbage, along with whole grains and legumes (beans, lentils, split peas). A 2002 study demonstrated that people who increased their intake of fruits and vegetables experienced a drop in blood pressure after six months. Many of these foods are rich in potassium and fiber, which can help lower blood pressure. (For more information on healthy dietary choices, see Basic Guidelines for the Juice Lady's Health and Healing Diet, page 290.)

Eat at least 60 percent of your fruits and vegetables raw. One study published in *South Medical Journal* (1985) shows that people who made 62 percent of their diet raw foods experienced a significant drop in blood pressure.

Increase your omega-3 fatty acids. According to a report in *Hypertension: Journal of the American Heart Association,* people who eat diets rich in fish, nuts, seeds, and oils that contain omega-3 fatty acids tend to have lower blood pressure. Several studies have shown that fish eaters tend to have lower blood pressures than even vegetarians. This has been attributed to eicosapentaenoic acid (EPA) and docosahexaenoic acid (DHA), two essential fatty acids found in fish. The body can also create EPA and DHA from EFAs found in such plant-based oils as flaxseed and hemp.

Eliminate or greatly reduce sugar and alcohol. Sugar requires an increase in the body's water stores; for every gram of sugar, three grams of water are needed for transport, storage, and metabolism. This increases fluid volume, which can lead to problems with urine elimination. Also, sugar increases levels of triglycerides and cholesterol, which increases blood viscosity, or stickiness. Alcohol, which acts like sugar in the body, causes similar problems.

Avoid all diet soda. Researchers have found a correlation between drinking diet soda and metabolic syndrome—the collection of risk factors for cardiovascular disease and diabetes, which include abdominal obesity, high cholesterol, elevated blood-glucose levels, and elevated blood pressure. In the study, scientists gathered dietary information on more than 9,500 men and women ages forty-five to sixty-four and tracked their health for nine years. The risk of developing metabolic syndrome was 34 percent higher among those who drank just one can of diet soda a day compared with those who drank none.

Use salt sparingly. Studies show that restricted use of sodium chloride, or common table salt, results in a fall in blood pressure and a reduction in the need for medication. If you eat out frequently, you may be ingesting much more salt than you realize, since restaurant food is often heavily salted for flavor. Request salt-free dishes so you can control your salt intake. Vinegar, lemon juice, and herbs make good substitute flavor enhancers. In addition, use potassium to offset the effects of sodium (see the Nutrient Recommendations). (The exceptions are Celtic sea salt and gray salt, which are very rich in minerals; you can use these in moderation in place of table salt.)

Juices help lower your blood pressure. Beetroot juice was proven in a 2008 study in the UK to lower blood pressure. Fresh juices are rich in the vitamins and minerals directly related to lowering high blood pressure and maintaining normal pressure. Many people have reported lowering their blood pressure simply by adding raw juices to their diets.

Limit or avoid caffeine consumption. Studies with coffee show that eliminating caffeine resulted in a significant reduction in blood pressure. Caffeine is also in green, white, and black tea, and soft drinks, chocolate, and some medications. If you have trouble giving up the taste of coffee, switch to water-processed decaf coffee. Or try decaf or herbal tea (see Herb Recommendations, page 179).

✳ Nutrient Recommendations

Calcium plays an important role in maintaining normal blood pressure. *Best juice sources of calcium:* kale, parsley, dandelion greens, watercress, beetroot greens, broccoli, spinach, romaine lettuce, string beans, celery, and carrots.

Magnesium. Multiple studies recommend that people who have high blood pressure (or who are at risk of developing it) maintain an adequate intake of magnesium. A Canadian study concluded that an adequate daily intake of calcium, potassium, and magnesium is essential in the management of high blood pressure. And studies have shown that people who consume more magnesium-rich foods have lower blood pressures than people who do not. *Best juice sources of magnesium:* beetroot greens, spinach, parsley, dandelion greens, garlic, blackberries, beetroot, broccoli, cauliflower, carrots, and celery.

Potassium-rich diets may allow significant reductions in hypertensive medication dosages. *Best juice sources of potassium:* parsley, Swiss chard, garlic, spinach, broccoli, carrots, celery, radishes, cauliflower, watercress, asparagus, and cabbage.

Vitamin C can keep blood pressure in the normal range. A study involving 39 participants showed that treatment with vitamin C significantly lowered blood pressure after thirty days, while placebo had no effect. *Best juice sources of vitamin C:*

kale, parsley, broccoli, Brussels sprouts, watercress, cauliflower, cabbage, spinach, lemons, limes, turnips, and asparagus.

✳ Herb Recommendations

Green tea has been shown in studies to lower blood pressure. It also comes decaffeinated.

Licorice should be avoided if you have high blood pressure.

✳ Juice Therapy

Beetroot juice. Volunteers recruited for a study at St. Bartholomew's Hospital in London were asked to drink approximately one British pint, equivalent to about 20 ounces in U.S. measurements, of beetroot juice or water. Those who drank the beetroot juice started to show reductions in blood pressure after an hour. At about 2.5 hours, participants who had drunk the juice showed significant reductions in both their systolic and diastolic readings.

Blackberry, carrot, cucumber, parsley, raspberry, and **spinach** juices are all traditional remedies for high blood pressure. Intake of parsley juice should be limited to a safe, therapeutic dose of one-half to one cup per day. Parsley can be toxic in overdose, and should especially be avoided by pregnant women.

Broccoli and **carrots** have a number of phytochemicals that are known to lower blood pressure.

Celery has long been recommended in Chinese medicine for lowering high blood pressure, and experimental evidence bears this out. Injecting laboratory animals with celery extract significantly lowered their blood pressure. In humans, eating as few as four celery stalks a day has done the same, so why not add celery to your juice recipes each day?

Garlic. In one study, people with high blood pressure were given one clove of garlic a day for twelve weeks. Afterward, they exhibited significantly lower blood pressure and cholesterol levels. You can add a clove of garlic to your juice, and surprisingly, it's quite good.

Pomegranates are known as one of the healthiest foods, largely because of their beneficial effects on cardiovascular health, according to recent studies.

Tomatoes are high in gamma-aminobutyric acid (GABA), a compound that can help bring down blood pressure.

✳ Juice Recipes

Spinach Power *(pg 341)*   **Afternoon Refresher** *(pg 326)*   **Magnesium-Rich Cocktail** *(pg 336)*   **Tomato Florentine** *(pg 343)*   **Beet-Cucumber Cleansing Cocktail** *(pg 328)*   **Calcium-Rich Cocktail** *(pg 329)*   **Colon Cleanser** *(pg 330)* **Ginger Twist** *(pg 332)*   **Happy Morning** *(pg 333)*   **Icy Spicy Tomato** *(pg 335)* **Morning Energizer** *(pg 337)*   **Orient Express** *(pg 338)*   **Salsa in a Glass** *(pg 340)* **Waldorf Twist** *(pg 345)*

Hypoglycemia

HYPOGLYCEMIA, or low blood sugar, occurs when too much insulin is secreted by the pancreas, generally in response to sugar consumption. Sugar circulates in the bloodstream as glucose, and excess insulin clears glucose from the blood, in this case, too quickly. This results in abnormally low blood-glucose levels. Hypoglycemia is usually diagnosed when an oral glucose tolerance test shows a glucose reading below 50 mg/dl, but some individuals have this condition even though their glucose levels are in the normal range. There is some debate about the nature of hypoglycemia. It is being diagnosed much less frequently than it was a few decades ago. Some doctors think the condition is caused by other medical problems and is not a disorder in itself. Others think that it is actually an early stage of diabetes.

The lack of glucose (hypoglycemia) as energy for the brain can cause symptoms ranging from headache, mild confusion, and abnormal behavior to loss of consciousness, convulsions, seizure, coma, and death. Hypoglycemia is usually characterized by milder symptoms, such as extreme tiredness, loss of alertness, loss of muscular strength and coordination, dizziness, double vision, increased heart rate, depression, staggering or inability to walk, craving for salt or sweets, allergies, ringing in the ears, inflammation of the skin, pain in the neck and shoulders, memory problems, and excessive sweating. Symptoms generally appear three to five hours after eating sugar or other refined carbohydrates.

Repeatedly eating refined carbohydrate foods, such as sweets and white-flour products, puts a great strain on the pancreas, as it is called on repeatedly to secrete insulin in response to high levels of sugar in the bloodstream. If this eating pattern continues, other organs begin to show signs of strain as well. As the presence of insulin causes blood-sugar levels to drop, the liver is signaled to release its glucose stores. The thyroid speeds up to aid the liver. The adrenal glands secrete hormones that cause even more glucose to be released. Eventually, all these glands and organs become overworked. Unless dietary changes are made, this condition can lead to diabetes in some individuals (see Diabetes Mellitus, page 131) and severe hypoglycemia in others.

✳ Diet Recommendations

Do not eat sugar-rich foods to relieve low blood-sugar symptoms. Eating something sweet may seem like the logical approach, and indeed this will cause your sugar levels to rise initially. But afterward your blood-sugar levels will plummet again as insulin is oversecreted in response to the sugar. This results in a Ping-Pong effect that leaves you feeling like you are bouncing off the walls.

Say good-bye to sweets such as cookies, candies, cakes, pies, doughnuts, and ice cream, along with refined white-flour products such as bread, rolls, pasta, and pizza; starchy vegetables like potatoes and winter squash; and milk (milk sugar). Avoid natural sugars, such as honey, maple syrup, dried sugar cane, brown rice syrup, and malt barley syrup as much as possible. Fruit is a source of simple carbohydrates, and you should eat no more than one or two pieces of fresh, whole fruit per day. (If your hypoglycemia is especially severe, do not eat even that.) Fruit sugar, or fructose, is very sweet—one and a half times as sweet as table sugar. Fruit juice is too high in fruit sugar and should be avoided, or at least consumed in very small quantities (no more than four ounces daily) and diluted fifty-fifty with water. Fructose is fructose no matter what the source and is not a good sugar substitute. Fructose causes insulin resistance, as proven in scientific tests. It is highly addictive, and many people find it difficult to give it up no matter how sick they become.

Avoid high-carbohydrate foods. When we continue to eat sugar, sweets, high-starch vegetables, and refined-flour products, the cells get resistant to this constant bombardment of glucose, and increasing levels of insulin are necessary to maintain a normal blood-glucose level. As the cells become resistant, the insulin assists in the conversion of the extra glucose into triglycerides, and they are deposited as body fat. Also, high insulin levels suppress two important hormones: glucagon and growth hormone. Glucagon promotes the burning of fat and sugar; growth hormone is used for muscle development and building new muscle mass.

Increase your consumption of essential fatty acids and protein. The body can maintain an ideal level of glucose by creating it in the liver from amino acids derived from protein and/or triglyceride fatty acids in a process called gluconeogenesis. Eat more protein and essential fatty acids (EFAs)—the "good fats" vital to your health. Raw nuts, seeds, and avocados make good snacks. They provide excellent sources of steady energy, and have a calming effect on hyperactive hypoglycemic states. Focus on eating complex carbohydrates, protein, and good fats together. For example, raw almonds, or other nuts or seeds, make a good, portable snack that has protein, fat, and carbohydrate in one source, and they're great combined with vegetable sticks.

People who have hypoglycemia often show signs of EFA deficiency, such as dry hair and skin, low body weight (although you can be both overweight and EFA deficient), depression, nervousness, aches and pains, and cramps. When you increase your intake of complex carbohydrates and protein and decrease your consumption of refined processed foods, your EFA levels will naturally increase. It is also beneficial to increase EFA levels by eating flaxseeds or hemp seeds (one to two tablespoons per day), taking cod-liver oil, and by eating cold-water fish such as salmon, halibut, tuna, cod, mackerel, and trout. Fish is an excellent protein source.

Eat plenty of nonstarchy, complex carbohydrates. Complex carbs include vegetables, whole grains, and legumes (beans, lentils, and split peas). Incorporating plenty of these foods is an important step in controlling hypoglycemia. Complex carbohydrates are high in fiber, which causes them to release sugar much more slowly into the bloodstream than simple carbohydrates do. Refined carbs are not only stripped of most of their fiber but also contain relatively few vitamins, minerals, and phytonutrients.

Why increase fiber in your diet? Fiber slows digestion and the release of sugars into the bloodstream. So eating more fiber helps you control blood sugar. It is important to eat the right type of fiber. Water-soluble fiber is the most beneficial for controlling blood sugar. Hemicellulose, mucilages, gums, and pectins are all water-soluble forms of fiber. And, you may be surprised to learn that these are the fibers found in fresh vegetable juice. Other sources of water-soluble fiber are legumes, oat bran, nuts, seeds, and vegetables. The fiber in flaxseed may help stabilize blood-sugar levels throughout the day, not only because the fiber slows the release of insulin, but also because they are a rich source of essential fatty acids. Pear and apple juices are very good sources of soluble fiber, but you should avoid them because of their sugar content. If you do decide to have a small amount, be sure to dilute it fifty-fifty with water.

Vegetable juice. According to a study in *The New England Journal of Medicine* (2000), a high intake of dietary fiber, particularly that of the soluble type, above the level recommended by the American Dietetic Association (ADA), improves glycemic control, decreases hyperinsulinemia, and lowers plasma lipid concentrations. Vegetable juice contains soluble fiber. It's also a storehouse of enzymes, which supports the pancreas and spares it from overwork.

Eat smaller, more frequent meals. You will do best eating smaller meals more often, rather than two or three large meals. Eating more frequently, and eating some protein at each meal or snack, helps keep blood sugar at a relatively constant level, as opposed to the big surges in blood sugar that occur after a large meal. One way to accomplish this is to save half a meal and eat it later as a snack. A protein snack before bedtime also helps keep blood sugar even throughout the night. This is important because low blood-sugar levels can cause you to sleep poorly or to wake up in the night hungry (nocturnal hypoglycemia).

Cleanse and support your liver. With hypoglycemia, the liver has been overworked. Support your liver by eating and drinking more liver-supporting foods and juices; beetroot and artichokes are especially helpful. Other beneficial foods include peas, parsnips, pumpkin, sweet potatoes, squash, yams, beans, broccoli, Brussels sprouts, cabbage, carrots, cauliflower, celery, chives, cucumber, eggplant, garlic, kale, kohlrabi, mustard greens, okra, onion, and parsley. The Liver Cleanse (page 310) can help improve liver function.

Avoid alcohol. Hypoglycemia is made far worse by alcohol consumption. Alcohol increases insulin secretion, thereby causing a drop in blood sugar. This state often creates a hunger for high-carb foods that can quickly raise blood sugar. These types of foods cause a greater craving for alcohol, and a dangerous spiral effect is created. Also, the work of breaking down alcohol puts an additional burden on the liver. Excessive alcohol consumption can also block the process of glucose production, depleting your body's stores of glycogen.

Avoid caffeine. Caffeine affects the brain in two ways: it drops the blood flow in the brain and at the same time it tells the brain to demand more glucose (sugar). So it has this dichotomy, and the end result is that the brain thinks it's getting less sugar than it actually is. It doesn't take a lot of caffeine to cause this response—only about two to three cups of coffee a day.

Eat more seaweed and microalgae. These foods, including spirulina, chlorella, and wild blue-green algae, help normalize blood-sugar metabolism. Seaweed, such as kelp and dulse, supply energy and contain high amounts of trace minerals, including iodine, silicon, and phosphorus.

✳ Nutrient Recommendations

General nutrients. Alpha-lipoic acid may improve the glucose-lowering action of insulin. Chromium, niacin, vitamins C and E, and vanadium (a trace mineral) are all essential nutrients that play important roles in regulating glucose levels in the body. Methyl sulfonyl methane (MSM) improves hypoglycemia, as it makes it easier for the body to introduce blood sugar through cell walls. (MSM is a compound found naturally in foods such as cow's milk, meat, seafood, fruits, and vegetables.)

Chromium is the most essential nutrient for blood-sugar control. It is a key part of glucose tolerance factor (GTF), which increases insulin's effectiveness in getting sugar into the body's cells. A chromium deficiency is thought to be an underlying contributor to both diabetes and hypoglycemia. Brewer's yeast is considered the best food source of chromium, and can be added to fresh vegetable juices. *Best juice sources of chromium:* green peppers, parsnips, spinach, carrots, lettuce, string beans, and cabbage. Chromium picolinate is the preferred form of supplemental chromium. Take 200 mg of chromium picolinate daily.

Magnesium may help reduce glucose-induced insulin secretion. *Best juice sources of magnesium:* beetroot greens, spinach, parsley, dandelion greens, garlic, beetroot, broccoli, cauliflower, carrots, and celery.

Vitamin B₃ (niacin) is another GTF component. *Best food sources of vitamin B₃:* brewer's yeast, rice and wheat bran, peanuts, turkey, chicken, and fish. It is not available in fruits and vegetables.

✴ Herb Recommendations

Dandelion root is a gentle tonic for the liver.

Licorice is used to support the adrenal glands. Licorice tea is sweet and can help you if you are having a difficult time cutting sweets out of your diet. Avoid licorice if you have high blood pressure, and do not use it for prolonged periods of time. Use a medicinal form of licorice, not licorice candy.

✴ Juice Therapy

Beetroot, celery, and **dandelion** juices have traditionally been used to cleanse and support the liver.

Jerusalem artichoke juice helps support the liver and pancreas, and helps normalize blood-sugar levels. It also helps curb cravings.

Parsley juice is rich in magnesium. Intake should be limited to a safe, therapeutic dose of one-half to one cup per day. Parsley can be toxic in overdose, and should be especially avoided by pregnant women.

String bean juice is a tonic for the pancreas and helps regulate blood sugar. One cup per meal is recommended (see Jack & the Bean, page 335).

Tomato juice, with a pinch of cayenne or a dash of hot sauce, can provide energy and help to revitalize the liver and adrenal glands.

Wheatgrass juice is especially rich in enzymes, which support the pancreas.

✴ Juice Recipes

Morning Energizer *(pg 337)*   **Sweet Dreams Nightcap** *(pg 342)*   **Liver Life Tonic** *(pg 336)*   **Weight-Loss Buddy** *(pg 345)*   **Jack & the Bean** *(pg 335)*   **Icy Spicy Tomato** *(pg 335)*   **Beautiful-Skin Cocktail** *(pg 328)*   **Spinach Power** *(pg 341)*   **Magnesium-Rich Cocktail** *(pg 336)*   **Memory Mender** *(pg 336)*   **Tomato Florentine** *(pg 343)*   **Peppy Parsley** *(pg 338)*

Indigestion

INDIGESTION (dyspepsia) is the term used to describe pain or discomfort in the upper abdomen or chest after meals. Heartburn is a burning pain caused by the stomach acid flowing back up your food tube (esophagus); this is called acid reflux. There are many symptoms associated with indigestion, including discomfort or burning pain in the upper abdomen following meals, belching, flatulence, bloating, or a feeling of fullness after eating.

The causes of indigestion are as varied as the symptoms themselves. Poor eating habits, eating too fast, eating too much, not chewing food well, eating a diet high in animal fat, eating fried or spicy foods, or eating under stressful conditions can cause indigestion. Food allergies and sensitivities may also contribute to the problem. Continually eating foods you are sensitive to can have a buildup effect, and can cause symptoms of indigestion. Also, a highly stressful lifestyle will affect how your digestive system functions. Stress can decrease secretions of digestive juices such as hydrochloric acid and enzymes, which aid in breaking down food, and can cause indigestion. Hydrochloric acid is produced by the cells lining the stomach, and is a key component of digestive juices. Either a deficiency or excess of this acid can cause indigestion. More serious problems can also cause indigestion, such as hernias and ulcers (see Ulcers, page 270).

Possibly one of the most prevalent reasons for indigestion is insufficient production or secretion of bile, a substance made by the liver and stored in the gallbladder. Bile aids in the digestion of fat and fat-soluble vitamins. Insufficient bile secretion is often due to liver and gallbladder congestion. When the liver is congested and stagnant, sediment often settles out of the bile and forms accumulations that resemble stones, sand, or mud. Over time, the amount of stones, sand, or mud increases, taking up significant space in the gallbladder and liver. When this happens, there is very little space to store new bile in the gallbladder. Since the body needs bile to help it digest fat and absorb nutrients like vitamins and minerals, gallbladder congestion results in malabsorption (poor absorption of nutrients) and poor digestion of food with symptoms of indigestion, along with a host of other symptoms (see Gallstones and Liver–Gallbladder Congestion, page 164).

✳ Diet Recommendations

By following the recommendations below, you can support your digestive system and bring relief for indigestion.

For immediate relief of acidity, mix one to two teaspoons of baking soda in eight ounces of water and drink.

Chew food well and sip juices slowly. This is perhaps one of the most important steps you can take to improve indigestion, along with cleansing your liver and gallbladder. Chewing begins the digestive process in your mouth by mixing food with saliva. Saliva contains the enzyme amylase, which starts the breakdown of starches into smaller molecules. There's a saying in natural medicine that you should juice your food (with your teeth) and chew your juice. This is because thorough chewing allows better assimilation and utilization of the nutrients contained in food. If the starting point of eating is rushed or inadequate, digestion suffers.

Eat smaller portions and more frequent meals. Overeating and/or mixing a lot of different food combinations can directly cause indigestion and acid reflux. Eating smaller meals and chewing the food thoroughly allows the digestive system to function optimally. Avoid drinking liquids during a meal as much as possible. Instead, consume plenty of liquids between meals. Also, avoid lying down directly after a meal.

Eat in a relaxed environment. Anxiety and stress while eating cause indigestion. Create a peaceful environment around mealtime. Sit down during meals. Don't watch TV while you eat. Focus on the enjoyment of eating, and grant yourself this time to set aside the worries and problems of the day.

Reduce your intake of irritating foods. Foods that irritate the lining of the stomach include fried, spicy, salty, and sweet foods, along with chocolate, animal fat, trans fats, and hydrogenated and partially hydrogenated oils (margarine). Alcohol and caffeine are also irritating to the gastrointestinal tract. Coffee can actually cause symptoms that can be mistaken for an ulcer. Therefore, both regular and decaffeinated coffee, as well as alcohol, should be reduced or eliminated from your diet. Heartburn, which is caused by stomach acid splashing into the esophagus, can often be controlled by eliminating these foods. The reason is that for some people these foods relax the muscle at the top of the stomach, letting stomach acid leak upward. Meals high in animal protein are difficult to digest, and consumption of foods containing chemicals, dyes, and additives can strain the digestive system.

Eat whole foods, with an emphasis on fresh fruits, vegetables, and vegetable juices. There is some evidence that people who suffer from chronic dyspepsia (acid indigestion) benefit from a low-carbohydrate diet. One study documented a 70 percent improvement in dyspeptic individuals who went on a low-carb diet. A good book on the low-carb diet with delicious recipes is my book *The Coconut Diet.*

Alkalinize your body. In conditions where acidity has accumulated in the tissues, as is the case with most chronic illness, or in cases where an acid-blocking medication such as Pepcid, Tagamet, Zantac, or Prilosec was utilized for management of stomach hyperacidity for more than a few isolated incidents, it becomes critical to return the body's acid/alkaline balance to a normal range. Acids are produced from such things as metabolic waste, acid-forming foods, and stress. Harmful acidity develops in the tissues of the body when the system's ability to eliminate the acids is reduced. Consequently, acids build up in the tissues and fluids of the body, where they interfere with normal cellular functions. This overly acidic condition creates an ideal breeding ground for harmful microorganisms like *Candida albicans,* creating an enormous burden on the immune system.

To counteract acidity, eat more alkaline foods. Foods are either alkaline or acid depending on the residue they leave behind after being metabolized by the body. The typical Western diet is high in acid-forming foods, which include muscle meats, sugar, alcohol, coffee, refined-flour baked goods, animal fats, hydrogenated and partially hydrogenated oil (margarine), some fruit, dairy, and eggs. Not surprisingly, these are the foods that should be consumed in moderation if you suffer from indigestion or heartburn. Focus on alkaline foods, which include all vegetables, vegetable juices, sprouts, seeds, nuts, legumes, beans, lentils, split peas, millet, olive oil, and sea vegetables like seaweed. Vegetable juices are very beneficial. You may need to eliminate fruit if your stomach acid is too high; if it's too low, lemon or lime juice mixed with water may be helpful. Surprisingly, acid indigestion may be caused by too little stomach acid in many individuals.

Eat raw almonds. Carry raw almonds with you for a snack. Chew them slowly to alleviate heartburn. (Raw almonds can be purchased at most health food stores.)

If you tend to put on weight, do not overindulge in almonds, since they are fairly high in calories.

Cleanse the liver and gallbladder. Cleansing your liver and gallbladder can help you dissolve stones and purge these organs. You may need to do several cleanses to make sure they are completely cleaned out. When they are, your digestion should greatly improve. These cleanses should be done at least twice a year (see The Liver Cleanse and The Gallbladder Cleanse, pages 310 and 318).

Go on short juice fasts. Give your digestive system a rest with a short one- to three-day vegetable-juice fast. You can quickly turn an acidic system around to one with a proper alkaline-acid balance by vegetable-juice fasting (see the Juice Fast, page 304).

Include Celtic sea salt or gray salt in your diet. Low-salt diets can make it very difficult if not impossible for the stomach to produce adequate amounts of hydrochloric acid. Health problems are not caused by all salt, but by refined sodium chloride (common table salt). Using unrefined, highly mineralized sea salt is healthful. This type of salt is grayish in color, and is produced by traditional methods used for hundreds of years. Available in most natural food stores, this healthier salt goes by names such as Celtic sea salt or gray salt. The common refined (white) sea salt sold in most stores does not have the same high mineral content.

✳ Things That Make Symptoms Worse

- Consuming a heavy meal
- Drinking excess alcohol
- Smoking
- Eating irregular meals; long gaps between meals give the acid more time to act (each meal neutralizes the acid for a while)
- Stress and anxiety
- Drugs such as aspirin and anti-inflammatory medicines used to treat arthritis
- Peptic ulcer (stomach or duodenal ulcer)

Avoid foods that cause allergies and sensitivities. If you have recurring indigestion, determine whether you have food allergies and sensitivities; then avoid those foods (see Allergies, page 27; also see the Elimination Diet, page 301).

✳ Nutrient Recommendations

Beta-carotene should be consumed liberally if you have chronic indigestion. It's converted to vitamin A according to the body's needs. Beta-carotene supports the mucus-secreting cells of the mucous membranes, which include the lining of the digestive tract, where it acts as an anti-inflammatory agent. When there is a vitamin A deficiency, the intestinal tract is much more susceptible to injury from such strong irritants as caffeine, alcohol, and spicy foods. Vegetable juices are some of the best sources of beta-carotene. *Best juice sources of carotenes in general:* carrots, kale, parsley, spinach, Swiss chard, beetroot with greens, watercress, broccoli, and romaine lettuce.

Betaine HCL. Individuals suffering with stomach and intestinal problems most frequently assume that heartburn, indigestion, gas, and reflux are caused by overproduction of stomach acid. But for most people, the opposite is true. Based upon the testing of sample groups, it has been theorized that well over half of the U.S. population beyond the age of fifty years is underproducing hydrochloric acid on a constant basis, leading to a host of digestive and immune problems.

You can take a test, known as the Heidelberg capsule test. Unfortunately, very few physicians have this test available. If it's not available to you, you can use a betaine hydrochloride supplement during your meals as a challenge, to see if digestive function improves.

Here's how to perform the challenge test: Purchase betaine HCL at your health food store. (HCL with pepsin is best.) Take one capsule at the beginning of a meal; eat a little food first, because it could burn if you take it on an empty stomach. Monitor how your stomach feels during and after eating. Should any burning or heaviness occur, or if burning has been present previously before taking the supplement, and it gets worse with the betaine HCL, discontinue. This is an indication that your stomach may be overproducing acid, or that your stomach lining may be damaged. If no noticeable stomach discomfort occurs, try taking two capsules at the start of your next meal and again monitor for burning and/or heaviness during and after eating. If taking two capsules produces some discomfort but one capsule does not, go back to one capsule at the start of each meal. If the two capsules produce no discomfort, try three at the start of your next meal. If digestion improves when taking three capsules at the start of each meal, stay with that dosage. Most people do not require increasing the dosage to four capsules.

Regular use of supplemental betaine HCL will, in most cases, retrain your stomach to produce higher concentrations of acid on its own. You may need to take betaine HCL for several weeks to several months, depending on your status. The most significant indication that acid production is improving is that betaine HCL supplementation will no longer be comfortably tolerated. If you do not reach that point, you may need to continue supplementing with betaine HCL.

Note: If your stomach acid is too high, you might benefit from taking an alkalinizing supplement called alkabase (sodium bicarbonate, potassium bicarbonate, sodium sulfate, calcium citrate, calcium lactate, sodium citrate, silica, sea salt).

✳ Herb Recommendations

Anise aids digestion through the action of volatile oils, which relax the bowels.

Chamomile tea has antispasmodic, anti-inflammatory, and gas-relieving effects.

Dandelion, gentian, and **goldenseal** are bitter herbs that have been used to aid digestion. Their action comes directly from properties that give them their bitter taste, which stimulates the central nervous system and eventually causes the release of gastrin, a digestive hormone. Avoid goldenseal if you are pregnant, and do not use it for more than ten days.

Gingerroot relieves gas and reduces bloating and pain; it also has anti-inflammatory properties.

Peppermint in tea contains menthol and has an antispasmodic effect on the digestive tract. It relieves gas and stomach cramps.

Slippery elm bark protects and soothes inflamed tissue in the stomach due to the action of the mucilage it contains.

✳ Juice Therapy

Cabbage juice, with its ulcer-healing factor, works for both indigestion and gastritis.

Fennel juice aids digestion and relieves gas.

Gingerroot has been used as a gas-relieving substance for thousands of years.

Lemon juice and water, consumed thirty minutes before a meal, is a traditional tonic for stimulating salivary and gastric secretions. For a refreshing lemon sparkler, try fresh lemon juice mixed with sparkling water. Or try one of the lemon-containing recipes. (Omit lemon from recipes if you have an overly acidic stomach or damaged stomach lining.)

Papaya and **pineapple** juices contain papain and bromelain, respectively, both protein-digesting enzymes that are helpful for indigestion and heartburn. These digestive enzymes increase digestive activity, tone the stomach, and directly soothe heartburn. They can be helpful sipped in small quantities with a meal. (Papaya does not juice very well, but it can be blended and makes a great addition to a smoothie. For my book of smoothie recipes, see *The Ultimate Smoothie Book.*

✳ Juice Recipes

Note: If you have an overly acidic stomach, omit the lemon juice in all recipes.

Triple C *(pg 344)*   **Mood Mender** *(pg 337)*   **The Ginger Hopper** *(pg 332)*   **Morning Energizer** *(pg 337)*   **Spinach Power** *(pg 341)*   **Antiulcer Cabbage Cocktail** *(pg 327)*   **Allergy Relief** *(pg 326)*   **Cabbage Patch Cocktail** *(pg 329)*   **Ginger Twist** *(pg 332)*   **Happy Morning** *(pg 333)*   **Hot Ginger-Lemon Tea** *(pg 334)*   **Liver Life Tonic** *(pg 336)*   **Mint Refresher** *(pg 337)*   **Orient Express** *(pg 338)*

Inflammation

INFLAMMATION is a natural bodily response to trauma and infection. It helps to rid the body of invading organisms and toxins, and also helps to "mop up" any dead cells and tissues. Without inflammation, injured tissues would not heal and infections would rage out of control. But chronic inflammation (also known as chronic systemic inflammation) is an inflammatory immune response of prolonged duration that eventually leads to tissue damage. One of the most destructive inflammatory molecules is called nuclear factor kappa B—a little molecule that creates a lot of damage. It can be activated by emotional stress, toxins, free radicals, and toxic, inflammatory, or allergenic foods. When it is activated, it can unleash the production of a host of inflammatory molecules—a steamroller of inflammation that affects your whole system.

In inflammation, the blood vessels become more permeable to allow immune cells and chemicals to enter spaces within the tissues. When the inflammation becomes chronic, this process can destroy healthy tissue surrounding the injured or infected area. Many ailments are associated with chronic inflammation, such as lupus, rheumatoid arthritis, fibromyalgia, atherosclerosis, inflammatory bowel disease, chronic pancreatitis, and chronic hepatitis. New research also links obesity with inflammation. Being overweight promotes inflammation, and inflammation promotes obesity in a continuous cycle.

It is estimated that more than half of Americans are inflamed, and most of them don't even know they are. Sometimes the rhythm of the immune system, which produces just enough inflammation to keep infections, allergens, toxins, and other stressors under control, is disrupted. And when it is, the immune system shifts into a chronic state of alarm, or *inflammation,* spreading rapidly throughout the body. When this "alarm" sounds in the heart it can cause heart disease; in the brain it can cause dementia or Alzheimer's disease; in the whole body, cancer; in the eyes, blindness; and in our fat cells, obesity.

Otherwise healthy individuals can be exposed through lifestyle and/or environment to substances the body perceives as irritants, such as low-grade infections from gum disease, viruses, bacteria, food allergens, toxins, and inflammatory foods such as sugar, alcohol, and trans fat. When we think of inflammation, it's usually an injured area that is swollen, red, and warm to the touch, but science is showing us that it can occur much more quietly and insidiously, without these kinds of obvious symptoms. Unless it's adequately dealt with, it can have dreadful effects on our health.

✳ Lifestyle Recommendations

Manage stress. Stress is a major contributor to the inflammatory response. As we learn to relax and let go of toxic emotions such as anger, resentment, rejection from others, self-rejection, worry, fear, and bitterness, we can move into a place of peace with ourselves and others. This is as necessary as an anti-inflammatory diet if we are to get rid of inflammation throughout the body. Our daily expressions hold clues to emotions that contribute to the destructive role of inflammation. How often do we use words such as "fiery temper, consumed with anger, burned out, worried sick, or afraid it won't work"? The war we wage in the body and mind releases powerful inflammatory hormones, acid in our stomachs, and pain in our joints and muscles to alert us to the problem. The solution is to let go of negative emotions, make peace with ourselves and others, and transform our emotional diet to one of joy, peace, love, and acceptance.

It's also very beneficial to implement an exercise program that produces those great feel-good endorphins that help the body release stress and elevate our mood. This can create a balance that will heal both mind and body.

✵ Diet Recommendations

"What you eat and how much you exercise are the most important factors governing inflammation," says Mark Hyman, M.D. Most of the factors for ridding yourself of inflammation lie within your control. You have the power to change them and heal your body. Here's what you can do:

Reduce your intake of meat. Animal products are the primary sources of arachidonic acid, a fatty acid that is converted to hormone-like substances called prostaglandins and leukotrienes—substances that can aggravate the inflammatory response.

Avoid sugar, refined carbohydrates, refined table salt, and junk food. We're in a destructive cycle eating the standard American diet. This diet causes inflammation and the production of cortisol, which causes elevated stress levels. This results in a craving for sweets, starch, refined-flour baked goods, salt, and junk food. Then the body produces more cortisol in response to the bad diet, which causes further inflammation, and more cortisol production—and on and on it goes. To break this cycle, avoid sugar; sweets; refined-flour products such as bread, pasta, rolls, and pizza; beef; pork; alcohol; coffee; black tea; dairy products (mucus forming); and junk food.

Eliminate food allergens. Food allergies can cause and/or contribute to the inflammatory process (see Allergies, page 27; see also the Elimination Diet, page 301).

Eliminate all hydrogenated and partially hydrogenated oils and trans fats. The American diet is loaded with omega-6 oils and trans fats as opposed to the anti-inflammatory omega-3 oils found in vegetables, certain seeds and nuts, and fatty cold-water fish. Omega-6 oils result in inflammatory chemicals circulating around the body, and reduce the ability of our cells to function normally. Polyunsaturated oils such as corn, soy, safflower, canola, and sunflower oils oxidize easily, especially when heated, meaning they react with oxygen, and form an oxide. Oxidized, vegetable oils can cause free-radical damage, and at high heat they form trans fats that generate even more free radicals that can damage thousands of cells. Partially hydrogenated oils, such as in margarine, are equally damaging. Use only healthy oils—extra-virgin olive oil for cold foods and salad dressings, and virgin coconut oil for cooking.

Eat more alkalinizing foods—they're anti-inflammatory. Fruits and vegetables are alkalinizing and contain many antioxidants that boost the immune system and prevent chronic inflammation. Also, fruits and vegetables are high in phytonutrients like bioflavonoids, which improve blood-vessel strength and reduce the tendency of capillaries to leak fluid. To shift the body in the direction of alkalinity, choose the following:

- Fruits and vegetables—six to nine servings a day (a serving is one-half cup cooked or one cup raw)
- Raw nuts and seeds, especially almonds, walnuts, and sunflower and pumpkin seeds
- Green tea and herbal tea
- Extra-virgin olive oil and virgin coconut oil
- At least sixty-four ounces of purified water to flush toxins and aid cellular metabolism.

Juice vegetables. Drink one to three glasses of freshly made vegetable juice each day. This can significantly help alkalinize your body and provides an abundance of antioxidants to bind free radicals.

Increase omega-3 fatty acids. Omega-3 fatty acids help reduce inflammation. An inappropriate balance of essential fatty acids (too much omega-6; too little omega-3) contributes to the development of disease, while a proper balance helps maintain and even improves health. A healthy diet should consist of roughly two to four times more omega-6 fatty acids than omega-3 fatty acids. The typical American diet, however, tends to contain fourteen to twenty-five times more omega-6 fatty acids than omega-3 fatty acids. Many researchers believe this imbalance is a significant factor in the rising rate of inflammatory disorders in the

United States. To increase your omega-3 fatty acids, choose cold-water fatty fish such as salmon, tuna, sardines, herring, mackerel, and trout, along with krill oil, cod-liver oil, flaxseeds, hemp seeds, and walnuts.

Cleanse your body. You can take anti-inflammatory drugs, swallow fish oil daily and faithfully gulp down supplements all year, but if you don't get rid of the cause of your inflammation, you'll simply be covering up the symptoms. Toxins cause inflammation. Detoxing your body is the best way to eliminate the cause. See the cleansing programs on pages 303 to 325.

Control parasites, fungus, yeasts, bacteria, and viruses. These pathogens can be hidden sources of inflammation. It's advantageous to periodically do a *Candida albicans* cleanse and a parasite cleanse (see Candidiasis, page 80).

✳ Nutrient Recommendations

Antioxidants are powerful free-radical quenchers. Free radicals, produced as part of the inflammatory process, are unstable molecules that damage cells. Damaged cells then become sources of even more free radicals, and a chain reaction is set in motion. Antioxidant nutrients bind to free radicals, preventing them from injuring healthy tissue and thereby reducing the inflammation process. The following antioxidants are quite helpful:

- **Selenium** is a powerful antioxidant. *Best juice sources of selenium:* Swiss chard, turnips, garlic, radishes, carrots, and cabbage.
- **Vitamin A** and **beta-carotene** are potent antioxidants. Beta-carotene is converted to vitamin A in the body as needed. *Best juice sources of carotenes in general:* carrots, kale, parsley, spinach, Swiss chard, beetroot greens, watercress, broccoli, and romaine lettuce.
- **Vitamin C** and **bioflavonoids** inhibit the release of histamine, a substance that is released in response to infections and allergies. In addition, vitamin C stabilizes cell membranes, and bioflavonoids enhance the action of vitamin C. *Best juice sources of vitamin C:* kale, parsley, broccoli, Brussels sprouts, watercress, cauliflower, cabbage, spinach, lemons, limes, turnips, and asparagus. *Best juice sources of bioflavonoids:* bell peppers, berries (blueberries, blackberries, and cranberries), lemons, limes, broccoli, cabbage, parsley, and tomatoes.

- **Vitamin E** is an anti-inflammatory antioxidant. *Best juice sources of vitamin E:* spinach, watercress, asparagus, carrots, and tomatoes.

Copper has been shown to decrease inflammation in laboratory animals. *Best juice sources of copper:* gingerroot, turnips, parsley, garlic, carrots, spinach, cabbage, lettuce, and cucumbers.

Zinc promotes anti-inflammatory activity. *Best juice sources of zinc:* gingerroot, turnips, parsley, garlic, carrots, grapes, spinach, cabbage, lettuce, and cucumbers.

✳ Herb Recommendations

Curcumin, a constituent of turmeric, has anti-inflammatory effects. Traditionally, it has been used on wounds, sprains, and inflamed joints to decrease inflammation. It is as effective as some prescription drugs in relieving the swelling and stiffness associated with arthritis. Curcumin is available in supplement form.

Devil's claw is similar in its anti-inflammatory effects to cortisone. It also helps relieve pain.

✳ Juice Therapy

Gingerroot juice has anti-inflammatory properties. It can also protect the stomach from the effects of nonsteroidal anti-inflammatory drugs (NSAIDs).

✳ Juice Recipes

The Ginger Hopper *(pg 332)* **Morning Energizer** *(pg 337)* **Spinach Power** *(pg 341)* **Spring Tonic** *(pg 342)* **Beautiful-Skin Cocktail** *(pg 328)* **Immune Builder** *(pg 335)* **Antiviral Cocktail** *(pg 327)* **Allergy Relief** *(pg 326)* **Ginger Twist** *(pg 332)* **Happy Morning** *(pg 333)* **Orient Express** *(pg 338)* **Wheatgrass Light** *(pg 345)*

Influenza

INFLUENZA, or the "flu," is a highly contagious viral infection that usually spreads throughout the upper respiratory tract and can go into the lungs. It is transmitted most often through coughing and sneezing. Symptoms may include fever (often higher than that which may accompany a cold), sore throat, dry cough, aching muscles, fatigue, weakness, nasal congestion, headache, nausea, and vomiting. Symptoms may appear suddenly after an incubation period of one to three days. Both colds and flu stem from viruses that infect the upper respiratory tract, but flu symptoms are more severe (see Colds, page 102). Flu epidemics, which tend to break out every two or three years, generally occur during the winter months.

Once you have the flu, there is no cure, though you can shorten the duration. Antibiotics don't work for viruses. In fact, not only do they have no impact on colds and flu, they also help create drug-resistant super-germs. They kill the good along with the bad gut bacteria, which often creates a bigger problem in the end known as candidiasis (an overgrowth of yeast; see Candidiasis, page 80). The flu must run its course. However, the recommendations noted below can shorten the length of illness by helping to strengthen your immune system. Studies confirm that this approach works. For example, a study in Newfoundland found that consumption of a multivitamin supplement for one year improved people's immune responses to influenza.

✳ Lifestyle Recommendations

Get plenty of bed rest. The body needs a lot of rest to fight off a virus. Deep sleep is one of the most important steps you can take because that is when the most healing hormones are released.

What about flu shots? If the average American were aware of the common components of flu vaccines, he or she might think twice before considering them. Here is a partial list of some of the preservatives and fillers that flu vaccines could contain: ethylene glycol (used in antifreeze), phenol (a chemical used as a disinfectant), formaldehyde, aluminum, mercury, and neomycin and streptomycin (antibiotics). If these fillers aren't enough of a deterrent, keep in mind that using flu vaccines can also negatively alter the way your immune system is designed to function. Manipulating your immune system through unnatural means, such as vaccines, can disrupt its balance and lead to malfunction. Vaccinations are increasingly implicated in the malfunctioning immune system due to overstimulus of the B cells and suppression of the T cells. This can lead to autoimmune diseases. Also, be aware that vaccinations cause brain inflammation, which has been linked with neurodegenerative diseases. Vaccine additives such as mercury and aluminum can adversely impact your brain health.

❋ Diet Recommendations

Consume only liquids for the first two days. Drink plenty of water, vegetable juices, vegetable smoothies, green and herbal teas, and vegetable broth. (For my vegetable smoothie recipes, see *The Ultimate Smoothie Book*.) Following the liquid diet, eat lightly and continue to drink plenty of fluids. Choose primarily vegetable juices. When you are ill, it is best to eat only small amounts of food.

Avoid all sugars. Sweets decrease the functioning of white blood cells, the body's main immune cells. Sugar and vitamin C compete for entry into white blood cells. If sugar is abundant, the cells' "docking sites" will be filled with sugar molecules and prevent vitamin C from entering. Therefore, avoid eating anything that contains sugar in any form while you are sick. This includes sucrose (table sugar), cane sugar, corn syrup, beet sugar, and such natural sugars as honey, maple syrup, molasses, fructose, fruit concentrate, dried fruit, and sugar alcohols like sorbitol, xylitol, and mannitol. Avoid aspartame (NutraSweet) and sucralose (Splenda) as well. Even fruit juice consumption must be minimized (except for lemon and lime) because of the concentration of fruit sugars. Orange juice is a poor choice when you are sick because it's high in fruit sugar. If you do drink any fruit juice, dilute it by half with water and drink no more than four ounces a day.

Eliminate all alcohol. Alcohol acts like sugar in the body. Studies show that the consumption of alcohol increases the susceptibility to infection by impairing immune function.

Eliminate all meat and junk food. Meat is difficult to digest. Junk food can contain high amounts of toxins. Also, nonfood additives such as dyes, synthetic sweeteners (such as aspartame), flavorings, preservatives, and oxidized oils can add to the body's toxic load and stress the mucous membranes. Avoid all artificial foods, such as margarine.

Eat chicken soup with lots of garlic. It really does help. Mom was right, but she probably didn't know that chicken soup has been shown to have natural antibiotic properties. Chicken noodle soup from a can is not what is recommended. Make your own or get someone to make it for you using lots and lots of garlic and vegetables.

✳ Nutrient Recommendations

Selenium deficiency may result in reduced antibody production and a decrease in the microbe-eating ability of white blood cells called phagocytes. Selenium-deficient phagocytes develop defective membranes, which results in the release of substances that further impair immune function. Selenium deficiency can also lead to the reduced activity of hormones produced by the thymus gland, a gland important to immune function. *Best juice sources of selenium:* Swiss chard, turnips, garlic, radishes, carrots, and cabbage.

Vitamin A and **carotenes** have been shown to enhance activity of immune-system components called natural killer (NK) cells. In one study, immune function was enhanced by 33 percent when participants had single servings of sweet potato, kale, and tomato juice every day for three weeks. These foods are rich in beta-carotene, lutein, and lycopene—substances that improve the ability of immune cells to multiply. Many carotenes are converted to vitamin A in the body as needed. *Best juice sources of carotenes in general:* carrots, kale, parsley, spinach, Swiss chard, beetroot greens, watercress, broccoli, and romaine lettuce.

Vitamin C and **bioflavonoids** are the first line of defense in neutralizing the attack of toxins called free radicals on immune cells. One study showed that vitamin C enhanced NK cell, T cell, and B cell activity up to tenfold in 78 percent of the participants after a single dose of the vitamin. Another study showed that dock-workers given 100 mg of vitamin C each day for ten months caught influenza 28 percent less than coworkers not taking vitamin C. And the average infection was 10 percent shorter in duration in those taking vitamin C. Other studies have reported that vitamin C in high doses (2 grams every hour for twelve hours) can lead to rapid improvement in infections. At the first sign of flu symptoms, take 500 mg of vitamin C with bioflavonoids or rose hips four to six times a day. The bioflavonoids and rose hips strengthen the vitamin C's infection-fighting power.

If you experience diarrhea, reduce the dosage of vitamin C until the diarrhea subsides. Use bioflavonoids along with vitamin C for their synergistic effect. *Best juice sources of vitamin C:* kale, parsley, broccoli, Brussels sprouts, watercress, cauliflower, cabbage, spinach, lemons, limes, turnips, and asparagus. *Best juice sources of bioflavonoids:* bell peppers, broccoli, cabbage, lemons, limes, parsley, and tomatoes.

Vitamin E, a potent antioxidant, is required for optimal functioning of lymphocytes and mononuclear cells. *Best juice sources of vitamin E:* spinach, watercress, asparagus, carrots, and tomatoes.

Zinc supports the immune system. Studies show zinc deficiency increases susceptibility to infections by impairing immune function. An adequate supply of zinc and other antioxidants will help prevent shrinkage of the thymus gland and will support thymus-hormone activity. *Best juice sources of zinc:* gingerroot, turnips, parsley, garlic, carrots, spinach, cabbage, lettuce, and cucumbers.

✳ Herb Recommendations

Garlic is known to kill the influenza virus in test tubes. It also stimulates the immune system and wards off complications such as bronchitis. It contains several helpful compounds, including allicin, which is one of the plant kingdom's most potent broad-spectrum antibiotics. Take several cloves of raw garlic per day during an infection. If you don't want garlic breath, try chopping it up into very small pieces; place them on a spoon, and swallow with a glass of water. Don't chew it. You can also add a clove or two to your vegetable-juice drinks.

Gingerroot. Make ginger tea. It is antiviral, and helps break up mucus and congestion. It's also excellent for stomach flu thanks to its antinausea compounds. To make the tea, boil two tablespoons of grated fresh gingerroot in two cups of purified water for fifteen minutes, then remove from the heat and steep for ten minutes. Drink a cup as needed (also see recipe for Hot Ginger-Lemon Tea, page 334). And add lots of gingerroot to your juice recipes.

Green tea has been shown to be effective in rendering the influenza virus inactive.

✳ Juice Therapy

Apple juice has antiviral properties. Use only green apples, such as Granny Smiths or pippins, since they have less sugar than other varieties. Always dilute apple juice fifty-fifty with water. It's even better added to vegetable juices, especially dark green, orange, and red-colored vegetables.

Beetroot (red) juice helps to inactivate the virus.

Gingerroot juice contains anti-inflammatory compounds, and is a traditional remedy for flu and colds.

Jerusalem artichoke juice is rich in inulin, which enhances the immune system by activating immunity defense mechanisms.

Wheatgrass juice is rich in chlorophyll, a blood purifier. Wheatgrass works best taken straight, but if your taste buds need a little help getting started, try the Wheatgrass Light recipe (see page 345).

✳ Juice Recipes

Waldorf Twist *(pg 345)* **The Ginger Hopper** *(pg 332)* **Hot Ginger-Lemon Tea** *(pg 334)* **Weight-Loss Buddy** *(pg 345)* **Morning Energizer** *(pg 337)* **Spinach Power** *(pg 341)* **Tomato Florentine** *(pg 343)* **Icy Spicy Tomato** *(pg 335)* **Colon Cleanser** *(pg 330)* **Immune Builder** *(pg 335)* **Salsa in a Glass** *(pg 340)* **Wheatgrass Light** *(pg 345)*

Insomnia and Jet Lag

INSOMNIA is a condition in which you have trouble falling or staying asleep. Some people with insomnia may fall asleep easily but wake up too soon. Others may have the opposite problem, or they have trouble with both falling asleep and staying asleep. The end result is poor-quality sleep that doesn't leave you feeling refreshed when you wake up. Insomnia and other sleep disorders affect about two-thirds of all Americans, with more women being affected more than men.

The most common causes of insomnia include general anxiety and stress, extreme temperatures, psychiatric problems such as depression, pain from arthritis or other diseases, and erratic work and sleep schedules. Other causes include substance abuse, caffeine intake, poor diet, nocturnal hypoglycemia (causes one to awaken during the night hungry), and abnormal limb movements such as restless leg syndrome.

Insomnia induced by jet lag frequently follows travel. Jet lag is characterized by sleeplessness, fatigue, and hunger at odd times. It occurs when the body's natural clock does not have a chance to adjust to time zone changes.

When we can't sleep, the question most of us have is, "What can I do about it, *now?*" Conventional medicine most often recommends nonbenzodiazepine hypnotic drugs such as Ambien, Rozerem, or Lunesta. There are many concerns surrounding these prescriptive medications, however, including dangerous activity during the night from driving a car or chopping food while still asleep to milder symptoms such as daytime drowsiness, dizziness, and fatigue. The very best thing you can do is get to the root of why you can't sleep and correct the problem. And research is showing that most of the issues with insomnia can be resolved with lifestyle and nutritional changes.

✳ Lifestyle Recommendations

Exercise. Numerous studies have shown that regular exercise does improve sleep—both quality and duration. Exercise relieves stress and allows the body to enter a more peaceful, restful sleep. And, it promotes the release of growth hormone, which leads to weight loss and better sleep.

Reduce stress. Stress is the primary reason for most sleepless nights. When stress continues nonstop in our lives, a troubling cycle is born—high stress leads to problems sleeping, which elevates our stress levels more, and makes us less able to deal with anxiety, and on it goes, with stress and insomnia worsening as time goes by. Nighttime comes, and worries fill our minds as soon as we place our heads on the pillow. What can we do to stop the cycle? Take charge in this situation. We're the manager of our mind and emotions, and we can tell the "worry thoughts" to leave. Stress reduction begins in our mind, with refusing to allow worrisome thoughts to trouble us. As soon as worry, fear, anxiety, anger, or any other stressful emotion or thought impinges on our peace of mind, we can let it go.

✻ Diet Recommendations

Diet makes a difference. Eat a high-complex-carbohydrate, varied-protein diet that's also rich in essential fats. One study found that this type of diet produces a significant increase in REM sleep, the sleep that is most refreshing. When it comes to protein, fish is an excellent choice. You get protein and omega-3s in one package. Complex carbohydrates include vegetables; whole grains such as millet, quinoa, rye, barley, oats, and brown rice; and legumes, such as beans, lentils, and split peas.

Drink plenty of vegetable juice and water. To avoid insomnia caused by jet lag, drink plenty of fluids when traveling. Eat high-water-content foods such as fruits, vegetables, and sprouts, and drink plenty of fresh vegetable juices. People who drink only raw juices and eat fresh fruit and vegetable snacks on the day they travel report feeling energized and free of the effects of jet lag.

Avoid caffeine, refined sugar, and alcohol. Caffeine is a stimulant; even a few cups of coffee in the morning can keep some people awake at night. Stimulants cause a decrease in serotonin levels. This decrease plays a direct role in the sleep cycle. The breakdown of caffeine occurs differently in each person. Some people break down caffeine quickly, while for others it may take more than twenty hours to breakdown one serving of caffeine. Caffeine is found not only in coffee and green and black tea but also in chocolate, soft drinks, aspirin, and other painkillers. (Caffeine and soda, along with a deficiency of magnesium, are also associated with restless leg syndrome.) Alcohol can interfere with the absorption of amino acids. Without good absorption of protein, we cannot make the neurotransmitters necessary for creating the brain chemicals that play a big role in the sleep cycle. Alcohol impairs the transport of L-tryptophan into the brain, which results in insufficient conversion of this amino acid into sleep-promoting serotonin. Sugar can cause a spike and then a sharp drop in blood levels of glucose, and a drop in blood glucose promotes awakening in the night. Alcohol, sugar, and caffeine are all very dehydrating. This affects the brain because it needs lots of water to detoxify.

Avoid substances that contain tyramine. Tyramine is an amino acid that increases levels of norepinephrine, an excitatory brain chemical that plays a role in insomnia and anxiety. When we awake, norepinephrine should be high, but it needs to fall all day for a good sleep cycle to occur. The following substances contain tyramine, and should not be eaten in the evening: cheese, chocolate, sauerkraut, bacon, ham, sausage, eggplant, potatoes, spinach, and tomatoes. In addition, avoid using tobacco, which also contains tyramine.

✳ Nutrient Recommendations

Amino acids can help balance neurotransmitters that influence sleep. Neurotransmitters are the natural chemicals manufactured in the body from the proteins we consume. They facilitate communication throughout the body and brain. Two neurotransmitters play very significant roles in a good sleep cycle. We need enough serotonin to fully convert to melatonin as well as enough norepinephrine. When we awake, our excitatory or stimulating neurotransmitters, such as norepinephrine, should be high. They need to fall all day long for a good sleep cycle to occur. Without both serotonin and norepinephrine, in balance, a good restful sleep cycle does not usually occur. If your serotonin is too low or your norepinephrine is too high or too low, you'll have insomnia. When they're balanced, you should get a good night's sleep, which means seven to nine hours of deep, restful sleep for most people.

Serotonin is converted from the amino acid L-tryptophan, which breaks down into 5-hydroxytryptophan (5-HTP) for the creation of serotonin. The body often needs larger amounts of this amino acid than we get from food. Additionally, other cofactors such as B vitamins and enzymes must be present for this to occur. Since L-tryptophan breaks down into 5-HTP at a very low percentage, 5-HTP is often taken as a supplement. Dosages should be based on testing, however. B vitamins are among the necessary nutrients for the creation and transport of L-tryptophan and conversion of 5-HTP into serotonin. They should also be taken as part of the complete brain-wellness plan. Also, omega-3 fatty acids and varied protein consumption are imperative. You may greatly benefit from an amino acid supplement program tailored to your body's specific needs. For testing and more information on this program, see Sources, page 351.

On a personal note: I've seen this amino acid program help people sleep well throughout the night when nothing else worked.

Calcium deficiency may cause you to wake up in the night and not be able to return to sleep. Low calcium levels may also lead to muscles that stay contracted and can't relax. *Best juice sources of calcium:* kale, parsley, dandelion greens, watercress, beetroot greens, broccoli, spinach, romaine lettuce, string beans, celery, and carrots.

L-tryptophan is a precursor to serotonin and melatonin, the body's main sleep hormone, and is considered the best amino acid for inducing sleep. *Best food sources of L-tryptophan:* tuna, turkey, and yogurt. Chlorella and blue-green algae are also sources of L-tryptophan.

Magnesium deficiency may cause you to wake up after a few hours of sleep and not be able to drift off again. This deficiency also contributes to restless leg syndrome. Magnesium-rich foods such as kelp, wheat bran and germ, almonds, and cashews can help induce sleep. *Best juice sources of magnesium:* beetroot greens, spinach, parsley, dandelion greens, garlic, blackberries, beetroot, broccoli, cauliflower, carrots, and celery.

Melatonin has been shown in studies to help readjust the sleep/wake cycle and reduce jet lag after traveling across time zones. The best way to use melatonin for jet lag is to take 2 to 5 mg in the evening thirty minutes before bedtime for five days before traveling to the new destination, and then continue taking it at the new destination. It is not recommended that you take melatonin on a long-term basis, however, because it can affect your body's own production of melatonin. If you have trouble sleeping other than when you travel across time zones, the amino acid program is far more effective and safe long-term. And it may be that when you have balanced your neurotransmitters effectively with the amino acid program, you may not need melatonin, even when you travel. (See Sources, page 351.)

Omega-3 fatty acids. Myelin is the protective sheath that surrounds neurons, and about 70 percent of it is composed of fat. Good fats provide a high-quality form of insulation that allows your neurons to operate at high speed. This insulation is necessary for good conduction since neurotransmitters conduct on the outside of this fatty acid coating.

Pantothenic acid deficiency can cause insomnia. *Best juice sources of pantothenic acid:* broccoli, cauliflower, and kale.

Vitamin B$_1$ (thiamine) deficiency may decrease the availability of serotonin. *Best food sources of vitamin B$_1$:* seeds, nuts, beans, split peas, millet, buckwheat, whole wheat, oatmeal, wild rice, lobster, and cornmeal. It can also be found, in lesser quantities, in sunflower and buckwheat sprouts, and in garlic. This nutrient is not available in appreciable amounts from fruits and vegetables.

✱ Herb Recommendations

Catnip, chamomile and **skullcap** soothe the nerves.

Valerian root has a sedating and tranquilizing effect.

✱ Juice Therapy

Celery juice contains silicon. This element strengthens nerve and heart tissue, and has a calming effect.

Lettuce juice has a sedative effect.

Parsley juice is a good source of both calcium and magnesium. Intake should be limited to a safe, therapeutic dose of one-half to one cup per day. Parsley can be toxic in overdose, and should be especially avoided by pregnant women.

✱ Juice Recipes

Sweet Dreams Nightcap *(pg 342)*   **Super Green Sprout Drink** *(pg 342)*   **Mood Mender** *(pg 337)*   **Jack & the Bean** *(pg 335)*   **Calcium-Rich Cocktail** *(pg 329)* **Magnesium-Rich Cocktail** *(pg 336)*   **Immune Builder** *(pg 335)*   **Afternoon Refresher** *(pg 326)*   **Pancreas Helper** *(pg 338)*

Menopause

COMMONLY REFERRED to as "the change of life," menopause is the end of menstruation. The word comes from the Greek *mens,* meaning monthly, and *pausis,* meaning cessation. Menopause is part of a woman's natural aging process, when her ovaries produce lower levels of the hormones estrogen and progesterone and she is no longer able to become pregnant. Unlike a woman's first menstruation, the changes leading up to menopause usually happen over several years. The average age for menopause is fifty-two, but menopause commonly happens anytime between the ages of forty-two and fifty-six. A woman has begun menopause, which usually lasts about five years, when she has not had a period for a full year.

During this period, female hormones do not disappear. Other organs take over for the ovaries. For example, the adrenal glands continue to produce androgens, the hormones responsible for the sex drive. However, levels of estradiol, the most common form of estrogen in the body, drop to one-tenth of their previous levels. It is falling levels of this hormone that are thought to be responsible for such menopausal symptoms as hot flashes, dizziness, night sweats, headache, difficulty breathing, shortness of breath, heart palpitations, vaginal dryness, nervousness, backache, and depression. If a woman is hypoglycemic (see Hypoglycemia, page 180), the symptoms are more pronounced. The decline in estrogen levels also makes a woman more prone to osteoporosis, in which the bones become more fragile, and to the buildup of cholesterol within the arteries, which can lead to heart disease.

Animal-based hormone replacement therapy (HRT) is normally prescribed by physicians, but it is not without risk for blood clots in the veins moving to the lungs (pulmonary embolism). It can also contribute to breast cancer. For hormone replacement, consider a plant-based estrogen instead. An estrogen derived from plants was shown in clinical trials to prevent osteoporosis at half the dose of the animal-based estrogen, and with fewer side effects, according to a study published in the *Archives of Internal Medicine* (1997). The plant estrogens (phytoestrogens) are found in sources like alfalfa sprouts and cereals. These substances may also offer protection against atherosclerosis, and may reduce cholesterol levels, reduce hot flashes, and decrease risk of breast cancer. Check with a natural medicine physician for more information as to what is right for you.

❋ Diet Recommendations

Eat a high-fiber diet. Your diet can make a big difference in how you feel during menopause. Include plenty of fresh vegetables and fruits, vegetable juices, whole grains, legumes (beans, lentils, split peas), seeds, and nuts in your meal plans. Eat animal proteins in small portions (choose a serving about the size of your fist). Make at least 50 to 60 percent of your diet raw fruits, vegetables, juices, sprouts, seeds, and nuts.

Juice, juice, juice! Juicing fresh vegetables offers a powerhouse of "help in a glass," so plug in your juicer and get going on a change for the better. Carrot and red beetroot juices are particularly helpful for the liver, and a well-functioning liver helps you get rid of menopausal symptoms. Drink fresh juice twice a day and you'll get a big boost. Go on periodic juice fasts. They can help you feel more vibrant and capable of coping with stress. Many people say they experience an improved sense of well-being after a juice fast. If you start juicing regularly, you may be among the many women who say they've had no menopausal symptoms at all (see the Juice Fast, page 304).

Cleanse your liver. The liver is the key organ for hormone metabolism. Your liver is involved in manufacturing hormones from cholesterol, converting thyroid hormones, and manufacturing, breaking down, and regulating sex hormones like estrogen, testosterone, DHEA, and progesterone. When it's not overburdened, the liver will prevent estrogen from changing into dangerous estrogen metabolites. These "daughter compounds" are called 2-hydroxyestrone, 4-hydroxyestrone, and 16-alphahydroxyestrone. These metabolites can have stronger or weaker estrogenic activity—and thus increase a woman's risk of breast, uterine, and other cancers—depending on how they are metabolized.

Properly metabolizing and excreting estrogen is crucial. Research strongly suggests that women who metabolize a larger proportion of their estrogen down the C-16 pathway, as opposed to the C-2 pathway, have elevated breast cancer risk. The estrogen metabolized down the C-16 route may be associated with direct toxic effects and carcinogenicity.

Estrogen is metabolized by a series of oxidizing enzymes in the cytochrome P 450 family (Phase I of liver detoxification). It is then sent on to Phase II for conjugation. Detoxification enzymes break down all manner of drugs, hormones, and environmental toxins into generally less-harmful metabolites. When Phase II slows down, there is a buildup of toxic intermediates. A healthy, uncongested liver is very important to the detoxification process. However, a healthy, uncongested liver is not the norm; there are too many toxins in our world for most people's livers to detoxify all of them without some assistance. Therefore, a liver cleanse at least twice a year could make a world of difference for you (see the Liver Cleanse, page 310).

Avoid substances that tend to dry the mucous membranes. These include alcohol, antihistamines, caffeine, and diuretics. Dry membranes contribute to vaginal dryness and irritation. One study also suggests that alcohol may influence the onset of menopause. Eliminate smoking and sugar consumption as well, since they can contribute to adverse menopausal effects.

✳ Nutrient Recommendations

Bioflavonoids and **vitamin C** have been shown in studies to reduce the frequency and intensity of hot flashes. Bioflavonoids (especially hesperidin and rutin) and vitamin C restore the structure of blood-vessel linings. This action helps reduce blood-vessel dilation, which reduces hot flashes. *Best juice sources of vitamin C:* kale, parsley, broccoli, Brussels sprouts, watercress, cauliflower, cabbage, spinach, lemons, limes, turnips, and asparagus. *Best juice sources of bioflavonoids:* bell peppers, berries (blueberries, blackberries, and cranberries), broccoli, cabbage, cantaloupes, lemons, limes, and tomatoes.

Essential fatty acids (EFAs) help to ease menopausal symptoms. Studies have found a decrease of 40 percent in hot flashes when women introduce EFAs into their diets. Fatty cold-water fish, fish oil, flaxseeds, walnuts, hemp seeds and hempseed oil are all good sources of omega-3 fatty acids. EFAs not only help reduce hot flashes, they also help decrease vaginal dryness. In addition, supplementation with evening primrose oil, another EFA-rich oil, has been shown to help the adrenal glands produce more estrogen. (For more information, see the fats and oils section in Basic Guidelines for the Juice Lady's Health and Healing Diet, page 290.)

Vitamin E can help reduce hot flashes and vaginal dryness. *Best juice sources of vitamin E:* spinach, watercress, asparagus, carrots, and tomatoes.

Avoid soy supplements and soy foods. Though soy supplements are still promoted as beneficial for reducing menopausal symptoms, one study found no significant changes in any symptoms tested using a concentrated isoflavone extract. However, there is abundant evidence that some of the isoflavones found in soy, including genistein and equol (a metabolite of daidzen), promote toxicity in estrogen-sensitive tissues and in the thyroid. Additionally, isoflavones are known inhibitors of thyroid peroxidase, which makes T3 and T4. This inhibition can generate thyroid abnormalities, including goiter and thyroiditis. Soy is also a goitrogen, meaning that it blocks iodine absorption, which can lead to low thyroid function. Animal studies also demonstrate carcinogenic effects of soy products. In addition, they can cause weight gain. (Cattle are fattened on soybeans.)

✳ Herb Recommendations

Black cohosh and **red clover** are used to help relieve hot flashes, depression, and vaginal atrophy.

Dong quai is a Chinese herb that has been studied for its potential to control hot flashes. Most Chinese herbalists use dong quai in combination with other herbs; you may want to consult an Oriental medicine doctor (OMD) for further recommendations.

Motherwort is used for menopausal symptoms.

✳ Juice Therapy

Gingerroot is a juice ingredient you may want to avoid if you suffer from hot flashes, since it raises body temperature. Otherwise, it could be very helpful.

✳ Juice Recipes

Spinach Power *(pg 341)*   **Salsa in a Glass** *(pg 340)*   **Spring Tonic** *(pg 342)*   **Sweet Dreams Nightcap** *(pg 342)*   **Happy Morning** *(pg 333)*   **Mood Mender** *(pg 337)* **Peppy Parsley** *(pg 339)*   **The Revitalizer** *(pg 340)*   **Beautiful-Skin Cocktail** *(pg 328)*

Menstrual Disorders

Disorders associated with the menstrual cycle are among the most prevalent female health problems. They include heavy menstrual bleeding (menorrhagia), amenorrhea (no menstrual bleeding), fibroids (noncancerous uterine tumors), dysmenorrhea (painful menstrual periods), and premenstrual syndrome (PMS). Some women experience a host of physical and/or emotional symptoms just before and during menstruation. From heavy bleeding and missed periods to unmanageable mood swings, women also battle with decreased energy, tension, irritability, depression, headache, breast tenderness, bloating, and water retention.

Menstrual disorders are brought on by lifestyle factors such as poor diet, stress, depression, lack of exercise or excessive exercise, and obesity or extremes in weight.

✳ Lifestyle Recommendations

In one study, women were asked to list up to three treatments they had tried and found most effective for treating PMS. They mentioned taking nutritional supplements, getting more exercise, and making dietary changes.

Get regular exercise. Exercising for at least twenty to thirty minutes three times a week can reduce the pain associated with menstrual cramps. Brisk walking, cycling, swimming, and step aerobics are good examples. It is also important to note that exercise produces endorphins, the feel-good chemicals, and helps to raise serotonin, the neurotransmitter associated with elevated mood.

Sleep consistent hours and get enough sleep; most people need seven to nine hours. Studies show that hormones get out of whack when you don't sleep enough or sleep well. This can cause carbohydrate cravings, weight gain, and bloating. Establish a bedtime routine to help your body and mind cue up for sleep. Also, when you are well rested, the body is less vulnerable to pain. Remember, too, that you may have different sleep requirements during your menstrual cycle (see Insomnia, page 202).

✳ Diet Recommendations

Eat a high-complex-carbohydrate diet. Eating fewer animal proteins decreases the amount of saturated fat in your body. This can help reduce PMS symptoms by reducing circulating estrogen levels and by removing sources of outside estrogen. Research shows that women with menorrhagia (excessive bleeding) have higher concentrations of an inflammatory substance called arachidonic acid in the uterine lining, which leads to excessive bleeding and cramping during menstruation. A high-fiber diet has been shown to result in a significant reduction in estrogen levels because fiber causes more estrogen to be excreted from the body. (For more information, see Basic Guidelines for the Juice Lady's Health and Healing Diet, page 290.)

Avoid sugar, caffeine, and alcohol. Alcohol is toxic to the liver. The liver is responsible for the breakdown of estrogen so that it can be excreted. Alcohol can increase the levels of estrogen, thus increasing pelvic congestion. Sugar causes constriction of blood vessels, which can worsen cramps. Both sugar and alcohol should be eliminated to avoid cramps and other symptoms. Sugar, especially when combined with caffeine, contributes to PMS and moodiness. Avoid all sweets, including artificial sweeteners. (You can use stevia or agave syrup, which are found at health food stores.) Caffeine is found in coffee, and green, black, and white tea, soft drinks, and chocolate—foods that promote anxiety, depression, and breast tenderness associated with PMS.

Juice vegetables and eat a high raw-food diet. Women who juice regularly and eat lots of raw foods often report that menstrual problems diminish or disappear on this diet. Use juice fasting and liver cleansing to help eliminate bloating and other menstrual difficulties. A short juice fast and a liver cleanse can help you improve most menstrual disorders (see the Juice Fast, page 304, and the Liver Cleanse, page 310).

✳ Nutrient Recommendations

B complex vitamins. The whole B complex is necessary for good health. Within the complex, there are two B stars. Vitamin B_6 plays a key role in the production of beneficial prostaglandins that relax the uterine muscles and keep cramps under control. B_6 stores are easily depleted, however. Stress and some medications, such as oral contraceptives, can easily cause a shortage. As a result, your body may not manufacture enough of the right kind of prostaglandins, leaving you feeling uptight and prone to cramps when your period comes. And if you're bothered by water retention or monthly weight gain, B_6 can help. Take between 200 and 300 mg daily as part of a B complex. Niacin is quite effective in helping to relieve cramps. To head them off before they start, try taking between 25 and 200 mg of niacin a day, beginning seven to ten days before your period is due and stopping the day your period starts. Niacin causes flushing; you could try niacinimide, which should not have that effect.

Calcium and **manganese** have been shown to work together to improve mood, concentration, and behavioral symptoms, as well as lessen pain, during the menstrual phase, and to reduce water retention during the premenstrual phase. Studies show that increasing calcium intake, without increasing manganese, did not improve mood and pain symptoms during the premenstrual phase. Most women reported much less severe symptoms when they followed a diet high in both calcium and manganese. Manganese's role is involved in blood clotting, and some research shows that a low intake is associated with a heavier menstrual flow. Women should get about 1,200 mg of calcium per day. If your diet is not rich in calcium, you could consider a calcium citrate supplement of 500 to 1,000 mg per day. The daily recommendation for manganese is 2 to 5 mg. *Best juice sources of calcium:* kale, parsley, dandelion greens, watercress, beetroot greens, broccoli, spinach, romaine lettuce, string beans, celery, and carrots. *Best juice sources of manganese:* spinach, beetroot greens, carrots, broccoli, cabbage, apples, tomatoes, and green beans.

Essential fatty acids (EFAs) are divided into two groups, omega-3 and omega-6 fatty acids. Studies have shown a correlation between low EFA levels and menstrual discomfort. Omega-3s are found in cold-water fish, such as salmon, tuna, trout, halibut, cod, and mackerel, cod-liver oil, and unrefined oils, such as hemp seeds and flaxseeds. One tablespoon of oil per day is recommended. (For more information, see the fats and oils section in Basic Guidelines for the Juice Lady's Health and Healing Diet, page 290.)

Vitamin C and **bioflavonoids** work together to lessen excessive bleeding. The capillaries in a woman's body weaken briefly just after ovulation and again for a few days before menstruation. Women who have heavy periods have considerably weaker capillaries than women whose flows are normal. Bioflavonoids taken with vitamin C over a period of several months can strengthen capillaries and reduce excessive bleeding. Studies show that pure ascorbic acid (vitamin C) is not as effective in treating capillary fragility as fruits and vegetables that contain both vitamin C and an abundance of bioflavonoids, which improve vitamin C storage in the body. Also, vitamin C enhances iron absorption, which is especially important since iron is lost during menstruation. *Best juice sources of vitamin C:* kale, parsley, broccoli, Brussels sprouts, watercress, cauliflower, cabbage, spinach, lemons, limes, turnips, asparagus, and cantaloupes. *Best juice sources of bioflavonoids:* bell peppers, berries (blueberries, blackberries, and cranberries), broccoli, cabbage, cherries, lemons, limes, parsley, and tomatoes.

✳ Herb Recommendations

American cranesbill is helpful in preventing excessive blood loss.

Black cohosh is a relaxant and "normalizer" of the female reproductive system. It is helpful for painful or delayed menstruation.

Black haw bark relaxes the uterus.

Cramp bark relaxes the uterus and relieves painful cramps associated with menstruation.

Motherwort stimulates delayed or suppressed menstruation, particularly when anxiety or tension is involved.

✳ Juice Therapy

Fennel juice is a uterine tonic.

Dark leafy greens, and **wheatgrass** juice, which are rich in chlorophyll and iron, help relieve excessive menstrual flow. Mustard greens are specifically recommended for PMS. Mustard greens are very strong tasting and should be mixed with generous amounts of such mild-flavored juices as carrot and apple.

Parsley juice is rich in bioflavonoids and vitamin C. Intake should be limited to a safe, therapeutic dose of one-half to one cup per day. Parsley can be toxic in overdose, and should be especially avoided by pregnant women.

✳ Juice Recipes

Bladder Tonic *(pg 329)*   **Cabbage Patch Cocktail** *(pg 329)*   **Natural Diuretic Cocktail** *(pg 338)*   **Liver Life Tonic** *(pg 336)*   **Mood Mender** *(pg 337)*   **Spring Tonic** *(pg 342)*   **Wheatgrass Light** *(pg 345)*   **Weight-Loss Buddy** *(pg 345)* **Tomato Florentine** *(pg 343)*   **Peppy Parsley** *(pg 339)*   **Pure Green Sprout Drink** *(pg 340)*   **Spinach Power** *(pg 341)*   **Calcium-Rich Cocktail** *(pg 329)* **Beautiful-Skin Cocktail** *(pg 328)*

Migraine Headaches

MIGRAINE HEADACHES are especially disabling. Attacks can last from two hours to three days, may cause severe, throbbing pain on one or both sides of the head, and may be accompanied by nausea and vomiting. Other symptoms include sensitivity to light, tingling, dizziness, ringing in the ears, chills, sweating, and drowsiness. Sufferers can sometimes do nothing but lie down in a darkened room until the symptoms abate. Symptoms are believed to start in childhood, but often do not show themselves directly as headaches. Rather, a child may experience colic, periodic abdominal pains, vomiting, and dizziness.

Although researchers have not yet determined one definitive cause of migraines, they have offered several theories:

Vascular theory. Blood vessels in the brain and head are supposed to contract and expand on command, thereby reducing or increasing blood flow to the brain at the appropriate times. The vascular theory argues that for migraine sufferers, the contraction-expansion mechanism in the blood vessels goes awry, interfering with blood flow in the brain and head. Eventually, these vessels become too relaxed and their walls too permeable, allowing fluid from the blood to leak into surrounding tissues, triggering pain and inflammation.

Serotonin theory. A neurotransmitter called serotonin helps control pain sensations, sleep, mood, and other bodily actions and feelings. A deficiency of this neurotransmitter can trigger migraines by encouraging inappropriate contraction and relaxation of the arteries. A lack of serotonin may also lower the pain threshold, making everything hurt more. Serotonin can be in a lower supply than the excitatory neurotransmitters, further exacerbating the migraine problem. Pain uses up inhibitory neurotransmitters, such as serotonin and GABA. As these neurotransmitters become in shorter supply, the migraine intensity often increases.

Hormonal imbalance theory. Often migraines begin when puberty is reached. Hormone levels are affected by neurotransmitter balance. Many patients report migraines at a certain time each month. This is much easier to diagnose in women than in men, though male hormonal imbalance can be a contributing factor.

Migraine Triggers

- Allergic reactions
- Bright lights; loud noises
- Physical or emotional stress
- Changes in sleep patterns or too much or too little sleep
- Smoking or exposure to smoke
- Skipping meals
- Alcohol or caffeine
- Sulfites
- Menstrual cycle fluctuations, birth control pills
- Tension headaches
- Foods containing tyramine (red wine, aged cheese, smoked fish, chicken livers, figs, and some beans), monosodium glutamate (MSG)
- Nitrates in processed meat like bacon, hot dogs, and salami
- Other foods such as chocolate, nuts, peanut butter, avocados, bananas, citrus, onions, dairy products, and fermented or pickled foods
- Pesticide-sprayed fruits/vegetables
- Perfumes or fragrances
- Weather
- Liver/gallbladder congestion
- Low serotonin levels

Neural theory. Migraines begin when certain regions of the brain become irritated. The body responds to the irritation by releasing chemicals that, among other things, cause the blood vessels to become inflamed and irritate the nerves.

Other causes include nutritional imbalances and deficiencies, toxicity, sinus congestion, and gallstones in the liver and gallbladder.

✳ Diet Recommendations

Eat more vegetables and other complex carbohydrates. Vegetables; whole grains, such as brown rice and millet; and legumes, such as beans, lentils, and split peas are good choices. Complex carbohydrates appear to help reduce migraines by normalizing serotonin levels. (For more information, see Basic Guidelines for the Juice Lady's Health and Healing Diet, page 290.)

Eliminate all food allergies and intolerances. Various food allergies, sensitivities, and intolerances are thought to underlie many migraine headaches. It is vital to determine which foods trigger an attack. In one study, eleven of the sixteen patients who followed an elimination diet had a significant decrease in headaches, and six became headache-free. In another study, seventy-eight of eighty-three children became headache-free when food allergens were eliminated. Some of the most common migraine-triggering foods are those that contain tyramine. This amino acid is found in alcoholic beverages, especially red wine and beer; yeast products (breads, rolls, crackers) and yeast concentrates found in prepared bouillons and gravies; sour cream; aged cheese, especially Stilton, cheddar, and blue cheese; red plums; figs; aged game; liver; canned and preserved meats and fish; Italian broad beans; string beans; eggplant; and soy sauce. Other foods that commonly trigger migraines include shellfish and fish; citrus fruit, especially oranges; wheat; tea; coffee (including decaf); meat, especially pork and beef; tomatoes; milk; rye; rice; oats; cane sugar; grapes; corn; nuts, especially walnuts; onions; and food additives, especially benzoic acid, sodium nitrate, MSG, NutraSweet, and tartrazine. Avoiding wheat, grains, and sugar seems to be particularly effective (see Allergies, page 27; see also the Elimination Diet, page 301).

Go on a juice fast before identifying your allergens. Before going on the Elimination Diet, follow a one- to three-day vegetable juice fast (see the Juice Fast, page 304). During a juice fast there may be some initial worsening of symptoms, but by the end there is usually a great measure of relief.

Eliminate all sources of monosodium glutamate (MSG). This food additive causes headaches in susceptible individuals. Glutamate is a neurotransmitter that is very excitatory in nature. The brain needs a certain amount of glutamate but too much can cause anxiety, irritability, and headaches. Added as a flavor enhancer, it is often found in packaged and processed foods, Chinese restaurant dishes, frozen foods, prepared meals, soups, chips, boxed dinners and helpers, canned gravy, and salad dressings, especially the "low-fat" ones. Items do not always list it as MSG; it can be called hydrolyzed vegetable protein, Accent, ajinomoto, or natural meat tenderizer, to name a few (for a complete list, see Epilepsy and Seizures, page 145).

Avoid all foods containing aspartame (NutraSweet). This artificial sweetener has been shown to cause severe headaches in some individuals.

Decrease your intake of animal fats. Saturated fats contribute to platelet stickiness, which is connected to migraines. Meat and fatty foods are often reported as triggers of migraine headaches.

Increase your intake of liver-supporting foods. Oriental medicine looks at migraines as being a result of liver problems, a condition known as liver heat. Liver heat is believed to be generated by a strained liver, generally due to overindulgence in rich foods. Overconsumption of meat, cheese, fats, eggs, alcohol, and sweets causes "liver stagnation," and migraines are among the conditions that result from this type of diet. Rye is a grain that Oriental medicine says is especially beneficial for the liver. Rye broth or a watery rye cereal called congee can be very helpful, unless you are allergic to rye or are gluten sensitive. Celery is another food that helps relieve liver heat. If you suffer from migraines, drink celery juice often.

Perform a liver/gallbladder cleanse. When the liver and gallbladder are congested, it can contribute to migraine headaches (see the Liver Cleanse, page 310 and the Gallbladder Cleanse, page 318).

On a personal note: I believe that stones and toxicity in the gallbladder and liver are significant contributors to headaches and migraines. Having suffered for more than ten years with occasional migraines, I can report that liver cleansing, along with the amino acid program (see below), has eliminated my migraines.

❋ Nutrient Recommendations

Amino acids can help balance neurotransmitters, which are the natural chemicals that facilitate communication between brain cells. The neurotransmitter serotonin helps control pain sensations. A deficiency can trigger migraines by encouraging inappropriate contraction and relaxation of the arteries. A lack of serotonin may also lower the pain threshold, making the pain worse. Neurotransmitters are manufactured in the brain from the amino acids (protein building blocks), which are produced in the body and extracted from food. Serotonin is converted from the amino acid L-tryptophan, which breaks down into 5-hydroxytryptophan (5-HTP) for the creation of serotonin. Other cofactors such as B vitamins and enzymes must be present for this to occur. Since L-tryptophan breaks down into 5-HTP at a very low percentage, 5-HTP often needs to be taken as a supplement. Dosages should be based on testing, however. B vitamins are among the necessary nutrients for the creation and transport of L-tryptophan and conversion of 5-HTP into serotonin. They should also be taken as part of the complete wellness plan. Also, varied protein consumption is imperative with this program so include nuts, seeds, beans, eggs, and muscle meats such as fish, chicken, turkey, and beef. (Choose organically fed, free-range/cage-free, with no hormones or antibiotics.) For information on neurotransmitter testing and the amino acid program, see Sources, page 351.

Coenzyme Q10 has been found to have a beneficial effect on the condition of some migraine sufferers. One study found that 61 percent of patients treated with coenzyme Q10 had a greater than 50 percent reduction in the number of days with migraines, making it more effective than most prescription drugs, and fewer than 1 percent reported any side effects. Coenzyme Q10 at dosages of 200 mg per day has been shown to significantly decrease the frequency of migraine headaches.

Essential fatty acids (EFAs), specifically the omega-3 fatty acids, have shown a significant ability to alleviate severe migraines. One study saw both migraine intensity and frequency decrease when individuals were given fish oils rich in omega-3s, which decrease platelet clumping. The best sources of omega-3 fatty acids include cold-water fish, such as salmon, tuna, halibut, cod, trout, and mackerel; flaxseeds, hempseed, and cod-liver oils; and walnuts. (For more information on omega-3 oils, see the fats and oils section in Basic Guidelines for the Juice Lady's Health and Healing Diet, page 290.)

Magnesium. People who suffer migraines often have low blood levels of this mineral. Magnesium helps muscles, including those surrounding arteries, to relax, and this may be why a deficiency of this mineral is linked to migraines. Researchers have learned that some of the same things that deplete the body's supply of magnesium—including stress, alcohol, and pregnancy—can trigger migraines in susceptible people. They also have discovered that certain medicines that successfully treat migraines mimic magnesium's actions. In one study, magnesium citrate reduced the frequency of migraines by almost 42 percent. Magnesium glycinate, the amino acid–bound form of magnesium, is the most absorbable form of magnesium. Less is needed in this format. The glycine is also helpful for calming the brain when it is "hot." *Best juice sources of magnesium:* beetroot greens, spinach, parsley, dandelion greens, garlic, blackberries, beetroot, broccoli, cauliflower, carrots, and celery.

Vitamin B$_3$ (niacin) causes blood-vessel dilation, and so is clearly useful in treating migraine headaches. Studies have found that intramuscular injections of vitamin B$_3$ help relieve migraine headaches. The current recommendation is 500 mg of B$_3$

(taken orally) at the onset of a headache. *Best food sources of this vitamin:* brewer's yeast, rice and wheat bran, peanuts, turkey, chicken, and fish. Vitamin B$_3$ is not available in fruits and vegetables.

✳ Herb Recommendations

Butterbur (*Petasites hybridus*) is a shrub native to Europe and parts of Asia and Africa. For the past thirty years, it has been prescribed for migraines in Germany. Butterbur contains substances that are believed to slow the body's production of leukotriene. With less leukotriene, blood vessels are less likely to become inflamed and migraines are less likely to develop.

Cayenne pepper contains capsaicin, which inhibits platelet clumping (connected to migraines) controls pain. This herb may be most effective in preventing, rather than alleviating, migraine attacks.

Feverfew is the herb most widely recommended for migraine headaches. One study showed that patients who ate fresh feverfew leaves, and who were then taken off feverfew and given an inactive placebo, had a significant increase in the frequency and severity of migraines. It may take up to one month for feverfew to bring relief, though it does not completely prevent attacks.

Lavender and **peppermint** incense and scents are shown to help. The smells of peppermint and lavender have been proven to help with migraines and other headaches—more so than most other scents.

Valerian is a sedative herb that is helpful in treating migraines brought on by stress. This herb will not alleviate the headaches but will lessen the pain.

✳ Juice Therapy

Cantaloupe, garlic, and **gingerroot** juices have all been shown to reduce platelet stickiness (which is connected to migraines).

Celery juice mixed with a little lemon is recommended for headaches.

Parsley juice contains magnesium. Intake should be limited to a safe, therapeutic dose of one-half to one cup per day. Parsley can be toxic in overdose, and should be especially avoided by pregnant women.

✳ Juice Recipes

Immune Builder *(pg 335)* **Ginger Twist** *(pg 332)* **Waldorf Twist** *(pg 345)*
Magnesium-Rich Cocktail *(pg 336)* **Spinach Power** *(pg 341)* **Allergy Relief** *(pg 326)*
Mint Refresher *(pg 337)* **Mood Mender** *(pg 337)* **Liver Life Tonic** *(pg 336)*

Multiple Sclerosis

MULTIPLE SCLEROSIS (MS) is a chronic, slowly progressing disease of the brain, spinal cord, and optic nerves. About 250,000 Americans are diagnosed with MS annually, with women being affected slightly more often than men. Worldwide, MS may affect 2.5 million individuals. In about two-thirds of patients, the disease begins between the ages of twenty and forty. The most common initial symptom is the sudden loss of vision in one eye and/or a tingling or feeling of numbness in one arm or leg. Weakness in a limb can cause fumbling or an unsteady gait. Other symptoms include mental changes; slurred speech; difficulties with bladder control; bowel dysfunction, particularly constipation; depression; difficulty concentrating; muscle weakness or stiffness; memory loss; and fatigue.

The causes of MS are not completely known, although it appears to be an autoimmune reaction in which the body's white blood cells, which normally fight infection, attack the myelin sheath that covers nerves in the spinal cord and brain, leaving scar tissue called sclerosis. Sometimes the nerve fiber itself is damaged or broken. Myelin not only protects nerve fibers; it makes their job possible. When myelin or the nerve fiber is destroyed or damaged, the ability of the nerves to conduct electrical impulses to and from the brain is disrupted, and this produces the various symptoms of MS.

There is not one single cause of MS, but rather a number of possibilities. This autoimmune reaction may occur as the result of an inborn hereditary abnormality being set off by a viral infection, by environmental factors like heavy metal toxicity, or by a psychological trigger such as trauma. Studies show a strong association between MS and a lack of winter sunshine. The disease becomes more prevalent as one moves away from the equator. Decreased sunlight exposure and possibly decreased vitamin D production may contribute to MS. This theory is bolstered by research into the biochemistry of vitamin D, which has shown that it is an important immune-system regulator. A large 2006 study by the Harvard School of Public Health reported a link between vitamin D deficiency and the onset of MS. Other data come from a 2007 study, which concluded that sun exposure during childhood reduces the risk of suffering MS. High meat, gluten (the protein found in bread), and dairy consumption, and a lower intake of fruits and vegetables, are also associated with MS. Dairy states, such as Wisconsin, Iowa, and Oregon, have up to 50 percent more MS cases than such states as Georgia and Tennessee. Dairy states also tend to be at greater latitude than other states, which means that either diet or latitude could be the bigger factor.

To some extent, the myelin can regenerate, allowing partial or complete recovery. Thus attacks may happen less frequently, or they may occur years apart. Conversely, an apparently mild case of MS can turn chronic and progressive, resisting all attempts at treatment. Currently there is no cure for MS, but flare-ups can be tamed or halted. Diet can play an important role in an overall treatment plan.

☀ Lifestyle Recommendations

Get plenty of sunlight. In a study of seventy-nine pairs of twins in which one twin had MS and the other did not, University of Southern California researchers found that sun exposure during childhood was associated with a reduced risk of MS. This study adds to the growing evidence that sun exposure (or vitamin D levels, including those produced by the body in response to sun) may help protect against the development of MS. Though the study doesn't state this, sun exposure might also help slow the progression of MS. Sunlight exposure also balances the secretion of the hormone melatonin. Too much melatonin may overstimulate the thymus gland, which can produce the autoimmune reaction that is believed to occur in MS.

☀ Diet Recommendations

Try the low-saturated-fat Swank diet. Roy Swank, M.D., and his colleagues have shown that diets low in fat cause the illness to go into remission and the symptoms to diminish. Beginning in 1948, Dr. Swank followed 144 MS patients. One group ate a diet very low in saturated fat—17 grams or less per day—while the rest ate more than 20 grams of saturated fat per day. In following patients over a thirty-five-year period, he has shown that those who follow this diet have lower disease-progression rates than those who do not. Most significantly, it has been shown that many patients are able to lead normal lives with dietary manipulation alone.

The low-saturated-fat Swank diet eliminated butter, margarine, hydrogenated oils, hydrogenated peanut butter, and shortening. Patients were allowed 10 to 40 grams of vegetable oils and 5 grams of cod-liver oil per day. During his thirty-five years of study, Dr. Swank observed that the patients who ate 10 to 15 grams or less of saturated fat a day showed the least fatigue and the least progression toward disability. Saturated fats are known to cause blood cells to stick together in clumps. This action may block small blood vessels in the central nervous system, starving some areas for oxygen and resulting in damage to myelin. To follow the Swank diet, avoid most animal products—no meat, poultry, eggs, or dairy. The only animal food permitted is fish, which provides essential fatty acids. Choose gluten-free whole grains, vegetables, fruit, and fresh juices, and eat or juice at least one serving of dark green vegetables every day.

Thomas Kruzel, N.D., observed that MS patients he's worked with begin to experience changes in the disease process within four to six weeks of starting the Swank diet, and often sooner. The longer the person continues with the diet, the more improvement occurs. He found that even people with severe manifestations of the illness receive some benefit. Inevitably, at some time in the process, a person will go off the dietary recommendations to see if in fact it is really helping or if he or she is just going through a period of remission. In every case, symptoms begin to return within a short period of time and resolve when the patient begins to follow the proper diet again.

Omit gluten-containing grains. The connection between MS and allergies may be the reason that the MacDougall treatment is effective for some people. Roger MacDougall was severely affected by MS. Confined to a wheelchair and almost blind, he created a diet for MS and, over the course of years, became virtually free of symptoms. Today, his eyesight is restored and he has full use of his legs. His diet forbids all gluten-containing cereals such as wheat, oats, rye, and barley. Like Swank, MacDougall also recommends severely limiting saturated fats, and strictly forbids dairy products, including butter, cream, and cheese. In addition, he recommends taking vitamins and minerals, including the B complex vitamins as well as vitamins C and E, calcium, magnesium, and zinc.

Use fresh juice and juice fasting in your treatment plan. Dr. Norman Walker, one of the great pioneers in juicing, recommended three quarts of fresh vegetable juice each day for MS. He observed that the juices, along with frequent colonics, slowly helped MS patients to recover. He specifically recommended carrot, celery, parsley, and spinach juices. Juices are rich in flavonoids. A survey of medical journal articles shows a preponderance of evidence that MS attacks occur during breakdowns of the blood–brain barrier. Some articles show that flavonoids can inhibit blood–brain barrier breakdown in rats under conditions that normally lead to such breakdowns. Flavonoids are also effective in reducing inflammation. Periodic juice fasts lasting from one to three days may also be beneficial (see the Juice Fast, page 304).

✳ Nutrient Recommendations

Alpha lipoic acid was shown to be helpful in a study of mice, and recently showed biochemical marker improvement in a human trial. A dose of 50 mg of alpha lipoic acid daily may be helpful.

Amino acids. Because depression is often a symptom associated with MS, and because serotonin is often low in MS, it can be beneficial to supplement the diet with amino acids tailored to your specific needs (for more information, see Depression, page 125).

Antioxidants. It appears that treatment with high levels of antioxidants can be helpful. The antioxidants include vitamin C, vitamin E, beta-carotene, and selenium. These antioxidants should be taken every day for the rest of your life. If you drink two to three quarts of vegetable juice daily, you'll be getting an abundance of these antioxidants and should not need additional supplementation.

Essential fatty acids (EFAs) can arrest or slow the deterioration of myelin. In parts of the world where EFA consumption is high, MS is rare. Since MS is a degradation of nerve tissue, make sure the most important omega-3 brain fats, eicosapentaenoic acid (EPA) and docosahexaenoic acid (DHA), are taken in adequate amounts. The best oils are cod-liver oil or hemp-seed oil; unrefined sesame oils are also helpful. In addition, evening primrose oil has been used in the treatment of MS, and octacosanol, present in wheat germ oil, may help nerves regenerate. Buy small amounts of these oils at a time, and keep them refrigerated at all times. These oils can go rancid quickly, which will do you more harm than good. Cold-water fish and fish oil are other good sources of omega-3s EFAs—especially the anti-inflammatory. Best choices are salmon, tuna, trout, mackerel, herring, sardines, and kippers. Another EFA, gamma-linolenic acid (GLA), can be found in black and red currant juices, but is most readily obtainable in capsule form. You should also decrease the omega-6 fats in your diet, which is very important in preventing and treating MS. Therefore, omit polyunsaturated oils like soy, canola, sunflower, corn, and safflower oil. You may use extra-virgin olive oil and virgin coconut oil. (For more information on omega-3 oils, see the fats and oils section in Basic Guidelines for the Juice Lady's Health and Healing Diet, page 290.)

Vitamin D appears to protect the body against MS. An analysis of the blood serum of more than 7 million U.S. military personnel, 257 of whom had MS, found that vitamin D is associated with a lower risk of MS. It has been observed that people in temperate latitudes may be more prone to MS because of a vitamin D deficiency. Insufficient exposure to sunlight may not allow the body to make enough vitamin D_3, the hormonal form of vitamin D. Studies show that administering vitamin D_3 completely prevents an MS-like disease in mice. The relative scarcity of MS in Japan and coastal Norway, and among Eskimo populations, could be explained by local diets that are rich in fish, an excellent source of vitamin D_3. *Best food sources of vitamin D:* cold-water fish, sunflower seeds, sunflower sprouts, and mushrooms. This vitamin is not found in appreciable amounts in fruits or vegetables. Cod-liver oil is an excellent source of both omega-3 fatty acids and vitamin D. Recommendation is one to two tablespoons per day.

Vitamin E helps prevent lipid peroxidation, which is free-radical damage to fats in cells. *Best juice sources of vitamin E:* spinach, watercress, asparagus, carrots, and tomatoes.

✳ Herb Recommendations

Curcumin. Preliminary studies in mice suggest that curcumin, a compound found in the curry spice turmeric, may block the progression of MS. According to researchers at Vanderbilt University, mice with an MS-like illness showed little or no signs of disease symptoms after being injected with curcumin, while animals without the treatment went on to severe paralysis.

Dandelion and **echinacea** are used as detoxification herbs. **Valerian** is used for its calming effect.

✳ Juice Therapy

Carrot, celery, parsley, and **spinach** juices. Drink three quarts of this juice combination each day. Other juice recipes can be added in place of some of this combination. Choose from the list below.

✳ Juice Recipes

Pure Green Sprout Drink *(pg 340)*   **Spinach Power** *(pg 341)*   **Spring Tonic** *(pg 342)*   **Morning Energizer** *(pg 337)*   **Salsa in a Glass** *(pg 340)*   **Allergy Relief** *(pg 326)*   **Beet-Cucumber Cleansing Cocktail** *(pg 328)*   **Gallbladder-Liver Cleansing Cocktail** *(pg 331)*   **Happy Morning** *(pg 333)*   **Mood Mender** *(pg 337)*   **Magnesium-Rich Cocktail** *(pg 336)*   **Peppy Parsley** *(pg 329)* **The Revitalizer** *(pg 340)*   **Wheatgrass Light** *(pg 345)*

Osteoarthritis

OSTEOARTHRITIS (OA) is also known as degenerative arthritis and degenerative joint disease. It is the most common form of arthritis, afflicting more than 46 million Americans (see also Rheumatoid Arthritis, page 255), with women outnumbering men after the age of forty-five. A significant percentage of all osteoarthritis commences in the knees; other common sites are the hips, hands, and spine. Osteoarthritis can begin as early as age thirty, and the number of people affected increases dramatically with age, with 80 percent of all persons over age sixty-five showing some signs of the disorder. Mild early-morning stiffness, stiffness following periods of rest, pain that gets worse on joint use, and loss of joint function are often the first symptoms. As the disease progresses, more joints may be affected, and the bone can become deformed.

Osteoarthritis causes the joints, especially the cartilage that lines the joints, to degenerate. Many people erroneously think that OA is due to wear and tear. This common misconception is due to the fact that OA typically does not show up in younger people. OA is actually caused by the water content of cartilage increasing while protein composition of cartilage degenerates. Besides aging, factors that may increase the risk of developing osteoarthritis include injury to joints, repetitive use of joints, being overweight, stressing the joints, and family history. There is some evidence that allergies—fungal, infectious, or systemically induced—may be a significant contributing factor to the appearance of OA in a synovial sac. People with OA have low-grade inflammation that results in pain in the joints, causing abnormal wearing of the cartilage that covers and acts as a cushion inside joints, along with destruction or decrease of the synovial fluid that lubricates those joints. Secondary osteoarthritis is associated with such predisposing factors as bone or joint abnormalities, injury, or inflammatory disease. OA can be halted and even reversed through dietary and lifestyle changes.

✳ Lifestyle Recommendations

Get physical therapy, use support devices, and get regular exercise. No matter what the severity, or where the OA lies, conservative measures, such as weight control, appropriate rest and exercise, and the use of mechanical support devices are usually beneficial. Knee braces, a cane, or a walker can be helpful aids for walking and support. See your doctor for a referral to a qualified physical therapist. The Arthritis Foundation states that physical therapy may be the single most valuable treatment for arthritis. In addition, you should engage in regular, low-impact exercise such as walking or swimming. Applying local heat before and cold packs after exercise can help relieve pain and inflammation, as can relaxation techniques. Weight loss can relieve joint stress and may delay progression of the disease.

Prayer and spirituality. Public opinion polls have shown that prayer is one of the most commonly used alternative therapies for arthritis. Research in behavioral medicine suggests that the interactions of the mind, body, and spirit can have powerful effects on our health. Only a few published scientific studies have examined the effects of prayer and spirituality on disease. Adding or deepening the spiritual aspects in your life could be good for you and your arthritis.

Reduce or eliminate the use of nonsteroidal anti-inflammatory drugs (NSAIDs) and aspirin. These drugs not only have gastrointestinal side effects, they also inhibit the creation of collagen, the main protein found in cartilage, and they increase joint destruction.

✳ Diet Recommendations

Eat a high-fiber diet. Include more raw foods—fruits, vegetables, vegetable juices, sprouts, nuts, and seeds—in your meal plans. Strive for a diet in which 50 to 60 percent of what you eat and drink consists of raw foods and juices. Following a high-fiber diet will also help you maintain a normal weight, especially if you exercise regularly. The Arthritis Center of Boston University says that being overweight is the most potent risk factor for osteoarthritis, especially of the knee and also the hips and hands (see Weight Loss, page 283; also see Basic Guidelines for the Juice Lady's Health and Healing Diet, page 290).

Avoid the nightshade family. Tomatoes, potatoes, eggplant, chili peppers, and bell peppers fall into this category, as does tobacco. Some researchers believe that the solanines in these plants either inhibit normal collagen repair in the joints or promote inflammatory degeneration. You may notice some improvement by eliminating this group of foods, and by not using tobacco. A number of doctors estimate that about a third of their patients are affected by the nightshade family. The best way to determine whether you are sensitive to the nightshades is to avoid this group of foods for about three months and see if you improve.

You might need to avoid citrus fruit. A certain percentage of people with OA notice improvement when they stop eating citrus fruit. Don't eat oranges, grapefruits, tangerines, lemons, and limes for three to four weeks, and see if you notice an improvement.

Reduce fats. A diet high in saturated animal fats or polyunsaturated vegetable oils (corn, soy, safflower, sunflower, and canola) can increase the inflammatory response, thereby contributing to joint and tissue inflammation. (Use extra-virgin olive oil and virgin coconut oil.)

Use cleansing programs, including juice fasting and liver cleansing. The removal of toxic substances from the joints through the lymphatic system can help reduce cartilage damage (see the Juice Fast, page 304, the Liver Cleanse, and the Gallbladder Cleanse, pages 310 and 318).

✳ Nutrient Recommendations

B vitamins, specifically vitamin B$_{12}$ (cobalamin), folic acid, and pantothenic acid, are important in treating osteoarthritis. Folic acid and vitamin B$_{12}$ have been shown in several studies to help arthritic hand joints, and pantothenic acid has provided relief from symptoms when as little as 12.5 mg was taken daily. Vitamin B$_{12}$ is not found in foods that can be juiced. *Best food sources of vitamin B$_{12}$:* meat, poultry, and fish. *Best juice sources of folic acid:* asparagus, spinach, kale, broccoli, cabbage, and blackberries. *Best juice sources of pantothenic acid:* broccoli, cauliflower, and kale.

Glucosamine is a naturally occurring substance found in joint structures that stimulates cartilage regeneration, protects against joint destruction, and alleviates the symptoms of osteoarthritis. As some people age, they lose the ability to manufacture sufficient levels of glucosamine. The result is that cartilage loses its gel-like consistency and its ability to act as a shock absorber. A substance derived from glucosamine is used to make certain components of cartilage and synovial fluid. Research indicates that supplemental glucosamine may improve symptoms of OA and delay its progression. The recommended dosage is 1,500 mg daily of glucosamine sulfate (divide into three doses of 500 mg each).

Phytoestrogens are estrogen-like factors found in plants that can help protect cartilage. *Best juice sources of phytoestrogens:* apples, celery, fennel, and parsley. Although soy foods are rich in phytoestrogens, it is not recommended that you use soy milk or processed soy products because they inhibit thyroid function, can contribute to breast cancer, and can cause weight gain. They are usually produced from genetically modified (GM) soybeans, which adds to the harmful effects of soy. It is still safe to use non-GM tofu, tempeh, or miso in small quantities.

SAMe (S-adenosylmethionine) in small-scale studies has been shown to be as effective as nonsteroidal anti-inflammatory drugs (NSAIDs) in reducing pain, although it takes about four weeks for the effect to take place. It also appears to be well tolerated by most people.

Vitamin C can promote collagen synthesis and repair. *Best juice sources of vitamin C:* kale, parsley, broccoli, Brussels sprouts, watercress, cauliflower, cabbage, spinach, turnips, and asparagus.

Vitamin D is needed for joint health. Studies show that low blood levels of vitamin D are associated with both the loss of cartilage and the development of bony outgrowths called osteophytes. In addition, low vitamin D levels present a risk factor for disease progression in osteoarthritic knees. Vitamin D in its active form is a hormone, and our bodies make it from sunlight. People who live in primarily overcast climates such as the Pacific Northwest should supplement their diets with vitamin D. This vitamin is not found in fruits and vegetables. *Best food sources of vitamin D:* cold-water fish, cod-liver oil, sunflower seeds, sunflower sprouts (can be juiced), and mushrooms.

Vitamin E has been shown to help fight OA, possibly because of its membrane-stabilizing effect and its ability to stimulate increased deposits of proteoglycans, substances that form part of the joint structure. *Best juice sources of vitamin E:* spinach, watercress, asparagus, and carrots.

✳ Herb Recommendations

Boswellia serrata is an herbal supplement known in Ayurvedic medicine to have antiarthritic effects. It is widely available in health food stores and online.

Devil's claw has anti-inflammatory and pain-relieving effects.

✳ Juice Therapy

Dandelion juice, half a cup in the morning and half a cup in the evening, has been used as a traditional remedy for osteoarthritis. Dandelion juice is very strong-tasting, so it helps to mix it with carrot or other mild-tasting juices, as in Liver Life Tonic (see page 336).

Gingerroot has been used in Ayurvedic (traditional Indian) medicine to ease inflammation. In one study of OA patients, more than 75 percent found varying degrees of relief from pain and swelling after using gingerroot. Some research has found that gingerroot extract may be helpful in reducing OA pain.

Parsley juice is an excellent source of phytoestrogens and vitamin C. Intake should be limited to a safe, therapeutic dose of one-half to one cup per day. Parsley can be toxic in overdose, and should be especially avoided by pregnant women.

✳ Juice Recipes

Liver Life Tonic *(pg 336)*   The Ginger Hopper *(pg 332)*   Ginger Twist *(pg 332)*
Calcium-Rich Cocktail *(pg 329)*   Pure Green Sprout Drink *(pg 340)*   Magnesium-
Rich Cocktail *(pg 336)*   Mood Mender *(pg 337)*   Peppy Parsley *(pg 339)*

Osteoporosis

OSTEOPOROSIS means "porous bone." It is normal for bones to lose density after age forty at a rate of about 2 percent per year. But in osteoporosis, the rate of bone loss exceeds that of bone creation. As a result, bone is lost gradually from the spine, hips, and ribs, which become more fragile and prone to fracture.

Osteoporosis is a major public health threat for an estimated 44 million Americans, or 55 percent of people fifty years of age and older. In the United States, 10 million individuals are estimated to already have the disease, and almost 34 million more are estimated to have low bone mass, placing them at increased risk for osteoporosis. Of the 10 million Americans estimated to have osteoporosis, 8 million are women and 2 million are men. Women are often more prone to osteoporosis at menopause, when their bodies produce less estrogen, which is involved with calcium in bone health. While osteoporosis is often thought of as an older person's disease, it can strike at any age.

A fracture, often after just a minor injury, may be the first sign that a person has osteoporosis. Back pain can occur when weakened vertebrae collapse. When a fracture does occur, it tends to heal very slowly. Risk factors for developing this condition include smoking, excessive use of alcohol, low calcium intake, vitamin D deficiency, lack of weight-bearing exercise, family history, low testosterone levels in men, estrogen deficiency as a result of menopause (especially early onset or surgically induced), and the use of certain medications, including steroids and barbiturates. There is also a strong association among cadmium, lead, and bone disease. Low-level exposure to cadmium or lead is associated with an increased loss of bone mineral density in both genders, leading to pain and increased risk of fractures, especially in the elderly and in females. Higher cadmium exposure results in osteomalacia (softening of the bone). People are exposed to cadmium by eating food grown in contaminated soil or fish from tainted water, but more extreme exposure comes from smoking or interaction with smelting, welding, or ship-building. Smoking doubles the average daily intake of cadmium.

✳ Lifestyle Recommendations

Exercise. Get at least thirty minutes of bone-strengthening activity at least five days a week. Muscle weakness can contribute to falls, so it is beneficial for people living with osteoporosis to strengthen muscles. Include both weight-bearing activities, like running or brisk walking, and resistance exercise.

Know your risk. Most guidelines recommend osteoporosis screening through bone mineral density (BMD) testing starting at age sixty-five or earlier for women who have health conditions or take medications that increase risk. To take the "Check Up On Your Bones" self-test, go to: www.niams.nih.gov/Health_Info/Bone/Optool/index.asp

Be aware of the depression connection. Research has found links between depression and bone loss. For example, women with a history of major depression have lower bone density and higher levels of cortisol, a hormone related to bone loss. If you're being treated for depression, ask your clinician whether you should have a BMD test. For information on how to nutritionally balance your body to alleviate those blues, see Depression, page 125.

How's your thyroid health? The thyroid makes a hormone called calcitronin that facilitates the absorption of calcium. If you're taking thyroid medication, that won't fix the underlying problem, and the calcium absorption will remain impaired. There is a high percentage of osteoporosis among people with hypothyroidism. It is very important to incorporate thyroid-supporting solutions into your bone-health program. For extensive information on this subject and a thyroid health quiz, see my book *The Coconut Diet*.

Maintain a healthy weight. If you lose a lot of weight during the menopausal transition, you're more likely to lose bone. Avoid extreme low-calorie diets.

Avoid falls. Keep floors clear of tripping hazards. Make sure stairways and entrances are well lit, use nonslide bath mats, and add grab bars to your bathtub or shower.

✳ Diet Recommendations

Eat a high-complex-carbohydrate diet with moderate protein intake. Diets high in animal proteins (which are high in phosphates) have been linked to increased loss of calcium. In research studies, high protein intake is known to encourage urinary calcium loss and has been shown to increase the risk of fracture. The best diet is one based on whole foods, rich in vegetables and fruit. (For more information on the healthy diet plan, see Basic Guidelines for the Juice Lady's Health and Healing Diet, page 290.)

Eat your vegetables and drink fresh green juices. Green vegetables such as kale, collards, parsley, and the darker green lettuces are rich in vitamins and minerals like vitamin K, calcium, magnesium, and boron; they are needed to support healthy joints and bones. Vegetables help preserve your bones. Researchers found that rats that ate common herbs and vegetables, such as onion, parsley, and salad greens, had significantly less bone loss than rats not on the special diet. A number of vegetables and vegetable mixtures, such as onion and Italian parsley, and a mixture of lettuce, tomato, cucumber, arugula, garlic, parsley, and dill, produced significant reduction in the rate of bone loss. One of the best ways to prevent bone loss is to normalize high body-acid levels with vegetables and vegetable juice. Vegetable juice, especially the green juices, is high in minerals and vitamin K that will actually anchor calcium into your bone matrix.

What about dairy? In a study with rats, soybeans and milk powder—foods thought to help slow the process of osteoporosis—had no effect on the rats' rate of bone reabsorption. Another study showed a major link between vegetable and fruit intake for increased bone density; no such effect was found for dairy products.

You may need to choose gluten-free. In one study, about 5 percent of people with osteoporosis also had celiac disease, compared with only 0.2 percent of people with healthy bones. Researchers say this occurrence was high enough to justify regularly screening patients with osteoporosis for celiac disease, and if the results come back positive, to put them on a gluten-free diet to treat both conditions. Gluten is found in wheat, rye, barley, and oats. You might benefit from omitting these grains. Try omitting them for three months and see if your bones strengthen.

Avoid alcohol, tobacco, caffeine, and aluminum. Studies show that bone loss is directly correlated with smoking and excessive alcohol use. (Smoking introduces damaging levels of cadmium into the body.) Smokers have been shown to lose bone faster and have higher rates of fracture. Studies have shown that even moderate coffee consumption, on the order of two to three cups daily, will cause calcium loss. Aluminum, which is used in baking powder, salt, cookware, antacids, processed cheese, and deodorant, to name a few places, can interfere with calcium absorption. Be sure to choose only aluminum-free products.

Avoid sodas. Some studies indicate that soft drinks (many of which contain phosphoric acid) may increase risk of osteoporosis. When phosphate levels are high and calcium levels are low, calcium is leached out of the bones. Sodas may be a major factor in osteoporosis because Americans consume such large quantities of them—about three quarts per week for every person in the country.

Avoid table salt. The much-used common table salt (sodium chloride) has additives such as aluminum to make it easy to pour. But aluminum interferes with calcium absorption. Also, this salt is devoid of minerals. Instead, use Celtic sea salt or gray salt, either of which is rich in minerals that are good for bone health. You'll find this type of salt at health food stores. These are different from the refined sea salt you'll find at most grocery stores.

✳ Nutrient Recommendations

There is scientific evidence to suggest that bone density is supported by a wide variety of nutrients in addition to calcium and vitamin D, which include boron, magnesium, zinc, copper, manganese, silicon, strontium, folic acid, and vitamins B_6, C, and K. One of the best ways to consume a wide array of vitamins and minerals is to juice lots of different vegetables. Add to that a few key supplements such as vitamin D and calcium, and follow the diet recommendations in this chapter, and you should be able to maintain healthy bones for life.

Boron can help prevent urinary loss of calcium. Boron is widely available in fruits and vegetables.

Calcium, when taken in adequate amounts, can slow the rate of postmenopausal bone loss by 30 to 50 percent. Adequate calcium intake has been shown to produce significant improvements in bone density more than five years after menopause. A large randomized controlled study found that the use of calcium, or calcium in combination with vitamin D supplementation, was effective in the preventive treatment of osteoporosis in people age fifty years or older. *Best therapeutic doses:* 1,200 mg of calcium daily (calcium citrate is a good choice); 800 IU of vitamin D$_3$ daily. *Best juice sources of calcium:* kale, parsley, dandelion greens, watercress, beetroot greens, broccoli, spinach, romaine lettuce, string beans, celery, and carrots. Vitamin D$_3$ is available in fish and fish oil, which is more absorbable and healthier than the vitamin D added to fortified products.

Copper deficiency can result in fragile bones. Copper is essential for the effectiveness of an enzyme that is involved in the creation of collagen, the major structural component of bone. *Best juice sources of copper:* carrots, garlic, gingerroot, and turnips.

Magnesium helps calcium get in and out of cells. An Israeli study revealed that women who consumed 250 to 750 mg of magnesium daily experienced bone density increases of up to 8 percent. Reduced amounts of magnesium can negatively affect the body's use of estrogen, which in turn affects the bones. *Best juice sources of magnesium:* beetroot greens, spinach, parsley, dandelion greens, garlic, blackberries, beetroot, broccoli, cauliflower, carrots, and celery.

Manganese is required for the creation of connective tissue, especially cartilage, and is generally deficient in the standard American diet. *Best juice sources of manganese:* spinach, beetroot greens, Brussels sprouts, carrots, broccoli, cabbage, beetroot, apples, and pears.

Potassium. Studies have shown that potassium helps your kidneys retain calcium, whereas low potassium intake leads to increasing losses of calcium in the urine. *Best juice sources of potassium:* sunflower sprouts, parsley, Swiss chard, garlic, spinach, broccoli, carrots, celery, radishes, watercress, and asparagus.

Silicon promotes the formation of bones and teeth. *Best juice sources of silicon:* bell pepper, cucumber, and root vegetables.

Vitamin C is important in the production of collagen. *Best juice sources of vitamin C:* kale, parsley, broccoli, Brussels sprouts, watercress, cauliflower, cabbage, strawberries, spinach, lemons, limes, turnips, and asparagus.

Vitamin D is associated with a significant reduction in the number of hip fractures among postmenopausal women. It's been shown to reduce fractures up to 25 percent in older people. Vitamin D deficiency can also cause muscle weakness. A large analysis of five clinical trials showed that 800 IU of vitamin D per day (plus calcium) reduced the risk of falls by 22 percent. Vitamin D supplementation can also help prevent bone loss and OA that occurs as the result of problems with the parathyroid glands (located in the neck). For those fifty and under, take between 400 and 800 IU daily, and those over fifty, take 800 to 1,000 IU daily. Vitamin D is not available in fruits and vegetables. *Best food sources of vitamin D:* cold-water fish, fish oil (especially cod-liver oil), sunflower seeds, sunflower sprouts (can be juiced), and mushrooms.

Vitamin K is found in plants, especially green leafy vegetables. It is important for converting a substance called osteocalcin (noncollagenous protein found in bone) to its active form, which anchors calcium in bone. *Best juice sources of vitamin K (K1 is the natural plant form of this vitamin):* kale, collard and turnip greens, broccoli, parsley, lettuce, cabbage, spinach, watercress, asparagus, and string beans.

Zinc can stimulate protein synthesis in bone. *Best juice sources of zinc:* gingerroot, turnips, parsley, garlic, carrots, grapes, spinach, cabbage, lettuce, and cucumbers.

✳ Herb Recommendations

Alfalfa, dong quai, and **licorice** all contain phytoestrogens that may be suitable alternatives to synthetic estrogen; you and your doctor can decide on the natural hormone replacement regimen that's best for you (see Menopause, page 207). Avoid licorice if you have high blood pressure, do not use it for prolonged periods of time, and use a medicinal form of the herb, not licorice candy.

✳ Juice Therapy

Kale is a good source of calcium and vitamins C and K, nutrients needed for good bone health.

Parsley juice is rich in calcium, magnesium, vitamin K, and zinc. Intake should be limited to a safe, therapeutic dose of one-half to one cup per day. Parsley can be toxic in overdose, and should be especially avoided by pregnant women.

✳ Juice Recipes

Calcium-Rich Cocktail *(pg 329)*   **Sweet Dreams Nightcap** *(pg 342)*   **Memory Mender** *(pg 336)*   **Pure Green Sprout Drink** *(pg 340)*   **The Ginger Hopper** *(pg 332)* **Immune Builder** *(pg 335)*   **Magnesium-Rich Cocktail** *(pg 336)*   **Jack & the Bean** *(pg 335)*   **Peppy Parsley** *(pg 339)*   **Happy Morning** *(pg 333)*   **Spinach Power** *(pg 341)*

Parasitic Infections

Parasites are creatures that feed off a host organism, and when the host is our bodies they can cause us considerable harm. Protozoa (single-cell organisms), such as Cryptosporidia, Giardia lamblia, Entamoeba histolytica, Blastocystis hominis, and Dientamoeba fragilis; helminths or worms, such as pinworms, roundworms, tapeworms, and hookworms; and flukes, such as blood and liver flukes, are a major cause of illness in the United States. And the problem is getting worse. Research suggests that three out of every five Americans will be infected by parasites at some point in their lives. Parasitic infections are often misdiagnosed, since health-care professionals, like most people, think these infections only occur in developing countries. This is simply not true.

Symptoms of parasitic infection include digestive problems like bloating, flatulence, abdominal pain, chronic constipation or diarrhea, anal itching, and mucus in the stool. Other parts of the body can also be affected, causing allergies, vaginal irritation, joint and muscle aches, brain or nervous system damage, immune dysfunction, night sweats, blood-sugar fluctuations, sudden food cravings, extreme emaciation or overweight, and chronic fatigue. The presence of one or more of these symptoms does not mean that one is infected, however, merely that it might be worth investigating the possibility.

Just as varied as the symptoms are the points of contamination, such as international travel, improperly washed or undercooked food, infected food handlers, contaminated water, household pets, day-care centers, and sexual partners. Another factor is the overuse of antibiotics that kill both good and bad bacteria, which disrupts the balance of the digestive tract and allows pathogens to multiply more freely.

Parasites depend on their host for survival. They leach nutrients that the host needs. Parasites can also cause nutritional deficiencies by impairing nutrient absorption and/or causing increased nutrient loss through the stool. Different organisms can cause malabsorption of different nutrients. For example, the tapeworm Diphyllobothrium lathum interferes with the absorption of vitamin B_{12}, which can cause pernicious anemia, and roundworm infection may interfere with the absorption of vitamin A. When an infection causes diarrhea, there may be serious nutrient losses that result in an impaired immune function.

✳ Lifestyle Recommendations

Follow safe food-preparation practices. Knowing how to head off parasites before they reach the dinner table is vital, especially if you are prone to parasitic infections. Wash your hands often, especially after handling raw meat, fish, or eggs. Disinfect cutting boards and utensils by soaking them in a gallon of water to which a teaspoon of chlorine bleach has been added or put them in the dishwasher. Cook animal protein thoroughly: meat and poultry until it is no longer pink inside and the juices run clear, fish until it is flaky and white, and eggs until the yolks are set.

✳ Diet Recommendations

Parasites invade bodily structures and inflict damage to those structures, so healing requires both elimination of the parasites and the regeneration of the affected structures through dietary and nutritional supplements.

Cleanse the colon. Parasites tend to become embedded in a mucus-encrusted intestinal wall. It is difficult to dislodge them until the mucus matter is removed. Mucus layers form as a result of eating devitalized, refined, or spoiled food; taking prescription or recreational drugs; and ingesting toxic or irritating substances, such as coffee, alcohol, and candy and other sweets. The body produces mucus to protect the intestinal tract from irritants. But when we consume irritating or toxic substances on a regular basis, the body's colon-cleansing processes become overwhelmed, and mucus layers build up (see the Intestinal Cleanse, page 307).

Eat your vegetables. This food group should make up about half of your daily diet, with a large percentage being raw. Vegetables contain a host of the nutrients you may be deficient in, and they promote the growth of beneficial intestinal bacteria. Especially choose vegetables rich in carotenes; they're the orange, red, and dark green veggies.

Drink vegetable juices and pure water. Vegetable juices can help heal the intestinal tract because of their high vitamin, mineral, and phytonutrient content. Minimize your use of fruit juices, which contain too much sugar. (Parasites like sugar.) Drink no more than four ounces of fruit juice daily, always diluted by half with pure water. Drink at least eight eight-ounce glasses of water a day. Use a water filter fine enough to catch extremely tiny parasites, such as cryptosporidia.

Eat only lean, well-cooked protein. Fish, white-meat turkey, chicken, eggs, and lamb are all good choices, especially if they're free-range/cage-free, and organically raised (no hormones, antibiotics, or pesticides). This food group should make up about a quarter of your daily diet. These foods provide the amino acid building blocks necessary to rebuild tissues and strengthen the immune system. At least 50 percent of your diet should come from vegetables, with an emphasis on raw veggies and vegetable juice. The other quarter of your diet can be made up of nuts, seeds, and legumes (lentils, split peas, and beans) with a small portion from whole grains (quinoa, rye, oats, brown and wild rice, and barley). Limit the grains, since they quickly turn to sugar, and omit wheat; many people are sensitive to this grain. Don't eat too much of any food that causes flatulence. This irritates the gastrointestinal tract, and compounds the malabsorption problem. The goal is to eat foods that will promote healing of the digestive system.

Choose healthy oils. Virgin coconut oil, hemp-seed oil, evening primrose oil, and black currant seed oil help lubricate the intestinal tract and serve as carriers of fat-soluble vitamins such as A and E. Virgin coconut oil may provide an effective defense against many parasites, including giardia. Research has confirmed that, like bacteria and fungi, giardia is destroyed by the medium-chain fatty acids (MCFAs) found in coconut oil. By using coconut oil and other coconut products every day, you may be able to get rid of giardia and possibly other protozoa. In one study, it was reported that treatment with dried coconut, followed by magnesium sulfate (a laxative), caused 90 percent parasite expulsion after twelve hours. (For more information, see the fats and oils section in Basic Guidelines for the Juice Lady's Health and Healing Diet, page 290.)

Completely eliminate sugar, alcohol, dairy, and unhealthy fat from your diet; parasites thrive on these foods. That means no sucrose (white sugar), brown sugar, corn syrup, fructose, dehydrated cane juice, fruit concentrate, honey, molasses, maple syrup, and brown rice syrup. Avoid not only all sweets and desserts, but also all dried fruit and full-strength fruit juices. Eat fresh fruit sparingly. Parasites love to dine on sugars. Sugar also suppresses the immune system, your much-needed ally in the battle with parasites. Also, be aware that alcohol and refined-flour products such as bread, rolls, pasta, and pizza dough turn to sugar quickly within the body, so avoid them along with dairy products and unhealthy fats and oils—most animal fats, trans fats, and hydrogenated and partially hydrogenated fats such as margarine, along with polyunsaturated vegetable oils such as corn, soy, safflower, sunflower, and canola oils, should be omitted.

Eat antiparasitic foods. Pumpkin and pumpkin seeds, garlic, onions, radishes, kelp, raw cabbage, ground raw almonds, and sauerkraut all act against parasites.

✳ Nutrient Recommendations

Carotenes and **vitamin A** are especially important nutrients, since they help increase resistance to the penetration of parasitic larvae into tissues. Vitamin A is only present in fruits and vegetables in the form of carotenes like beta-carotene, which the body can convert to vitamin A as needed. *Best juice sources of carotenes:* carrots, kale, parsley, spinach, Swiss chard, beetroot greens, watercress, broccoli, and romaine lettuce.

Digestive enzymes. Proteases are digestive enzymes that break down protein. They're responsible, along with other digestive secretions, for keeping the small intestine free of parasites. Use undiluted pancreatic extract (8-10X USP), 750 to 1,000 mg ten to twenty minutes before meals. Bromelain (pineapple enzymes) and papain (papaya enzymes) are digestive aids that can also act against parasites. Because of the sugars in the fruits, the supplement form is best.

Hydrochloric acid, a digestive fluid normally found in the stomach, can destroy many parasites. After age forty, hydrochloric acid secretion diminishes, which lowers resistance to parasites. Some people are genetically prone to low hydrochloric acid levels, as are people who are under a lot of stress. Supplemental betaine HCl with pepsin can be helpful; take one to three 10-mg tablets or capsules with meals. Always eat some food first before taking betaine HCL.

Thymus extract improves thymus gland activity. The thymus gland is responsible for many immune functions, including production of T cells. These white blood cells are responsible for what is called cell-mediated immunity, an immune function that is very important for parasite resistance. If you suffer from parasites, it is a good indicator that your immune system is not functioning well. Use predigested calf thymus extract in a recommended dose of 750 mg per day.

✳ Herb Recommendations

Barberry, goldenseal, and **Oregon grape root** can be effective against different types of parasites. Do not use any of these herbs if you are pregnant, and do not use them for more than ten days at a time.

Clove oil is excellent for a variety of parasites, but it must be from cloves that have not been irradiated. Irradiation destroys its medicinal properties.

Grapefruit seed extract is highly effective against bacteria, protozoa, yeast, and viruses.

Green hulls of black walnut in tincture work against tapeworms.

Pinkroot is especially effective against roundworms.

✳ Juice Therapy

Cabbage and **radish** juices are antiparasitic.

Garlic juice is effective against roundworm, pinworm, tapeworm, and hookworm.

Green juices are particularly helpful for all types of parasites.

✳ Juice Recipes

Orient Express *(pg 338)* **Triple C** *(pg 344)* **Turnip Time** *(pg 344)* **Morning Energizer** *(pg 337)* **Immune Builder** *(pg 335)* **Spinach Power** *(pg 341)* **Afternoon Refresher** *(pg 326)* **Garlic Surprise** *(pg 332)* **Salsa in a Glass** *(pg 340)* **Sinus Solution** *(pg 341)* **Pure Green Sprout Drink** *(pg 340)* **Colon Cleanser** *(pg 330)*

Prostate Enlargement, Benign (BPH)

THE PROSTATE is a chestnut-size gland that surrounds the urethra, the narrow tube through which both sperm and urine flow. This gland secretes the milky white fluid that transports and protects sperm. As a man ages, the prostate can start to enlarge, creating a condition known medically as benign prostatic hyperplasia (BPH). The early stages of BPH may be symptom-free. But symptoms generally develop as the enlargement continues, and include an increased need to urinate, nighttime awakening to urinate, and reduced flow of urine. Urination can become painful. If left untreated, BPH can eventually obstruct the bladder outlet. This causes retention of urine, which can lead to bladder infection and possibly kidney damage.

BPH is very common, and affects more than 50 percent of all men at some time in their lives. It is thought to be the result of hormonal changes associated with aging. Levels of testosterone decrease, but levels of other hormones, including estrogen and prolactin, increase. Scientists note that many older men continue to produce and accumulate high levels of DHT (a substance derived from testosterone) in the prostate gland, which can encourage the growth of cells. The increase in DHT is largely due to a decreased rate of removal of DHT combined with an increase in the activity of the enzyme 5-alpha-reductase, which converts testosterone to DHT. Scientists have noted that men who do not produce significant amounts of DHT do not develop BPH.

BPH is not malignant, but its symptoms are similar to those of prostate cancer. If you are experiencing any BPH-related symptoms, it is very important to see your doctor as soon as possible.

✳ Diet Recommendations

Because diet plays an important role in prostate health, the following suggestions should help you prevent or correct BPH.

Choose organic, whole foods as often as possible. It is suspected that the tremendous increase in chemicals in our food such as pesticides and other pollutants is contributing to the massive increase in BPH in recent decades. Pesticides and other contaminants are known to increase the actions of 5-alpha-reductase, which converts testosterone to DHT.

Limit consumption of animal fat and vegetable oils. Lipid peroxidation, meaning free-radical damage to cholesterol and other fats, is particularly toxic and carcinogenic to the prostate gland. Damaged fat and cholesterol, which occur in high-heat cooking of meat like charbroiling and frying foods, are believed to play a role in abnormal cell growth and can contribute to BPH. Lower your intake of cholesterol and saturated fats by reducing consumption of fatty meats, fried foods, dairy products, and greasy snacks such as chips. (Follow the Basic Guidelines for the Juice Lady's Health and Healing Diet, page 290.)

Avoid polyunsaturated vegetable oils. Some research has indicated that the omega-6 fatty acids that dominate polyunsaturated vegetable oils (corn, safflower, soybean, canola, and sunflower oil) may increase the risk of prostate cancer. Also, these oils oxidize easily (meaning the fat is damaged) when heated and can contribute to abnormal cell growth. These oils constitute most of the oil that is consumed in the United States. Choose extra-virgin olive oil for cold food preparation, like salad dressings, and virgin coconut oil for cooking, which is the least likely to oxidize when heated.

Eat more lycopene-rich foods such as tomatoes, spinach, kale, mangos, broccoli, and berries. When consumed daily, they promote prostate health and play a role in preventing prostate cancer. In a Harvard Study (July 2003), it was found that men who ate 10 or more servings of tomatoes (sauce, juice, and whole tomatoes) daily were 45 percent less likely to develop prostate cancer.

Avoid alcohol, caffeine, and sugar, as they have an adverse effect on the way testosterone is metabolized and cleared from the body. Beer, in particular, can raise prolactin levels. Elevated prolactin levels, which cause impotence, may also cause enlargement of the prostate.

❋ Nutrient Recommendations

Bioflavonoids are among the phytonutrients used as the first-line BPH treatment in Germany and Austria. A review of the scientific literature shows that these compounds have provided significant benefits in 70 percent of the BPH patients who took them. *Best juice sources of bioflavonoids:* bell peppers, berries (blueberries, blackberries, and cranberries), broccoli, cabbage, lemons, limes, parsley, and tomatoes.

Increase omega-3 fatty acids. Some research has suggested that omega-3 fatty acids may be protective against BPH. Omega-3 fats are found in plants like flaxseed and hemp seed, certain nuts (particularly walnuts), and fish oil and fish, including salmon, sardines, halibut, swordfish, trout, and tuna. Some studies have reported a lower risk for prostate cancer in men who ate fish frequently (two or more times a week). Boosting EFA levels has led to significant improvements for many people with BPH. Gamma-linolenic acid (GLA), derived from evening primrose and borage oils, is particularly beneficial; this fatty acid appears to be a powerful inhibitor of 5-alpha-reductase.

Vitamin B$_6$ (pyridoxine) is important to hormone metabolism and works with zinc to reduce prolactin levels. *Best juice sources of vitamin B$_6$:* kale, spinach, turnip greens, and bell peppers.

Zinc has been shown to reduce the size of the prostate and to lessen symptoms for most BPH patients. Zinc inhibits the activity of 5-alpha-reductase. *Best juice sources of zinc:* gingerroot, turnips, parsley, garlic, carrots, spinach, cabbage, lettuce, and cucumbers.

✳ Herb Recommendations

Saw palmetto has the most documented benefits of any natural treatment for BPH. It has been shown in clinical studies to significantly diminish the signs and symptoms of BPH. About 90 percent of men who have mild to moderate BPH experience some improvement in symptoms during the first four to six weeks of using saw palmetto. All major symptoms of BPH have been relieved, especially nighttime urinary frequency. The recommended dosage is 320 to 640 mg daily. Saw palmetto may work best when combined with pygeum extract. (Pygeum africanum is an evergreen tree native to Africa.) Recommended dosage of saw palmetto is 50 to 100 mg twice per day.

✳ Juice Therapy

Asparagus juice has been used for prostate problems. Combine asparagus juice with carrot and lettuce or carrot, cucumber, and beetroot juices.

Tomato juice has been shown to inhibit the activity of adenosine deaminase (an enzyme), which is connected to BPH, in prostate tissue.

✳ Juice Recipes

The Ginger Hopper *(pg 332)* **Calcium-Rich Cocktail** *(pg 329)* **Cherie's Quick Energy Soup** *(pg 330)* **Sweet Dreams Nightcap** *(pg 342)* **Memory Mender** *(pg 336)*

Psoriasis

PSORIASIS is a common and chronic skin disease. A person with psoriasis generally has patches of raised red skin with thick silvery scales. The affected skin may be red and scaly or have pustules, depending on the type of psoriasis. The lesions appear most often on the knees, elbows, and scalp, and nail pitting is common. Psoriasis can also affect the joints (psoriatic arthritis). Psoriasis tends to occur in cycles, with flare-ups followed by periods of remission.

Evidence from research studies strongly suggests that psoriasis is a disorder of the immune system. Normally, the immune system defends the body from infection by bacteria, viruses, and other invaders. Sometimes, however, it mistakenly attacks the cells, tissues, and organs of a person's own body. When this happens, the resulting disease is called an autoimmune disease. Scientists have found some evidence indicating that this is the case in psoriasis.

Heredity is one factor in the cause of psoriasis. Several factors appear to contribute to or trigger this condition, including streptococcal infection, bowel toxins, poor protein digestion, poor liver function, excess alcohol and animal-fat consumption, and nutritional imbalances. Stress seems to worsen the eruptions. Up to 80 percent of patients report an emotional trauma prior to a flare-up. Obesity, skin injuries, and some drugs can aggravate the condition.

When someone experiences a psoriasis flare-up, a cascade of immunological events takes place in the skin, and results in an increase in inflammation. When inflammatory cells increase, it leads to a chain of events that causes psoriatic skin lesions. The goal is to eliminate the triggers as much as possible.

✳ Diet Recommendations

With psoriasis, the cells reproduce every three to four days. Before cells can mature and shed, new cells appear and form plaques on the surface of the skin.

Cyclic adenosine monophosphate (cAMP) and cyclic guanidine 5 monophosphate (cGMP) control cell division. Higher levels of GMP increase the rate of cell division, while the right levels of AMP decrease it. AMP and GMP levels can be rebalanced through the help of dietary and lifestyle changes, thus bringing psoriasis flare-ups under control. Following the guidelines herein can bring relief and make significant improvements in skin health.

Eat a high-fiber diet. Eat more vegetables, in particular. They are very anti-inflammatory. At least 50 percent of your diet should consist of raw fruits, vegetables, sprouts, and vegetable juices. Another 25 percent should come from whole grains and legumes. (It's a good idea to omit gluten—wheat, barley, rye, and oats. A percentage of psoriasis sufferers are sensitive to gluten and this can cause a flare-up.) One study documented a decrease in psoriasis symptoms with an increase in fruit and vegetable consumption. A low-fiber diet contributes to an increase in intestinal toxins, which include bacteria and yeast overgrowths (see Candidiasis, page 80) and parasites (see Parasitic Infections, page 238). These microbes can promote an increase in cGMP levels within skin cells, causing rapid division. (For more information on healthy eating, see Basic Guidelines for the Juice Lady's Health and Healing Diet, page 290.)

Include more psoralen-containing foods before going into the sun. (Substances from plants that are sensitive to light or can be activated by light, psoralens are used together with UV light to treat psoriasis.) These foods include celery, citrus, carrots, figs, fennel, and parsnips. They can contribute to making the skin more sun-sensitive to the positive effects of ultraviolet light. These foods can be juiced.

Limit red meat, dairy, and animal fats. With psoriasis, there is excessive production of the inflammatory compound known as leukotriene, formed from a fat component called arachidonic acid, which is found in meat and other animal fats. Reduce arachidonic acid levels by limiting meat, poultry, and dairy products. Also be aware that today meat, poultry, dairy, and eggs are not the same as the animal proteins human beings ate a hundred years ago. Today, these animals are given supplemental hormones and antibiotics, which show up in the flesh. Also, the animals are fed genetically modified (GM) grains. All of this has an impact on us when we eat them. When you consume *any* animal protein, make sure it is organic, free-range/cage-free, and antibiotic- and hormone-free. Some people have also benefited from eliminating gluten (wheat, rye, oats, and barley) and other allergenic foods from their diet.

Eliminate alcohol and tobacco. Alcohol consumption and smoking worsen psoriasis. They should be completely eliminated.

Complete a liver and colon cleanse. These cleansing programs will aid the healing process. A connection has been made between a sluggish liver and psoriasis. This is not surprising, since a poorly functioning liver cannot easily clear toxins from the body. The Liver Cleanse (page 310) can promote healing, along with the Intestinal Cleanse (page 307).

Juice-fast to remove toxins. Going on short vegetable-juice fasts from one to three days several times a year can be very beneficial in clearing toxins from the body. This can help heal psoriasis. According to one study, fasting and a vegetarian diet have helped some people heal psoriasis (see the Juice Fast, page 304).

✳ Nutrient Recommendations

Beta-carotene has been shown in studies to benefit people with psoriasis. Vitamin A, created from beta-carotene within the body, is of primary importance for healthy skin. *Best juice sources of carotenes in general:* carrots, kale, parsley, spinach, Swiss chard, beetroot greens, watercress, broccoli, and romaine lettuce.

Folic acid. A study published in the *British Journal of Dermatology* found that sixteen of fifty-eight patients with psoriasis had a deficiency in folic acid. Apparently, even a mild folic-acid deficiency can affect some people with this disease. *Best juice sources of folic acid:* asparagus, spinach, kale, beetroot greens, broccoli, and cabbage.

Lecithin helps clear cholesterol from tissues. Psoriasis-affected skin typically contains abnormally high levels of cholesterol. Out of 155 psoriasis patients in one study, 118 either controlled or improved their symptoms by taking lecithin. Lecithin can be purchased at most health food stores; add lecithin granules to juice or smoothies, or take lecithin in capsule form.

Omega-3 fatty acids appear to reduce the amount of inflammation associated with psoriasis. One study involved eighty-three patients who had such severe cases of psoriasis, they were hospitalized. Each individual was randomly assigned either omega-3 treatments or omega-6. Those who received the omega-3 fatty acids significantly improved when compared to those who received the omega-6 fats. Increase your intake of fish, nuts, flaxseed, and fish-oil supplements. Eat cold-water fish, such as salmon, tuna, trout, mackerel, halibut, cod, and sardines, at least three times a week. You should also increase the amount of green leafy vegetables you eat.

Zinc can help people with psoriasis. A zinc-copper imbalance has been observed in psoriasis patients (the ratio of zinc and copper is off, with too little zinc and too much copper). *Best juice sources of zinc:* gingerroot, turnips, parsley, garlic, carrots, grapes, spinach, cabbage, lettuce, and cucumbers.

✳ Herb Recommendations

Milk thistle (silymarin) is used in the treatment of psoriasis. This herb can help improve liver function, inhibit inflammation, and reduce excessive skin-cell proliferation.

✳ Juice Therapy

Beetroot juice is excellent for liver detoxification. Many people with psoriasis have congestion in their bowels and liver. Drink at least one glass of beetroot juice per day. You may want to combine beetroots with carrots, celery, and cucumbers, since beetroot juice is quite strong by itself.

Carrot juice provides both beta-carotene and zinc.

✳ Juice Recipes

Morning Energizer *(pg 337)*   **Beautiful-Skin Cocktail** *(pg 328)*   **Colon Cleanser** *(pg 330)*   **Liver Life Tonic** *(pg 336)*   **The Ginger Hopper** *(pg 332)*   **Spring Tonic** *(pg 342)*   **Allergy Relief** *(pg 326)*   **Beet-Cucumber Cleansing Cocktail** *(pg 328)*   **Gallbladder-Liver Cleansing Cocktail** *(pg 331)*   **Immune Builder** *(pg 335)*   **Super Green Sprout Drink** *(pg 342)*   **Wheatgrass Light** *(pg 345)*

Respiratory Disorders

THE RESPIRATORY TRACT, from the nose to the lungs, is subject to a number of disorders. Colds and flu are two of the more common respiratory problems (see Colds, page 102 and Influenza, page 198), but inflammation can occur anywhere in the respiratory tract.

Sinusitis is an inflammation of the sinuses, the open spaces in the facial bones. The most common cause of acute sinusitis is infection, whether viral, bacterial, or fungal in nature. When a sinus is blocked for any length of time, it fills with a thin fluid that becomes a host to microbial growth. Chronic sinusitis can occur as the result of food allergies; dental infections; bacterial, viral, and fungal infections; polyps; and reflux disease. Symptoms include nasal congestion, profuse discharge (usually yellow or green), fever, chills, a foul smell, and frontal headaches that worsen when lying down or bending over.

Laryngitis, an inflammation or irritation of the larynx, is usually caused by a viral infection of the upper airways or such irritants as cigarette smoke or other inhaled irritants, alcohol, or an allergic reaction. It is marked by hoarseness or loss of voice and often begins with postnasal drip and constant throat clearing.

Bronchitis is a respiratory disease in which the mucous membrane in the lungs' bronchial passages becomes inflamed. As the irritated membrane swells and grows thicker, it narrows or shuts off the tiny airways in the lungs, resulting in coughing spells accompanied by thick phlegm, sore throat, fatigue, nasal discharge, muscle aches, and breathlessness. The disease comes in two forms: acute (lasting less than six weeks) and chronic (reoccurring frequently for more than two years). In addition, people with asthma also experience an inflammation of the lining of the bronchial tubes called asthmatic bronchitis. Causes range from lung infections (most are viral) to industrial pollution and cigarette smoking.

Pneumonia is an infection or inflammation of the lungs most commonly caused by a bacteria, virus, or fungus. The air sacs in the lungs fill up with fluid and dead white blood cells, reducing the amount of air space. The symptoms are fever and chills, followed by cough with lots of phlegm, chest pain, difficulty breathing, and shortness of breath.

❊ Diet Recommendations

Drink plenty of fluids. For all respiratory tract conditions, it is very important to drink plenty of fluids. Fluids keep the mucous membranes moist and better able to repel viral infections. Keeping mucous membranes from becoming dry and inflamed prevents a breeding ground for infection. Drink only nutritious liquids, such as vegetable juice, broth, herbal tea, and pure water. Do not drink any soda; the chemicals and sugar or artificial sweeteners can weaken your immune system. Even fruit juice, became of its fruit sugar, is not recommended.

Drink lots of hot fluids. Cold viruses multiply fast when the temperature around them is about 90°F. However, they are far less likely to replicate as quickly when their environment heats up. Hot fluids will warm your throat, which should help to impair viral replication. As a bonus, hot fluids have a mild decongestant effect, which helps relieve nasal stuffiness. Hot herbal drinks such as ginger tea are doubly helpful because of their antiviral effect.

Juice-fast. Going on a vegetable-juice fast for one to three days can be very beneficial (see the Juice Fast, page 304).

Eat light, and include plenty of vegetables in your diet. A very light diet is recommended for the days you don't juice-fast. Vegetable soup, stew, vegetable juice, and broth are recommended. Vegetables rich in beta-carotene and vitamin C are particularly helpful; they are the yellow, orange, red, and dark green vegetables.

Avoid foods that contain sugar. Simple sugars, including natural sugars such as honey and fruit sugar, impair immune function. That's because sugar competes with vitamin C for the same route of transportation into white blood cells, the body's main infection fighters. Consuming too much sugar decreases vitamin C levels in these cells, which impairs their effectiveness. Therefore, avoid all sugary foods. Eat whole fruit in moderation, and avoid fruit juice (except for lemon and lime). If you drink fruit juice, have no more than four ounces daily, diluted by half with pure water.

Reduce your intake of dairy products and refined-flour baked goods, such as breads, rolls, pasta and pizza. These foods, along with sugar, contribute to mucus production. Ridding the body of excess mucus is part of the healing process for all respiratory conditions.

Increase your consumption of spicy foods. Hot, spicy foods such as cayenne pepper, chili pepper, horseradish, and mustard can help ease respiratory symptoms. Spicy foods help to open air passages and bring some relief for bronchitis sufferers. Cayenne pepper is often used to increase circulation and to help produce a clearing effect in the mucous membranes. Cayenne also acts as an antibiotic. Hot water with lemon and a dash of cayenne is helpful.

Perform liver/gallbladder detox. Though not appropriate for any upper respiratory condition when in the acute phase, liver and gallbladder cleanses can be very beneficial for chronic conditions or when you are on the mend and to prevent infections in the future. Allergies and sinus conditions will often disappear after the liver has been cleansed (see the Liver Cleanse, page 310, and the Gallbladder Cleanse, page 318).

✳ Nutrient Recommendations

Bromelain, a digestive enzyme found in pineapple, has been shown to alleviate symptoms and lessen mucous membrane inflammation, especially in acute and chronic sinusitis. It makes bronchial secretions more fluid and helps to decrease the amount of secretions. One study showed an improvement in nasal inflammation and breathing difficulties in 87 percent of patients taking bromelain. Because pineapple juice has a lot of fruit sugar, it is best to take a bromelain supplement when fighting a respiratory infection.

Vitamin A and **beta-carotene** are recommended for combating respiratory illnesses. Vitamin A contributes to the health of the epithelial cells that coat the respiratory tract. It is also capable of stimulating various immune processes, including natural killer cell activity and antibody response. Beta-carotene and other carotenes are the only form of pro-vitamin A found in fruits and vegetables; they are converted to vitamin A within the body as needed. *Best juice sources of carotenes in general:* carrots, kale, parsley, spinach, Swiss chard, beetroot greens, watercress, broccoli, and romaine lettuce.

Vitamin C and **bioflavonoids** are important immune-system stimulators. Vitamin C is found in great quantities in white blood cells, and the supply needs to be constantly replenished when the body is fighting infection or inflammation. One study showed that if vitamin C levels were low, the individual was more likely to develop bronchitis. Bioflavonoids make vitamin C more effective. *Best juice sources of vitamin C:* kale, parsley, broccoli, Brussels sprouts, watercress, cauliflower, cabbage, spinach, lemons, limes, turnips, and asparagus. *Best juice sources of bioflavonoids:* bell peppers, broccoli, cabbage, parsley, and tomatoes.

Vitamin E is another strong ally in supporting the immune system. It plays a role in a broad range of defense mechanisms on the cellular level. *Best juice sources of vitamin E:* spinach, watercress, asparagus, carrots, and tomatoes.

Zinc is an important immune-stimulating mineral. Studies have shown that zinc lozenges can soothe sore throat and reduce a cold's duration. *Best juice sources of zinc:* gingerroot, turnips, parsley, garlic, carrots, spinach, cabbage, lettuce, and cucumbers.

✳ Herb Recommendations

Echinacea contains several compounds that make it a good immune-system support herb. For example, two components of the herb are key. Inulin directly affects important cellular processes involved in fighting infection and inflammation. Caffeic acid is antibacterial and contains compounds that help to keep mucous membranes strong.

Goldenseal contains a compound that is an effective antibiotic. This herb also enhances the immune system by increasing blood flow to the spleen, the organ responsible for releasing many important immune-stimulating compounds. Avoid goldenseal if you are pregnant, and do not use it for more than ten days.

Lobelia is an herbal expectorant that propels mucus from the lungs. It does this while also relaxing the muscles of the respiratory system, which reduces wheezing and chest discomfort. It is especially helpful for bronchitis.

Yarrow promotes sweating, thereby helping the body deal with fevers.

✳ Juice Therapy

Carrot and **radish** juices are best combined. Fresh radish juice is similar in effect to horseradish, but milder. It's too strong, however, to take straight, and should be mixed with carrot juice (five ounces of radish juice with eleven ounces of carrot juice).

Celery juice will help you relax and sleep better.

Cranberries contain one of nature's most potent vasodilators, which opens up congested bronchial tubes and helps restore normal breathing.

Garlic juice is a strong immune-system stimulant, and is both antibacterial and antiviral. It also helps reduce bronchial secretions.

Lemon juice is rich in vitamin C and bioflavonoids and helps clear mucus. Mix it with a little horseradish to help dissolve mucus in the sinuses and bronchial tubes quickly and effectively.

Parsley juice contains beta-carotene, bioflavonoids, vitamin C, and zinc. Intake should be limited to a safe, therapeutic dose of one-half to one cup per day. Parsley can be toxic in overdose, and should be especially avoided by pregnant women.

Pear juice, diluted by half with water and served at room temperature, helps loosen congestion in the lungs.

Persimmons (very ripe ones) soothe sore throats.

Radish juice is a traditional remedy for sinus disorders.

Watercress and **turnip** juices help ease bronchitis and pneumonia.

✳ Juice Recipes

Sweet Dreams Nightcap *(pg 342)* **Mood Mender** *(337)* **Morning Energizer** *(pg 337)* **Sinus Solution** *(pg 341)* **Ginger Twist** *(pg 332)* **Afternoon Refresher** *(pg 326)* **Spinach Power** *(pg 341)* **Tomato Florentine** *(pg 343)* **Orient Express** *(pg 338)* **Turnip Time** *(pg 344)* **Calcium-Rich Cocktail** *(pg 329)* **Cranberry-Apple Cocktail** *(pg 331)* **Hot Ginger-Lemon Tea** *(pg 334)* **Wheatgrass Light** *(pg 345)* **Liver Life Tonic** *(pg 336)*

Rheumatoid Arthritis and Other Autoimmune Diseases

RHEUMATOID ARTHRITIS (RA) is an autoimmune disease that causes chronic inflammation of the joints. It can also cause inflammation of the tissue around the joints, as well as other organs in the body. Symptoms include fatigue, low-grade fever, weakness, insomnia, lack of appetite, muscle and joint aches, and stiffness. There is often severe joint pain, with increasing inflammation beginning in the small joints and progressively affecting all the joints. Eventually, deformities can develop that limit range of motion in the joints, with the ends of the bones becoming enlarged. More women than men are affected.

Unlike osteoarthritis, RA is an autoimmune reaction in which the body's immune system produces antibodies that attack its own tissues. It is suspected that certain infectious agents, such as viruses, bacteria, and fungi, or toxic factors in the environment might trigger the immune system to attack the body's tissues. The result is an immune system that is geared up to promote inflammation in the joints and occasionally other tissues and organs such as the lungs or eyes. What causes this reaction is unknown, but investigation has centered on lifestyle and nutritional factors, food allergies, abnormal bowel permeability, smoking, and genetic factors. Also, overactivity of B-cells is thought to be responsible for debilitating or chronic autoimmune disorders such as RA, lupus, multiple sclerosis, and myasthenia gravis.

There are several studies that point to diet therapy as a promising way to reduce inflammation, ease symptoms, and heal the body. Even though there is no known cure, you can still heal from RA and reverse symptoms, with the exception of areas that have permanent damage.

In addition to RA, there are several other autoimmune diseases that affect connective tissue, including lupus, ankylosing spondylitis, and scleroderma. From a nutritional perspective, the treatment for any autoimmune disease is the same as the one used for RA.

✳ Lifestyle Recommendations

Avoid or reduce nonsteriodal anti-inflammatory drugs (NSAIDS). These agents, including aspirin and ibuprofen, can damage the intestines, allowing allergy-causing particles to leak into the system and thereby contributing to the worsening of RA.

Treat *Candida albicans*. Eliminate any small intestine bacterial and yeast overgrowth. Many people with RA have bacterial and yeast overgrowth in the small intestine. This condition is connected with both severity of symptoms and disease activity. There are numerous reports that treatment of yeast infections has eased rheumatic symptoms (see Candidiasis, page 80; see also the Intestinal Cleanse, page 307).

Release unhealthy thinking such as jealousy, hate, greed, worry, fear, or unforgiveness. These can affect the joints and tissues. Also, let go of all unhealthy situations. For example, avoid staying in circumstances where your energy is being drained by others who are codependent or who feed off your energy to replenish their own.

✳ Diet Recommendations

It has been proven that certain foods increase pain, while others reduce it. Combining natural remedies to rebuild cartilage, avoiding foods that cause joint pain, and adding other treatments such as supplements can substantially lessen pain and heal the body.

Eat a whole-foods diet with an emphasis on vegetables. Mackerel is an excellent protein choice; include omega-3–rich salmon, sardines, trout, or herring at least two times a week. Eat only small amounts of meat and poultry occasionally, and avoid all meat and poultry that is not free-range/cage-free and raised without antibiotics and hormones. (Free-range has omega-3 fatty acids.) Include plenty of green vegetables, such as kale, okra, celery, parsley, and watercress, and wheatgrass juice, along with seaweed, carrots, barley, avocados, pecans, and spirulina. And increase consumption of sulfur-containing foods such as legumes, garlic, onions, Brussels sprouts, and cabbage.

Eat a high-raw-foods diet (more than 60 percent) and go organic. A Finnish study showed that an uncooked vegan diet (also called a living-foods or raw-foods diet) and adding *Lactobacillus acidophilus* decreased subjective symptoms of RA. A return to an omnivorous diet aggravated symptoms. Choose organic fruits and vegetables because they have a higher nutritional content and far fewer toxins for the liver to detoxify. Also, they contain more of the live plant enzymes that are necessary in the digestive process.

Increase omega-3 fatty acids. Studies have shown that diets rich in omega-3 fatty acids help reduce the pain, stiffness, and inflammation associated with RA. Evidence suggests that about 6 grams of omega-3 fatty acids a day seems to have an anti-inflammatory effect. Take fish-oil capsules or cod-liver oil (doses of up to three tablespoons a day), and eat two or three meals of fatty fish (salmon, mackerel, trout, herring, sardines) each week. Give yourself time to measure results because it might be up to four months before you notice any improvement in your condition.

Note: It is best not to mix cod-liver oil with other supplements that contain vitamins A and D because you can get too much of these fat-soluble vitamins, and over a long period of time, that can be toxic.

Avoid animal fats. Fats compete with each other for use in the production of prostaglandins. When the body selects omega-3–rich fats, as it does when fish oil is abundant, the prostaglandins produced are anti-inflammatory. When arachidonic acid from animal fats is abundant, the prostaglandins produced are pro-inflammatory. Cut way back on fat from meat (completely avoid luncheon meat), dairy products (especially ice cream, cheese, and butter), mayonnaise, and baked goods, and use only salad dressings made with olive oil. Avoid margarine, trans fats, hydrogenated oil, and polyunsaturated oils—safflower, sunflower, soy, canola, and corn oils.

Choose good fats. The most nutritious oil is extra-virgin olive oil for cold foods such as salad dressing; the safest oil for cooking is virgin coconut oil, which does not easily oxidize when heated.

Limit simple carbohydrates. Sugary foods; white rice; white-flour baked goods, such as bread, crackers, pizza, and pasta, and other refined carbohydrates set up a state of inflammation in the body, causing increases in cytokines and other pro-inflammatory compounds. Grains, even whole grains, are high in omega-6 fatty acids, which are pro-inflammatory and should be eaten very sparingly. Multiple sclerosis, lupus, and rheumatoid arthritis are rare in populations where very few grain products are consumed. Limit all these foods if you want the best chance of reducing arthritis pain and progression of the disease.

Juice-fast. Studies have shown that juice fasts decrease joint pain and reverse RA. In one scientific review, the authors concluded that fasting may be the most rapid means of inducing relief of arthritic pain and swelling for persons with RA. Four controlled studies investigated the effects of fasting and subsequent vegetarian diets for at least three months. These studies showed a significant beneficial long-term effect, suggesting that fasting followed by a vegetarian diet is beneficial in the treatment of RA. One study followed 27 RA patients for a four-week stay at a health farm where they fasted. At the end of the four weeks, they showed significant signs of improvement. They continued with a vegetarian program, and after one year, benefits were still present. You can start with a two- or three-day vegetable-juice fast (see the Juice Fast, page 304).

Avoid alcohol and caffeine. Consumption of both coffee and alcohol has been shown to release adrenaline and/or noradrenaline, which can contribute to RA. Consumption of alcohol can also result in the release of histamine, and certain red wines have a high concentration of histamine, which may explain the frequently reported red wine intolerance among people with RA. One study showed coffee consumption to be a risk factor for RA.

Avoid the nightshade family. Tomatoes, eggplant, potatoes, sweet peppers, paprika, chili peppers, and tobacco frequently have a negative effect on arthritis. In a study with five thousands arthritics, more than 70 percent of those who avoided nightshades reported a gradual improvement over the seven years of the study. Some species of nightshade foods contain the alkaloid solanine, which is a glycoalkaloid poison. Solanine has natural fungicidal and pesticidal properties, making it one of the plant's natural defenses. Several doctors have found that about one-third of their patients are sensitive to the nightshade family and that eating these foods causes RA symptoms. Try avoiding these foods for three months and see if your symptoms improve. Then add one back and see if symptoms get worse.

Eliminate food allergies. Research is looking at the possibility that some people develop antibodies against proteins they eat and that those antibodies then attack similar proteins in the body. Foods most likely to cause intolerance: wheat, pork (including bacon), oranges, milk, oats, rye, eggs, beef, coffee, malt (beer), cheese, grapefruit, tomatoes, peanuts, sugar, butter, lamb, lemon, corn, and soy. If you are allergic to citrus fruits, omit them from the recipes (see Allergies, page 27; see also the Elimination Diet, page 301).

✳ Nutrient Recommendations

Antioxidants are substances that fight the actions of toxic free radicals. Several studies have indicated that the risk of RA is highest among people with the lowest levels of antioxidants—vitamins C and E, beta-carotene, and selenium.

Beta-carotene and **vitamin A** help fight RA. Consumption of foods rich in beta-carotene is associated with a lowered risk of RA. Beta-carotene (provitamin A) is the only form of vitamin A found in fruits and vegetables, and is converted by the body to vitamin A as needed. *Best juice sources of carotenes in general:* carrots, kale, parsley, spinach, Swiss chard, beetroot greens, watercress, broccoli, and romaine lettuce.

Pantothenic acid may be helpful, as deficiencies of this nutrient have been found to be directly related to RA symptoms. *Best juice sources of pantothenic acid:* broccoli, cauliflower, and kale.

Selenium is thought to be helpful for RA because it fights inflammation. It is used for the production of glutathione peroxidase, an enzyme that works inside joints to round up free radicals. *Best juice sources of selenium:* Swiss chard, turnips, garlic, radishes, carrots, and cabbage.

Vitamin C and **bioflavonoids** play vital roles in fighting RA. Vitamin C promotes anti-inflammatory activity. People with RA have been shown to have low levels of vitamin C in their blood. Bioflavonoids help make vitamin C more effective. *Best juice sources of vitamin C:* kale, parsley, broccoli, Brussels sprouts, watercress, cauliflower, cabbage, strawberries, spinach, lemons, limes, turnips, and asparagus. *Best juice sources of bioflavonoids:* apricots, bell peppers, berries (blueberries, blackberries, and cranberries), broccoli, cabbage, parsley, lemons, limes, and tomatoes.

Vitamin E has provided some benefits for people with RA. *Best juice sources of vitamin E:* spinach, watercress, asparagus, carrots, and tomatoes.

Vitamin K may stabilize cell membranes in rheumatoid tissue. *Best juice sources of vitamin K:* turnip greens, broccoli, lettuce, cabbage, spinach, watercress, asparagus, and string beans.

✳ Juice Therapy

Blackberry, blueberry, and **cherry** juices, all rich in anthocyanidins and proanthocyanidins, have been shown to be effective in reducing inflammation associated with arthritis.

Dandelion juice is a traditional remedy for healing RA. The recommendation is to drink one-half cup in the morning and evening. Dandelion juice is very strong-tasting; you may want to dilute it with water or other juices. Or you can try Liver Life Tonic (page 336) and add extra dandelion juice.

Gingerroot contains anti-inflammatory compounds, and inhibits production of prostaglandins and leutkotrienes. In one study, Indian researchers gave 3 to 7 grams of gingerroot a day to twenty-eight people with RA. More than 75 percent of those participating in the study reported at least some relief from pain and swelling. Even after more than two years of taking high doses of gingerroot, none of the people reported side effects. One of the easiest ways to get high doses of gingerroot is to juice it.

Parsley juice is effective in combating and flushing uric acid from the tissue, which eases painful limbs and joints. Take one teaspoon of parsley juice three times daily for six weeks. Wait three weeks before taking again.

Raw potato juice, which has been used as a folk medicine for centuries, is considered a successful treatment for RA (provided you are not sensitive to the nightshade family*). Juice four to six ounces and drink on an empty stomach, diluted fifty-fifty with water. *If your symptoms worsen, discontinue immediately.

Sprouts should be included in food preparation and added to juice recipes because they are rich in sterols and sterolins, which are plant fats present in all fruits and vegetables. There is clinical proof that they significantly moderate the effects of the immune system. Without sterols and sterolins, the immune system may become too stressed to produce enough invader-fighting T-cells or may over-produce the B cells responsible for the autoimmune response.

Wheatgrass juice. A 1999 Finnish study of rheumatoid arthritis patients treated to a living-foods diet (raw foods), which included wheatgrass juice, reported improvements significant enough to suggest that a living-foods diet that includes wheatgrass juice may lead to a lessening of not just RA symptoms but also several other health risk factors, including those for cardiovascular diseases and cancer. For therapeutic effects, drink two to four ounces per day. Juice should be taken on an empty stomach at least one hour before meals or two hours after eating.

✳ Juice Recipes

Liver Life Tonic *(pg 336)* The Ginger Hopper *(pg 332)* Magnesium-Rich Cocktail *(pg 336)* Cherie's Quick Energy Soup *(pg 330)* Triple C *(pg 344)* Spinach Power *(pg 341)* Allergy Relief *(pg 326)* Cabbage Patch Cocktail *(pg 329)* Ginger Twist *(pg 332)* Immune Builder *(pg 335)* Peppy Parsley *(pg 339)* Pure Green Sprout Drink *(pg 340)* Wheatgrass Light *(pg 345)* (Use only if you can't drink wheatgrass juice alone. Remember, it's most effective when consumed by itself.)

Stress

S TRESS is the emotional and physical strain caused by our response to pressure from the outside world. Common stress reactions include tension, irritability, inability to concentrate, and a variety of physical symptoms that include headache and a fast heartbeat.

Modern life is filled with stressors—job pressures, relationship problems, and financial worries, to name a few. Actually, a stressor can be almost anything that creates a bodily disturbance, such as environmental or microbial toxins, physical trauma, or exposure to heat or cold. Symptoms can include headache, fatigue, tension, irritability, inability to concentrate, insomnia, digestive disturbances, neck and back pain, difficulty breathing, frequent urination, sweaty palms, tight muscles that may cause pain and trembling, and either loss of appetite or overeating.

There are three stages of the stress response, called the general adaptation syndrome. The first is the alarm stage. This fight-or-flight response triggers the adrenal glands to release adrenaline and other hormones that prepare the body to either fight a perceived danger or run away. The second stage is the resistance stage. The body begins to adapt to the stressor(s) by releasing adrenal hormones that convert protein into energy. This elevates blood-sugar levels and sets up a cascade of hormonal and chemical changes with adverse affects. There may be depression of the immune system, decreased bone strength, poor memory, and decreased energy. Coping abilities can diminish, causing feelings of insecurity and inadequacy. The third and final stage is exhaustion. The body is depleted of energy by loss of both potassium and such adrenal hormones as cortisol. When adrenal hormones become depleted, hypoglycemia can result because cells are not receiving enough fuel. There is a complete loss of resistance, and the exhaustion will affect any inherently weak organ or system, such as the heart, blood vessels, adrenal glands, or immune system. If the stress continues, there is an increased risk of diabetes, high blood pressure, and cancer.

Many addictions are linked to a stressful lifestyle, such as overeating, smoking, drinking, excessive television watching, too much shopping, inappropriate sexual activity, and drug abuse. These are used as an escape or a temporary way of "switching off," but they do not address the underlying problem. Negative coping behaviors offer only temporary diversion and can create more stress in the long run than they relieve. To fight stress, you need to recognize and eliminate coping behaviors. Instead, come up with your own stress-management program that works for you. Include comfort choices, other than comfort foods, that are really good for you. Nutrition plays an important role in this program, as a variety of nutrients and herbs can help support overworked adrenal glands, immune system, and organs. This, in turn, helps you deal more effectively with stress.

✳ Lifestyle Recommendations

You can develop your own comprehensive approach to stress management. This involves: (1) learning ways to calm your body and mind, such as meditation, prayer, relaxation, and breathing techniques; (2) dealing with such lifestyle factors as time management and relationship issues; (3) exercising on a regular basis; (4) eating a healthy diet and juicing regularly; and (5) using nutritional supplements that support the body during stress. The effects of stress on your body are to some extent affected by your perception of the stress. If you can let go of the "self" that says "I want my life to turn out this way," you can use stress creatively.

Exercise to increase endorphins. Get thirty to sixty minutes of aerobic exercise at least three times a week, and take a ten- to thirty-minute walk every day. And while you walk, smile. It's the ultimate stress reliever.

Place stressful events in perspective. Realize that life is a school and you are here to learn. Problems are simply part of the curriculum that appear and fade away like algebra class—but the lessons you learn will last a lifetime. So, no matter how bad a situation is, it will change. But always remember—you are "too blessed to be stressed" over anything. And holding grudges is extremely stressful; forgive everyone—including yourself—for everything, no matter what. When you do, you come out the winner.

✳ Diet Recommendations

Eat a high-fiber, high-complex-carbohydrate diet that includes adequate protein. When faced with stressful situations, get the best nutrition possible. This means eating fewer refined foods, and eating more whole grains, vegetables, fruits, sprouts, nuts, seeds, and fish. You should get 25 to 30 grams of fiber each day. (For more information, see Basic Guidelines for the Juice Lady's Health and Healing Diet, page 290).

Drink plenty of fresh vegetable juice and go on short juice fasts. Your body needs extra nutrition during times of stress, and juice provides a concentration of nutrients in an easily digestible, easily assimilated form. Juice-fasting gives your digestive system a rest so it can concentrate on other functions, like repair and rejuvenation. Juicing foods with high concentrations of vitamins (especially C and the B complex) and minerals will help protect you against the negative effects of stress. In addition, studies show that fasting may be helpful during times of stress (see the Juice Fast, page 304).

Identify food allergies. Controlling food allergies and intolerances can be helpful in managing stress, because anxiety and fatigue are among the symptoms of food allergies (see Allergies, page 27; also see the Elimination Diet, page 301).

Avoid caffeine, which can contribute to stress. Excess caffeine consumption is characterized by depression, nervousness, irritability, recurrent headaches, heart palpitations, and insomnia. Caffeine is found in coffee, tea, chocolate, and soda.

It causes the release of adrenaline, thus increasing the level of stress. Consuming too much caffeine has the same effect as long-term stress.

Stop smoking. Tobacco's harmful effects on the body are well-known. It can cause stress in the body.

Avoid alcohol. Alcohol is a major cause of stress. The irony of the situation is that most people drink as a way to combat stress. But, in actuality, they make their situation worse by consuming alcohol. Alcohol causes the secretion of adrenaline, resulting in nervous tension, irritability, and insomnia. Excess alcohol will increase fat deposits in the liver and decrease immune function. It also limits the ability of the liver to remove toxins from the body. In the absence of efficient filtering by the liver, toxins continue to circulate through the body, resulting in additional stress on the body.

Avoid sugar and refined carbohydrates such as sweets and white-flour baked goods; they affect blood sugar and can lead to hypoglycemia—a blood-sugar dysfunction that results in irritability and depression (see Hypoglycemia, page 180). When we're stressed we often experience cravings for carbohydrate-rich comfort foods like mashed potatoes, ice cream, candy bars, or pizza. These foods do provide temporary emotional comfort by increasing blood-sugar levels and serotonin (the feel-good chemical) in your brain. But two or three hours after eating these foods, your insulin levels will soar, causing your blood-sugar levels to plunge. This forces your body to increase cortisol production to maintain adequate blood-sugar levels to the brain. Then, you'll wind up increasing your production of cortisol, which, in turn, will generate more stress and require another cycle of self-medication with carbohydrates while your overall biochemical imbalance worsens.

✳ Nutrient Recommendations

Amino acids. An inability to handle stress may be the result of shortages of key brain chemicals that can be restored naturally. Low serotonin levels are often the cause of long-term stress. Mood, behavior, and brain biochemistry are intricately linked. Inability to handle stress may be the result of flawed message transmission in the brain—flawed because key brain chemicals known as neurotransmitters are in short supply. They're short because the body's amino acid pool from which they're made is itself low. We tend to use up these important brain neurotransmitters faster than we can create them from our diet. As stress increases over time, it can be very difficult to make adequate quantities of the neurotransmitter serotonin to meet demands, which is why our unhealthy responses to stress tend to increase as we age. Gamma–aminobutyric acid (GABA) is an amino acid that can be taken for temporarily relief, but most GABA only crosses the blood–brain barrier at a rate of 10 percent. Beta phenyl GABA, however, crosses at a 90 percent rate. You may be surprised at how well you can handle stress when you get the amino acids your body needs and your neurotransmitters are balanced. You should also be able to sleep better (see Insomnia, page 202).

B vitamins, omega-3 fatty acids, and varied protein consumption are imperative with the amino acid program; therefore, include three or four different protein selections each day. Choose from nuts, seeds, beans, eggs, and muscle meats such as fish, chicken, turkey, and beef while on the amino acid program. (Choose organically fed, free-range or cage-free animal products with no hormones or antibiotics.) Also add a good fish-oil supplement and a B complex vitamin. For information on brain neurotransmitter testing and the amino acid program, see Sources, page 351.

Magnesium is considered the antistress mineral. It's needed during times of stress. A deficiency can interfere with nerve and muscle impulses, causing irritability and nervousness. Low levels of this mineral are associated with behavioral problems. *Best juice sources of magnesium:* beetroot greens, spinach, parsley, dandelion greens, garlic, blackberries, beetroot, broccoli, cauliflower, carrots, and celery.

Omega-3 fatty acids. The two primary mediators of emotions are cytokines (hormones that are involved in inflammation) and eicosanoids (hormone-like compounds produced from essential fatty acids). Fish oil such as cod-liver oil or krill oil gives your body the ability to control both cytokines and eicosanoids, and thus can help you deal with the wide variety of emotional issues that take place in your life.

Pantothenic acid is known as the antistress vitamin. A deficiency results in adrenal atrophy, characterized by fatigue, headache, sleep disturbances, nausea, and abdominal discomfort. *Best juice sources of pantothenic acid:* broccoli, cauliflower, and kale.

Potassium intake should be increased during times of stress to support the adrenal glands. Every effort should be made to maintain adequate potassium levels, and drinking fresh juices is one of the best ways to get potassium. *Best juice sources of* *potassium:* parsley, Swiss chard, garlic, spinach, broccoli, carrots, celery, radishes, cauliflower, watercress, asparagus, and cabbage.

Selenium may help protect the body against infections during times of stress. *Best juice sources of selenium:* Swiss chard, turnips, garlic, radishes, carrots, and cabbage.

Vitamin C and **bioflavonoids** are important for both adrenal gland and immune system functioning. Vitamin C levels can drop during times of stress. Bioflavonoids work with vitamin C, allowing the body to absorb this vitamin more effectively. *Best juice sources of vitamin C:* kale, parsley, broccoli, Brussels sprouts, watercress, cauliflower, cabbage, strawberries, spinach, lemons, limes, turnips, and asparagus. *Best juice sources of bioflavonoids:* bell peppers, berries (blueberries, blackberries, and cranberries), broccoli, cabbage, parsley, lemons, limes, and tomatoes.

✳ Herb Recommendations

California poppy, kava kava, lavender, and **valerian** all have a sedative effect. California poppy, kava kava, and valerian also help fight insomnia.

Catnip, hops, and **mugwort** help you fall asleep faster, wake up less often, and go into a deeper sleep.

Chamomile and **Saint-John's-wort** reduce nerve and muscle pain. Saint-John's-wort is also effective against depression and insomnia.

Ginseng exerts beneficial effects on adrenal functioning, and enhances stress resistance. Korean or red ginseng (Panax ginseng) and Siberian ginseng (Eleutherococcus senticosus) are effective. Avoid Siberian ginseng if you have an autoimmune disease such as rheumatoid arthritis.

✳ Juice Therapy

Celery juice has a calming effect and supports the nervous system.

Fennel juice helps promote the release of endorphins, the feel-good brain chemicals.

Lettuce juice calms digestion.

✳ Juice Recipes

Sweet Dreams Nightcap *(pg 342)*   Mood Mender *(pg 337)*   Immune Builder *(pg 335)*   Ginger Twist *(pg 332)*   Beautiful-Skin Cocktail *(pg 328)* Spinach Power *(pg 341)*   Liver Life Tonic *(pg 336)*   Turnip Time *(pg 344)* Cherie's Quick Energy Soup *(pg 330)*   Happy Morning *(pg 333)*   Calcium-Rich Cocktail *(pg 329)*   Wheatgrass Light *(pg 345)*

Tuberculosis

TUBERCULOSIS (TB) is a bacterial infection caused by *Mycobacterium tuberculosis.* It most commonly affects the respiratory system but can spread to other areas of the body, such as the gastrointestinal and genitourinary tracts, bones, joints, nervous system, lymph nodes, spleen, and liver. TB symptoms include coughing (usually an early-morning cough) and flu-like symptoms with chest pain, difficulty breathing, coughing up blood, decreased appetite, low-grade fever, sweats that worsen at night, and weight loss. Sometimes symptoms do not appear for up to two years after the initial infection occurs.

TB rates have risen as the AIDS epidemic has spread. People infected with the HIV virus, especially those who are homeless, are at greater risk of developing this disease. International travel to areas where TB is rampant, and immigration from these areas, has contributed to the increase in TB. Unfortunately, a form of TB that is resistant to drugs has appeared, making this disease more difficult to treat. Diet changes and juicing can work miracles when it comes to healing TB.

✳ Diet Recommendations

Eat a high-fat diet. Odd as this may sound, studies show that a high-fat diet helps heal TB. A study done in 2001 showed that a cholesterol-rich diet accelerated the sterilization rate of sputum cultures in pulmonary tuberculosis patients, suggesting that cholesterol should be used as a complementary measure in antitubercular treatment. This is not a newly discovered treatment, however. As late as the 1940s, a high-fat diet, along with bed rest and exercise, was the treatment of choice for TB. A high-fat diet consisted of butter, cream, eggs, and other animal products. You could add to that shellfish and virgin coconut oil. Make sure all the animal products are cage-free or free-range, organically fed, and free of antibiotics and hormones. For more than seventy great recipes incorporating coconut oil, see my book *The Coconut Diet*.

Make 50 percent of your diet raw food. Choose vegetables, fruit, vegetable juice, sprouts, seeds, and nuts. It is whole, unprocessed, and largely uncooked food that will give your body the nutrients it needs to heal. Raw foods are "alive" with nutrients in their most effective state. You also need adequate protein, such as fish, poultry, meat, legumes (beans, lentils, and split peas), unsweetened yogurt, and eggs, along with whole grains. Also, include plenty of garlic and onions in your meal plans. (For more information, see Basic Guidelines for the Juice Lady's Health and Healing Diet, page 290.)

Drink plenty of fresh juices. You may find trying to chew plateful after plateful of raw vegetables exhausting and impossible. But fresh, raw juice is already broken down and easy to digest, and doesn't require chewing. You can drink these life-giving juices throughout the day and your digestive system will not be overtaxed, while at the same time you'll receive a concentration of nutrients. Just be sure to drink your juices at room temperature. Chilled juices and foods are hard on weakened lungs.

✳ Nutrient Recommendations

Antioxidants fight free radicals that damage cells and they support the immune system. It is very important that you build your immunity by consuming the following antioxidants:

- **Selenium** plays a key role in the activity of glutathione peroxidase, a vital enzyme that affects a wide variety of immune-system components. *Best juice sources of selenium:* Swiss chard, turnips, garlic, radishes, carrots, and cabbage.
- **Vitamin A** and **beta-carotene** are vital for the development and maintenance of immune cells. The body uses beta-carotene to create vitamin A. *Best juice sources of carotenes in general:* carrots, kale, parsley, spinach, Swiss chard, beet-root greens, watercress, broccoli, and romaine lettuce.
- **Vitamin C** and **bioflavonoids** work together to support the immune system. Vitamin C helps stimulate immune-cell activity, particularly that of the germ-eating neutrophils, and increases production of white blood cells.

Bioflavonoids act against viruses and have the ability to increase levels of vitamin C within cells. *Best juice sources of vitamin C:* kale, parsley, broccoli, Brussels sprouts, watercress, cauliflower, cabbage, strawberries, spinach, lemons, limes, turnips, and asparagus. *Best juice sources of bioflavonoids:* lemons, limes, parsley, cabbage, bell peppers, tomatoes, broccoli, and berries (blueberries, blackberries, and cranberries).

- **Vitamin E** is found in especially high concentrations in immune-cell membranes. This vitamin is essential for normal immune functioning, as it can help prevent free-radical damage to immune cells, which weakens their ability to perform. *Best juice sources of vitamin E:* spinach, watercress, asparagus, carrots, and tomatoes.

Essential fatty acids (EFAs), especially the anti-inflammatory omega-3s, are needed for a strong immune system. Flaxseed or hemp seed and cod-liver oil are all good sources of omega-3 fatty acids, as well as such cold-water fish as salmon, tuna, trout, sardines, mackerel, and halibut. (For more information, see the fats and oils section in Basic Guidelines for the Juice Lady's Health and Healing Diet, page 290.)

✳ Herb Recommendations

Echinacea is an immune-system builder.

Elecampagne, horehound, marshmallow, and **mullein** are expectorants and decongestants.

✳ Juice Therapy

Note: Drink all juices at room temperature; chilled liquids and foods are hard on weakened lungs.

Dandelion leaf juice contains various phytochemicals that are believed to deactivate the TB bacterium.

Fenugreek and **alfalfa** sprout juices help heal the lungs.

Garlic juice has antiviral properties.

Mint juice. One teaspoon of mint juice, mixed with two teaspoons of pure malt vinegar and a teaspoon of honey (optional), should be mixed in one-half cup (about 120 ml) of carrot juice. This should be taken as a tonic three times a day. It liquefies the sputum, nourishes the lungs, increases body resistance against infection, and prevents the harmful effects of antitubercular drugs.

Pear juice can help heal the lungs.

Pineapple juice is beneficial in the treatment of tuberculosis. It has been found to be effective in dissolving mucus and aiding recovery. This juice was used regularly in the past in treating this disease when it was more common than it is at present. One glass is recommended daily.

Potato juice is a traditional remedy for TB.

Turnip juice has been used as a traditional remedy for lung diseases, especially TB. Combine with watercress and garlic juice for best results.

Wheatgrass juice is rich in enzymes and blood-purifying chlorophyll. You must have an abundance of enzymes for your body to heal. Wheatgrass juice works best taken straight, but if you need a little help getting it down to start with, try Wheatgrass Light (see page 345).

✳ Juice Recipes

Liver Life Tonic *(pg 336)*   **Pure Green Sprout Drink** *(pg 340)*   **Immune Builder** *(pg 335)*   **Turnip Time** *(pg 344)*   **Wheatgrass Light** *(pg 345)*   **Spinach Power** *(pg 341)*   **Morning Energizer** *(pg 337)*   **Tomato Florentine** *(pg 343)*   **Sweet Dreams Nightcap** *(pg 342)*

Ulcers

AN ULCER is an erosion of tissue that leaves an open wound. A peptic ulcer is a sore in the lining of the stomach or duodenum—the first part of the small intestine. If peptic ulcers are found in the stomach, they're called gastric ulcers. If they're found in the duodenum, they're called duodenal ulcers. You can have more than one ulcer. Duodenal ulcers are more common and affect about 10 percent of Americans, with more men suffering from them than women.

Symptoms include a burning pain in the gut that occurs forty-five to sixty minutes after eating, or at night, feels like a dull ache, comes and goes for a few days or weeks, starts two to three hours after a meal or comes in the middle of the night when your stomach is empty, and usually goes away after you eat. Other symptoms include weight loss, lack of appetite, pain while eating, feeling sick to your stomach, and vomiting.

The body makes strong acids that digest food, and a lining protects the inside of the stomach and duodenum from these acids. If the lining breaks down, the acids can damage the walls. Both Helicobacter pylori (*H. pylori*—a bacteria) and nonsteroidal anti-inflammatory drugs (NSAIDs) such as aspirin or ibuprofen can weaken this lining, so acid can reach the stomach or duodenal wall. Elements that can increase the production of stomach acid and worsen the situation include stress and anxiety, taking aspirin or other NSAIDs over a long period of time, steroid use, smoking, or drinking too much coffee or alcohol.

Typical medical treatments for ulcers are either antacids or prescription drugs such as Tagamet and Zantac. Both of these prescription drugs are associated with a number of side effects including digestive disturbances, nutritional imbalances, liver dysfunction, disruption of bone metabolism, and breast development in men. The other medical treatment for ulcers is antacids; however, many popular antacids also have side effects. The calcium carbonate antacids (e.g., Tums, Alka-2) actually produce a "rebound" effect on gastric acid secretion and may cause kidney stones. The sodium bicarbonate antacids (e.g., Rolaids, Alka-Seltzer, Bromo Seltzer) tend to cause systemic alkalosis, and interfere with heart and kidney function. Aluminum-magnesium compounds (e.g., Maalox, Mylanta, Di-Gel) may cause calcium and phosphorus depletion as well as possible aluminum toxicity.

✳ Diet Recommendations

Eat a high-fiber, complex-carbohydrate diet. A high-fiber diet has been associated with a reduced rate of ulcers. A study of 47,806 men found that consumption of the fiber found in fruits, vegetables, and legumes (beans, lentils, and split peas) was associated with a reduced risk of duodenal ulcer. The researchers found that soluble fiber, such as the pectins found in fruits, vegetables, and juice, are more strongly associated with this reduction in risk than insoluble fiber (the type of fiber ejected when juicing). The researchers also found that diets that contained a lot of refined foods, such as white flour and white rice, were associated with a higher rate of duodenal ulcers. Therefore, eat only brown rice and whole-grain baked goods. Add plain yogurt to your diet; it has been shown to protect the stomach against irritants. (For more information, see Basic Guidelines for the Juice Lady's Health and Healing Diet, page 290.)

Increase omega-3 fatty acids. Some studies suggest that omega-3 fatty acids, which are found in fatty fish like salmon, mackerel, sardines, trout, and herring, and supplemental fish oil such as cod-liver oil or krill oil may help reduce the risk of ulcers. Omega-3 fats increase the production of prostaglandins, compounds that help to protect the lining of the entire digestive tract, including the lining of the stomach and intestines.

Eat small meals frequently throughout the day. This helps relieve stress on your digestive system.

Eat more unripe bananas, if you have *H. pylori*. One study found that substances called protease inhibitors, which are concentrated in unripe bananas, protect against such bacterial infections as those caused by *H. pylori*. Researchers say this may be why unripened bananas have traditionally been used to cure stomach ulcers.

Avoid foods that increase stomach-acid production or aggravate the condition, which include fried foods, black tea and coffee (includes decaffeinated), chocolate, strong spices, black pepper, red or hot pepper, chili powder, citrus fruits and juices, tomato products, animal fat, peppermint, and carbonated drinks. These items typically increase the acidity of the stomach or aggravate it and therefore can contribute to ulcer development or aggravate symptoms of existing ulcers. Milk also falls into this category, despite the persistent belief among some people that milk soothes the stomach. (Avoid all dairy, which includes cheese, ice cream, and yogurt.)

Eliminate food allergies. Clinical and experimental evidence points to food allergies as a primary cause of ulcers. The link between allergies and ulcers has been investigated in several studies. In one study, 98 percent of patients with radiographic evidence of ulcers had coexisting lower and upper respiratory tract allergic disease. In another, twenty-five of forty-three allergic children had X-ray–diagnosed ulcers. A diet that eliminates food allergies has been used with great success in preventing and treating recurrent ulcers.

If food allergy is the cause, the ulcers will continue to recur until the offending food or foods are eliminated from the diet. Ironically, many people with ulcers soothe themselves by drinking a lot of milk, a highly allergenic food.

Reduce your intake of sodium. An American study has linked high intakes of salt and soy sauce to a higher risk of stomach ulcers. Avoid adding salt to your food and use food labels to check for added sodium. Foods commonly high in sodium include canned soup, tortilla chips, potato and corn chips, salted nuts, salted meats (e.g., bacon, pastrami, salami, corned beef), blue cheese, and cornflakes. Switching to a diet containing fewer packaged or processed foods will definitely reduce your sodium intake. Completely avoid common table salt; choose Celtic sea salt or gray salt, either of which is rich in minerals, and use sparingly.

✳ Nutrient Recommendations

Bioflavonoids help reduce stomach acid levels. They also counteract the production and secretion of histamine, a chemical known to stimulate the release of gastric acid. In addition, bioflavonoids help make vitamin C more effective. *Best juice sources of bioflavonoids:* apricots, bell peppers, berries (blueberries, blackberries, and cranberries), broccoli, cabbage, and parsley.

Vitamin A and **carotenes** protect the mucous membranes of the stomach and intestines. Vitamin A is available in fruits and vegetables in the form of carotenes, which are converted by the body into vitamin A as needed. *Best juice sources of carotenes in general:* carrots, kale, parsley, spinach, Swiss chard, beetroot greens, watercress, broccoli, and romaine lettuce.

Vitamin C promotes wound healing and protects against infections. *Best juice sources of vitamin C:* kale, parsley, broccoli, Brussels sprouts, watercress, cauliflower, cabbage, strawberries, spinach, turnips, and asparagus.

Vitamin E promotes healing and aids in reducing levels of stomach acid. *Best juice sources of vitamin E:* spinach, watercress, asparagus, carrots, and tomatoes.

Vitamin K aids healing and neutralizes stomach acid. It can also prevent bleeding. *Best juice sources of vitamin K:* turnip greens, broccoli, lettuce, cabbage, spinach, watercress, asparagus, and string beans.

Zinc helps increase production of the protective substance gastric mucin, and it may help heal ulcers. *Best juice sources of zinc:* gingerroot, turnips, parsley, garlic, carrots, spinach, cabbage, lettuce, and cucumbers.

✳ Herb Recommendations

Aloe vera, in a dosage of four ounces daily, can help stop ulcer bleeding and speed the healing process. Do not use aloe bitters.

Bilberry, calendula flower, goldenseal, and **myrrh** all have antiulcer properties. They also inhibit the growth of *H. pylori* bacteria. Avoid goldenseal if you are pregnant, and do not use it for more than ten days at a time.

Licorice, in the form of deglyrrhizinated licorice (DGL), promotes healing of gastric and duodenal ulcers. DGL is available in chewable tablets from most health food stores; take between meals or twenty minutes before meals. Unlike other forms of licorice, DGL can be taken indefinitely.

✳ Juice Therapy

Alfalfa and **wheatgrass** juices are good sources of vitamin K and blood-purifying chlorophyll. These juices prevent bleeding, aid healing, and neutralize stomach acid. Barley grass juice is another good choice.

Cabbage juice has been found to be very successful in treating peptic ulcers. Research has shown that drinking one quart of raw cabbage juice each day for at least a week resulted in the healing of an ulcer within an average of three weeks. Cabbage juice has been well documented in medical literature as having remarkable success in treating ulcers. Dr. Garnett Cheney from Stanford University's School of Medicine and other researchers have performed several studies using fresh cabbage juice. They have found that the majority of patients with ulcers experienced complete healing, sometimes in as little as seven days. Cabbage juice contains mucinlike compounds believed by researchers to be the healing agents. Celery also contains these compounds, so you can add some celery juice to the cabbage, with some carrot for flavor.

Parsley juice is rich in beta-carotene, bioflavonoids, vitamin C, and zinc. Intake should be limited to a safe, therapeutic dose of one-half to one cup per day. Parsley can be toxic in overdose, and should be especially avoided by pregnant women.

Pineapple juice contains bromelain, an enzyme that improves digestion and relieves symptoms of ulcers.

Purple grape juice with seeds contains substances that act as anti-inflammatory agents and strengthen tissues.

✳ Juice Recipes

Omit the lemon and lime from all recipes until your ulcer has healed.

Pure Green Sprout Drink *(pg 340)*   **Wheatgrass Light** *(pg 345)*   **Morning Energizer** *(pg 337)*   **Antiulcer Cabbage Cocktail** *(pg 327)*   **Calcium-Rich Cocktail** *(pg 329)*   **Magnesium-Rich Cocktail** *(pg 336)*   **Beautiful-Skin Cocktail** *(pg 328)*   **Spinach Power** *(pg 341)*   **Triple C** *(pg 344)*

Varicose Veins and Hemorrhoids

VARICOSE VEINS are enlarged veins that can be flesh-colored, dark purple, or blue. They often look like cords, and appear twisted and bulging. They are swollen and raised above the surface of the skin, and are commonly found on the backs of the calves or on the insides of the legs. Defects in the vein walls lead to dilation of the veins and damage to the valves, which causes blood to pool in the veins. The veins then bulge, becoming widened, distended, and sometimes twisted. This condition may be without symptoms, or it may be associated with tender or sore legs, feelings of heaviness, or pain in the legs. Fluid retention, discoloration, and ulceration of the skin can develop.

Hemorrhoids are varicosities located in the rectal and anal areas. Symptoms may include pain, rectal itching or bleeding, and blood in the stool. Hemorrhoids are usually caused by a low-fiber diet, constipation (see Constipation, page 114), or liver dysfunction.

If the affected veins are near the surface, they pose very little danger. However, this condition can be more serious if it involves obstruction and valve defects of the deeper veins of the legs. This type of varicose vein can lead to thrombophlebitis, an inflammation of the veins that in turn can lead to blood-clot development. Varicose veins are caused by a variety of factors, including a low-fiber diet, obesity, pregnancy, straining in defecation such as in constipation, and standing for long periods of time. This condition affects about half of all middle-aged adults in the U.S.

✳ Diet Recommendations

Eat a high-fiber diet. A high-fiber diet is one of the most important components in the prevention and treatment of varicose veins and hemorrhoids. At least 50 percent of your diet should consist of raw foods—fruits, vegetables, juices, sprouts, seeds, and nuts. Consume at least 30 grams of fiber a day. Eating more fiber and fewer refined and starchy carbohydrates will help you maintain a healthy weight. This is another important consideration, since being overweight can contribute to varicose vein and hemorrhoid development. (For more information, see Basic Guidelines for the Juice Lady's Health and Healing Diet, page 290.)

Eat more gingerroot, garlic, and onions. People with varicose veins have a decreased ability to break down the fibrin surrounding the affected veins. These foods help break down fibrin.

Enjoy a juice day once a week. Juicing vegetables every day can be very beneficial. In addition, choosing a vegetable-juice diet one day a week will help relieve constipation, give the digestive system a rest, and provide abundant nutrients that support blood-vessel health.

Avoid these foods: sugar, ice cream, and other sweets; refined salt; alcohol; fried foods; processed and refined foods (e.g., white-flour baked goods); coffee; black tea; excess animal protein and fat; and cheese. Sugar (especially fructose) and fat may cause an elevation in enzymes that break down collagen and open holes in capillary walls.

✳ Nutrient Recommendations

Anthocyanidins and **proanthocyanidins.** In numerous studies, people with various circulation problems, including hemorrhoids and varicose veins, given supplemental anthocyanidins, experienced dramatic and sometimes total improvement in their conditions. Researchers did not find side effects in any of the published studies. Similar compounds known as proanthocyanidins—derived from grape seeds or pine needles—support skin and blood vessels. They increase the amounts of intercellular vitamin C and collagen (fibrous protein bundles that form the connective tissue that supports blood vessels, ligaments, and cartilage). A small, preliminary trial found that supplementation with 150 mg of proanthocyanidins per day improved the function of leg veins after a single application in people with widespread varicose veins.

Essential fatty acids (EFAs) can be helpful in maintaining blood-vessel health. Take one tablespoon of cod-liver oil daily. (For more information, see the fats and oils section in Basic Guidelines for the Juice Lady's Health and Healing Diet, page 290.)

Vitamin C and **bioflavonoids** work together to strengthen blood vessels. *Best juice sources of vitamin C:* kale, parsley, broccoli, Brussels sprouts, watercress, cauliflower, cabbage, strawberries, papaya, spinach, citrus fruits, turnips, mangoes, asparagus, and cantaloupes. Among the bioflavonoids, rutin is used routinely to treat varicose veins. It is present in many foods, including citrus fruits, apricots, blueberries, blackberries, cherries, rose hips, and buckwheat. Another bioflavonoid, quercetin, has also shown promise in treating varicose veins. *Best juice sources of bioflavonoids:* apricots, bell peppers, berries (blueberries, blackberries, and cranberries), broccoli, cabbage, cherries, lemons, limes, parsley, and tomatoes.

Vitamin E improves circulation and helps prevent the typical heavy feeling in the legs associated with varicose veins. *Best juice sources of vitamin E:* spinach, watercress, asparagus, carrots, and tomatoes.

Vitamin K is helpful for bleeding hemorrhoids. *Best juice sources of vitamin K:* turnip greens, broccoli, lettuce, cabbage, spinach, watercress, asparagus, and string beans.

Zinc is an anti-inflammatory that aids healing. *Best juice sources of zinc:* gingerroot, turnips, parsley, garlic, carrots, spinach, cabbage, lettuce, and cucumbers.

✳ Herb Recommendations

Gotu kola helps strengthen tissue structure around frail veins and also improves blood flow.

Horse chestnut seed extract has been shown to reduce inflammation associated with varicose veins and stimulate regeneration of damaged veins. The active ingredients in horse chestnut appear to be a group of chemicals called saponins, of which aescin is considered the most important. Aescin appears to reduce swelling and inflammation. It's not exactly clear how aescin works, but theories include "sealing" leaking capillaries, improving the elastic strength of veins, preventing the release of enzymes (known as glycosaminoglycan hydrolases) that break down collagen and open holes in capillary walls, and decreasing inflammation. In a study of 240 people with varicose veins (194 of them women), taking 50 milligrams of aescin twice a day for twelve weeks reduced swelling in the lower legs by 25 percent. It also has been used effectively for treating varicose veins as a poultice contained in compression stockings. (To learn how to make and use a poultice, see "How to Make an Herbal Poultice" at www.ehow.com/how_2127630_herbal-poultice.html.)

✳ Juice Therapy

Blackberry, blueberry, cherry, and **raspberry** juices contain anthocyanidins and proanthocyanidins, pigments that help strengthen vein walls and increase the muscular tone of the veins.

Carrot and **spinach** juices may be beneficial for varicose veins.

Garlic and **gingerroot** juices help break down fibrin.

Parsley juice is an important source of several nutrients, including bioflavonoids, vitamin C, and zinc. Intake should be limited to a safe, therapeutic dose of one-half to one cup per day. Parsley can be toxic in overdose, and should be especially avoided by pregnant women.

Pineapple juice contains the enzyme bromelain, which promotes fibrin breakdown. Bromelain can also help prevent the formation of the hard, lumpy skin that forms around varicose veins.

Purple grapes are actually beneficial because of the compounds in their seeds, which improve the support structure of vein walls.

✳ Juice Recipes

Immune Builder *(pg 335)* **The Ginger Hopper** *(pg 332)* **Spring Tonic** *(pg 342)* **Spinach Power** *(pg 341)* **Beautiful-Skin Cocktail** *(pg 328)* **Magnesium-Rich Cocktail** *(pg 336)* **Allergy Relief** *(pg 326)* **Wheatgrass Light** *(pg 345)* **Garlic Surprise** *(pg 332)* **Ginger Twist** *(pg 332)* **Happy Morning** *(pg 333)* **Morning Energizer** *(pg 337)* **Natural Diuretic Cocktail** *(pg 338)* **Peppy Parsley** *(pg 339)* **Pure Green Sprout Drink** *(pg 340)*

Water Retention

WATER RETENTION, also known as edema, is an abnormal accumulation of fluid in the spaces between the cells or within body cavities. Fluid is always moving in and out of cells, between cells and tissue spaces, and between the blood and the tissues. The force of blood pressure tends to push water out of the blood and into tissue spaces, and to pull water into the blood from the tissues. Normally, there is a dynamic balance between the "push and pull" forces, but when an imbalance occurs, edema is the result.

Pitting edema can be demonstrated by applying pressure to the skin of a swollen leg, for example, and depressing the skin with a finger. If the pressing causes an indentation in the skin that persists for some time after the release of the pressure, the edema is referred to as pitting edema. In nonpitting edema, which usually affects the legs or arms, pressure that is applied to the skin does not result in a persistent indentation.

Water retention can be confined to a localized area, such as the lower legs and ankles, or generalized, affecting the whole body. Localized water retention in the lower extremities is often the result of poor venous return. This means that blood is pumped to the extremities, but the body does not do an efficient job of moving it from the extremities back to the heart.

There are many possible causes of water retention. Some are serious, such as congestive heart failure, and some are lifestyle-related, such as standing or sitting all day. The most common systemic diseases associated with edema involve the heart, liver, kidneys, and thyroid, and high or low blood pressure. In these diseases, edema occurs primarily because of the body's retention of too much salt. The excess salt holds water in the interstitial tissue spaces, where the retained surplus of fluid is recognized as edema. Hormonal changes that occur in women just prior to each menstrual period can cause bloating. Also, varicose veins and thrombophlebitis (a blood clot with inflammation of the veins) of the deep veins of the legs can cause inadequate pumping of the blood by the veins (venous insufficiency). The resulting increase of "back pressure" in the veins forces fluid to leak into the interstitial tissue spaces, where it is retained. A contributing factor is poor capillary structure, known as poor vascular integrity. If the walls of the capillaries are not strong and resilient, they become more permeable. This makes it easier to push water out of the blood into tissue spaces. One sign of poor vascular integrity is easy bruising (see Bruises, page 63).

✳ Diet Recommendations

Drink plenty of water. Although it might seem counterintuitive, drinking plenty of water helps reduce water retention. The reason has to do with your body's response to water retention. As water is lost from your blood into the tissue spaces, the non-water parts of your blood (cells, minerals, protein) become more concentrated. This signals your body to hold on to the water it has, so that your blood can maintain proper dilution. Your body does this by changing the way your kidneys filter your blood so that less water is released into the urine. Drinking plenty of water will help keep your body from concentrating urine and retaining more water. Most people don't drink enough water. You should drink eight to ten eight-ounce glasses of purified water each day. Herbal tea can count toward your water quota. Coffee, black tea, soda, and alcohol do not; they are dehydrating, and you should avoid them as much as possible. (If you do drink any of these occasionally, drink an extra glass of water for every cup or glass of them that you drink.)

Eat adequate protein. Protein deficiency is a known cause of edema. Plasma osmotic pressure is one of the forces that pulls water from tissues back into the blood, and is directly related to the amount of protein in the blood. This means you should eat high-quality, low-fat protein, such as fish, skinless chicken, or other free-range meat with plenty of vegetables and legumes. It is not advisable to increase your protein intake if you have kidney disease. Consult with your doctor in that case before eating more protein (see also the Kidney Cleanse, page 322).

Choose plenty of foods and juices that support your liver. The liver plays an important role in regulating the protein content of your blood. Foods that support liver function can be helpful in dealing with many conditions, including water retention.

Liver-friendly foods such as beetroot and artichokes can help the liver function optimally. Other liver-friendly foods include peas, parsnips, potatoes, pumpkin, sweet potatoes, squash, yams, beans (green and yellow), broccoli, Brussels sprouts, cabbage, carrots, cauliflower, celery, chives, cucumber, eggplant, garlic, kale, kohlrabi, okra, onion, and parsley. Bitter greens and herbs, such as mustard greens and dandelion leaves, are especially helpful in stimulating the liver (see the Liver Cleanse, page 310).

Eat and juice your vegetables. Vegetables contain a lot of water. They also contain plenty of bioflavonoids and vitamin C—substances that help improve tissue integrity and can help reduce the tendency of capillaries to leak fluid into the surrounding tissue spaces. Eat plenty of the fruits and vegetables that have the most bioflavonoids, which are those that are brightly colored orange, yellow, red, purple, blue, or dark green. Berries and cherries are especially high in bioflavonoids, and blueberries are particularly good for maintaining blood-vessel integrity. Eat fruit and use fruit juice sparingly, however, to avoid consuming too much fruit sugar. (Limit fruit juice to no more than four ounces daily, and dilute it by half with water or vegetable juices.)

Avoid sweets and refined carbohydrates. In Chinese medicine, water retention is considered a "damp" condition. Foods that are cold, sweet, or mucus-forming contribute to this dampness, and should be avoided as much as possible. Foods that combine one or more of these qualities, such as ice cream (cold, sweet, and mucus-forming), are the worst for damp conditions, and should be completely avoided. Foods that are thought to "dry up" damp conditions are celery, lettuce, pumpkin, scallions, turnips, corn, and legumes (beans, lentils, split peas). Bitter herbs and salad greens are also helpful.

Use salt sparingly. High levels of sodium in the body will cause the body to retain water in order to dilute the sodium. This is why low-sodium diets are often prescribed for people who have water-retention problems or high blood pressure. Completely avoid common table salt (sodium chloride). Use Celtic sea salt or gray salt sparingly; they are rich in helpful minerals (found at health food stores).

✳ Nutrient Recommendations

Vitamin B₆ (pyridoxine) may help ease water retention by acting against sodium retention. *Best juice sources of vitamin B₆:* kale, spinach, turnip greens, bell peppers, and prunes.

Vitamins E and **C with bioflavonoids** can help maintain blood-vessel integrity, which helps to keep fluid from leaking out of the blood vessels. *Best juice sources of vitamin E:* spinach, watercress, asparagus, carrots, and tomatoes. Vitamin C strengthens capillary walls by playing a role in the formation and maintenance of collagen, the basis of connective tissue. Healthy collagen is important in maintaining the integrity of blood vessels. *Best juice sources of vitamin C:* kale, parsley, broccoli, Brussels sprouts, watercress, cauliflower, cabbage, strawberries, spinach, lemons, limes, turnips, and asparagus. **Bioflavonoids** enhance the activity of vitamin C. *Best juice sources of bioflavonoids:* bell peppers, broccoli, cabbage, parsley, and tomatoes.

✳ Herb Recommendations

Burdock and **yellow dock** stimulate liver function. Burdock is also mildly diuretic.

Corn silk is a good diuretic.

Dandelion root can help remove water and improve overall liver function.

Nettle is known to alleviate fluid retention.

✳ Juice Therapy

Asparagus juice, a diuretic, helps cleanse the kidneys.

Cantaloupe (with the seeds), cucumber, lemon, parsley, and **watermelon** juices are all diuretics. Parsley juice intake should be limited to a safe, therapeutic dose of one-half to one cup per day. Parsley can be toxic in overdose, and should be especially avoided by pregnant women.

Dandelion leaf juice helps fight water retention.

✳ Juice Recipes

Afternoon Refresher *(pg 326)*   **Liver Life Tonic** *(pg 336)*   **Triple C** *(pg 344)*
Peppy Parsley *(pg 339)*   **Beautiful-Skin Cocktail** *(pg 328)*   **Tomato Florentine** *(pg 343)*   **The Ginger Hopper** *(pg 332)*   **Allergy Relief** *(pg 326)*
Bladder Tonic *(pg 329)*   **Natural Diuretic Cocktail** *(pg 338)*   **Garlic Surprise** *(pg 332)*   **Turnip Time** *(pg 344)*   **Wheatgrass Light** *(pg 345)*

Weight Loss

BEING OVERWEIGHT is generally defined as exceeding the recommended weight for one's height and build. Under revised guidelines set by the federal government, 65 percent of all Americans over the age of twenty are overweight or obese. The body mass index (BMI) is a measurement that uses height and weight to determine the amount of body fat. The panel that set the revised standards defined overweight as having a BMI of 25.0 to 29.9 and obesity as having a BMI of 30.0 and above. (The National Institutes of Health publishes a BMI table; see the Appendix, page 355). A high BMI is especially troublesome for people who carry their weight around the middle. Waist circumference is associated with abdominal fat, which in turn is associated with an increased risk for such disorders as heart disease and diabetes. A waist circumference of more than forty inches in men and thirty-five inches in women signifies a problem in persons with a BMI of 25 or over.

Since the mid-1970s, the prevalence of overweight and obesity has increased sharply for both adults and children. Data from two NHANES surveys show that among adults ages twenty to seventy-four years the prevalence of obesity increased from 15.0 percent (in the 1976–1980 survey) to 32.9 percent (in the 2003–2004 survey). The two surveys also show increases in overweight among children and teens. For children ages two to five years, the prevalence of overweight increased from 5 percent to 13.9 percent; for those ages six to eleven years, prevalence increased from 6.5 percent to 18.8 percent; and for those ages twelve to nineteen years, prevalence increased from 5.0 percent to 17.4 percent.

Health risks for obesity include diabetes, hypertension, hypercholesterolemia, heart disease, certain cancers, stroke, and arthritis. Among children, there is also an increased risk of being overweight or obese in adulthood. In overweight and obese insulin-resistant individuals, even modest weight loss has been shown to improve insulin resistance. Thus, weight loss is recommended for all individuals who have or are at risk for diabetes.

What has contributed to the ever-growing waistline of Americans? A great change came to the American diet several decades ago. We were told to stop eating animal products and start eating carbohydrates. The food pyramid told us to eat a staggering number of grain servings each day (six to eleven). Americans were glad to comply with bagels and muffins for breakfast, sandwiches or pasta for lunch, and pizza or pasta for dinner. Lots of high-carb snacks filled the day, and the weight, like the sun, kept on rising. People became insulin-resistant and craved more and more carbs. Now we know the culprit. The carbs packed on the pounds, and most people are aware of this. But many people are also addicted to those carbs. If you're one, you can change that. This program has worked for hundreds of people I've worked with. And it can work for you as well.

✳ Lifestyle Recommendations

Get out and exercise. To lose one pound per week, you need to take in 500 fewer calories a day than you burn off. That means eating less and exercising more. As an example, taking a brisk walk for one hour and fifteen minutes will burn 500 calories. But if you eat 250 fewer calories a day, you can take a shorter walk and still lose a pound. Strength training to build your muscles is also important because muscle tissue burns more calories per pound than fat. More muscle means more fat-burning potential, even when you're at rest.

Get plenty of sleep. Research shows that when we don't get enough deep, restful sleep five major appetite-influencing hormones (leptin, ghrelin, insulin, growth hormone, and cortisol) get out of whack, causing us to want to eat more food. Ghrelin goes up; it's the hormone that causes us to crave carbs. And leptin, a hormone produced by fat, goes down; this hormone curbs our appetite. Leptin tells the body and brain how much energy it has, whether it needs more energy (saying "be hungry"), whether it should stop being hungry, and what to do with the energy it has (reproduce, regulate cellular repair). Most people need seven to nine hours sleep a night to keep the appetite hormones in balance. For more information, see my book *Sleep Away the Pounds*.

✳ Diet Recommendations

Choose a high-alkaline diet. Achieving a 75/25 (alkaline/acid) balance in foods and beverages and regulating your body's alkaline/acid chemistry through simple dietary changes can result in weight loss, increased energy, and a greater sense of well-being. Many of the foods and beverages we choose are acidic or turn acidic in our body. Culprits include sweets, junk food, trans fats and oxidized oils, coffee, alcohol, meat, poultry, eggs, dairy, fish, most grains, and some fruit. The body must maintain a healthy pH balance; in the blood between 7.35 and 7.45. To deal with excess acid, the

Alkaline Foods

Vegetables	Sesame seeds	Tahini
Vegetable juices	Flaxseed	Fats and oils
Fruits	Buckwheat groats	• Flax
• Lemon	Spelt	• Hemp
• Lime	Lentils	• Avocado
• Avocado	Cumin seeds	• Virgin coconut
• Tomato	Any sprouted seed	• Palm
• Grapefruit	Sprouts (soy, alfalfa, mung	• Virgin olive
• Watermelon (neutral)	bean, wheat, radish,	• Evening primrose
• Rhubarb	chickpea, broccoli)	• Borage
Almonds	Bragg Liquid Aminos (soy	
Pumpkin seeds	sauce alternative)	
Sunflower seeds	Hummus	

body will store it in fat cells. It will even make more fat cells in which to store acid to keep it from damaging delicate tissues and organs. The same is true of toxins (see The power of detoxification, page 286.) Many people have noticed that their weight begins dropping off when they increase alkaline foods such as vegetables, sprouts, essential fats, and vegetable juices. The body can finally let go of the fat cells containing the acid because there's plenty of alkaline buffer to neutralize and carry the acid out of the system. Acid levels may rise in the system at this time, which would indicate that fat is melting away with the acid it contains. You can measure pH with color pH indicator strips (found at most drugstores).

Make 75 percent of your diet alkaline foods, with at least half your vegetables raw in the form of salads, sprouts, raw food dishes, dehydrated food (dehydrated at 118° F or below), and vegetable juices, along with a little alkaline fruit, seeds, nuts, and good oils. Make the other 25 percent of your diet animal proteins, whole grains, and nuts (not on the alkaline list).

Drink two to three glasses of fresh vegetable juice daily and use juice fasting. Vegetables in particular are wise juice choices because your body can make virtually every calorie count for metabolism, rather than storage in fat cells. They help immensely in alkalinizing the body. Fruit juice contains fruit sugar, so always dilute fruit juice by half with water or vegetable juices to dilute the sugar and prevent appetite stimulation. (Do not use more than four ounces of fruit juice a day.) A great weight-loss and maintenance program is to juice-fast one day, or at least half a day, a week (see the Juice Fast, page 304). *On a personal note:* I have received scores of letters and calls from people who have lost ten, twenty, seventy, and even one hundred fifty pounds by following my weight-loss program, which includes two to three glasses of fresh juice each day in addition to replacing one meal with a glass of vegetable juice. Personally, I have found that short vegetable-juice fasts provide a great jump-start for any weight-loss program. They help you not only to lose a pound or two, but also to feel energized and renewed. I followed this program for nearly two decades and have maintained about the same weight year after year.

Know the power of detoxification. Just as acids are stored in fat cells, so are toxins (which are acidic). As you detoxify your body with intestinal, liver, and gallbladder cleansing, along with lots of fresh vegetable juices each day, you'll notice the weight melting away. And get into a sauna or do aerobic exercises that make you sweat. Sweating is the only way to get rid of plastic toxins (see the intestinal, liver, and gallbladder cleanses, pages 307–325).

Increase the fiber in your diet. Eat more high-fiber foods, such as vegetables, low-sugar fruit, and legumes (beans, lentils, split peas). Add a fiber supplement such as psyllium, guar gum, or pectin. (Avoid fiber products that contain sugar or other sweeteners.) When taken with juice or water before a meal, fiber supplements form a gelatinous mass in the digestive tract that creates a feeling of fullness. As a result, you will be more likely to eat less food. An added bonus is that fiber supplements have been shown to enhance blood-sugar control and insulin sensitivity, and to actually reduce the number of calories your body absorbs. A high-fiber diet also supports good colon function and helps eliminate the toxins released during weight loss.

Add virgin coconut oil. Coconut oil is known as *slimming oil* because it's rich in medium-chain triglycerides (MCTs). MCTs promote weight loss because the liver likes to burn them rather than store them in fat cells. They act a lot like kindling in a fire. Coconut oil also helps improve your thyroid function, which will greatly facilitate weight loss. You can read more about the amazing coconut diet weight-loss plan in my book *The Coconut Diet,* which has more than seventy delicious recipes.

Avoid sugars and artificial sweeteners. Sweets stimulate the appetite. They also contain empty calories that tend to be stored as fat rather than used for energy. Artificial sweeteners such as aspartame (NutraSweet) and sucralose (Splenda) are not better for weight loss or your health; they are worse. A recent study followed fourteen dieting women and found that those drinking a beverage sweetened with aspartame ate significantly more food than those drinking a beverage sweetened with sucrose (refined sugar). Neither sweetener is a good choice, but artificial sweeteners are worse for your health and for appetite stimulation and obesity. If you want to see a graphic example of what aspartame (NutraSweet) can do (e.g., obesity and tumors), take a look at the photos of one woman's experiment with this sweetener and rats. Go to http://articles.mercola.com/sites/articles/archive/2008/3/11/one-womans-astonishing-experiment-with-aspartame.aspx.

Avoid all diet soda. Researchers have found a correlation between drinking diet soda and metabolic syndrome—the collection of risk factors for cardiovascular disease and diabetes, which include abdominal obesity, high cholesterol, high blood-glucose levels, and elevated blood pressure. Scientists gathered dietary information on more than 9,500 men and women ages forty-five to sixty-four and tracked their health for nine years. The risk of developing metabolic syndrome was 34 percent higher among those who drank just one can of diet soda a day compared with those who drank none.

Recognize sugar and other carbohydrate cravings. If you desire sweets, refined grains (breads, crackers, pasta), and such starchy vegetables as potatoes, winter squash, and corn, there's a good chance you have a carbohydrate craving. This can contribute to a condition known as insulin resistance. Being insulin-resistant means your body stops responding to insulin, and instead grabs every calorie it can and deposits it as fat. So no matter how little you eat, you will gradually gain weight. Your cells cannot absorb the glucose they need, so they signal your brain that you need more carbohydrates, in particular sugars. The result is persistent food cravings and weight gain (see Cravings, page 118).

Drink at least eight glasses of water daily. Drinking a glass of water before a meal can help you feel full more quickly, so you'll eat less. Water also helps your body use its stored fat, promotes good colon function, and flushes away the toxins released during weight loss.

✳ Nutrient Recommendations

Chromium, a trace mineral, can significantly improve your body's sensitivity to insulin, the main sugar-control hormone. Proper insulin function is the key to maintaining normal blood-sugar levels and to promoting thermogenesis—the burning of calories by raising body heat. When chromium is deficient in the diet, insulin activity is blocked, blood-sugar levels become elevated, thermogenesis diminishes, and cravings for sweet foods develop. Several studies using chromium combined with exercise have shown significant weight loss, increased muscle mass, and improved insulin response in the participants. *Best juice sources of chromium:* green peppers, apples, parsnips, spinach, carrots, lettuce, string beans, and cabbage.

Magnesium is involved in energy regulation. In one study, a deficiency of this mineral was associated with higher levels of body fat. *Best juice sources of magnesium:* beetroot greens, spinach, parsley, dandelion greens, garlic, blackberries, beetroot, broccoli, cauliflower, carrots, and celery.

Pantothenic acid, a B vitamin, plays a role in fat metabolism. This vitamin was shown to facilitate weight loss in one study. *Best juice sources of pantothenic acid:* broccoli, cauliflower, and kale.

Vitamins C and **E** play important roles in fat metabolism. Deficiencies of these vitamins have been associated with higher body-fat levels. *Best juice sources of vitamin C:* kale, parsley, broccoli, Brussels sprouts, watercress, cauliflower, cabbage, strawberries, spinach, lemons, limes, turnips, and asparagus. *Best juice sources of vitamin E:* spinach, watercress, asparagus, carrots, and tomatoes.

Zinc deficiency has been associated with higher body-fat levels. *Best juice sources of zinc:* gingerroot, turnips, parsley, garlic, carrots, spinach, cabbage, lettuce, and cucumbers.

✳ Herbal Recommendations

Bladderwrack and **hawthorn** are used to stimulate the adrenal glands and improve thyroid function. Bladderwrack is a species of kelp (a seaweed) that contains significant amounts of iodine. Limit consumption to once a week to avoid ingesting too much iodine.

Chickweed is a traditional herbal remedy that has been used to suppress the appetite.

Juniper berries act as a diuretic that also facilitates detoxification. To avoid kidney irritation, do not take juniper berries for long periods of time.

✳ Juice Therapy

Alfalfa, asparagus, cucumber, dandelion, lemon, and **parsley** juices are good diuretics; in addition, alfalfa and dandelion are good detoxification agents. Parsley juice intake should be limited to a safe, therapeutic dose of one-half to one cup per day. Parsley can be toxic in overdose, and should be especially avoided by pregnant women.

Daikon radish has been used in traditional Chinese medicine to help eliminate excess fat. You can juice daikon radishes.

Gingerroot juice can stimulate thermogenesis.

Jerusalem artichoke and **parsnip** juices are traditional remedies that help curb cravings for sweets and junk food. The key is to sip the juice slowly when you have a craving for high-fat or high-sugar food.

Radish has been used as a traditional remedy to help promote healthy thyroid function. A healthy thyroid gland is important in weight loss and weight maintenance.

✳ Juice Recipes

Skinny Sip *½ small or medium lemon, washed, or peeled if not organic;* 1 cup unsweetened mineral water
Weight-Loss Buddy *(pg 345)*   **Orient Express** *(pg 338)*   **Spring Tonic** *(pg 342)*
Liver Life Tonic *(pg 336)*   **Radish Care** *(pg 340)*   **Magnesium-Rich Cocktail** *(pg 336)*   **Pure Green Sprout Drink** *(pg 340)*   **Ginger Twist** *(pg 332)*
Afternoon Refresher *(pg 326)*   **Beautiful-Skin Cocktail** *(pg 328)*

Basic Guidelines for the Juice Lady's Health and Healing Diet

JUICING FRESH PRODUCE can help you achieve and maintain optimal health. You can attain the best results when you combine daily juice with an overall healthy diet plan. In this section, you'll learn about the most important principles of the health and healing diet, along with daily serving recommendations and food suggestions. To help you plan your day, a sample menu follows based on those recommendations.

✴ Principle 1: Drink fresh vegetable juice each day and eat more of your foods raw.

To help you move to a state of vibrant health and high-level wellness, nutritional experts now recommend that you eat nine to thirteen servings of vegetables and fruit a day—two or three servings being fruit and the rest vegetables. This new guideline of nine a day may seem staggeringly high until you consider that juicing, which is fast and easy, can make up half of that amount. Juicing enables you to quickly consume a lot of vegetables and a little fruit in a glass. When you include a couple of glasses of fresh juice each day, you can reach the nine-a-day goal each and every day.

Along with your fresh juice, eat at least half your vegetables raw in the form of salads, sprouts, raw food creations, dehydrated foods (dehydrated at 118°F. or below is considered raw—enzymes and vitamins are preserved), and vegetable juices.

Raw foods, especially if they are organically grown, contain an abundance of vitamins, minerals, enzymes, and phytonutrients. And when they're picked at the peak of ripeness, they're particularly rich in health-promoting vitamins and minerals. Plants make vitamins and take in inorganic minerals from the soil and convert them to organic minerals that our bodies can use.

Plants also provide energy through a series of actions known as photosynthesis—a process in which plants use the energy from sunlight to produce carbohydrates, which cellular respiration converts into ATP, the "fuel" used by all living things. Sunlight energy combined with carbon dioxide from the air and water from the soil is converted into usable chemical energy, a process made possible by chlorophyll, the substance that makes plants green. This energy, abundant in raw foods, gives us vibrant health and energy.

Eating a large portion of vegetables and fruit raw is so important because vitamins and enzymes are destroyed in cooking. Enzyme deficiencies can hinder the chemical reactions necessary for our optimal health. And cooking not only destroys nutrients, it also wipes out some of the flavor. Just one more reason to choose raw foods—they taste delicious, especially when they're organically grown.

✳ Principle 2: Make about 75 percent of your diet alkaline foods.

Achieving a 75/25 (alkaline/acid) balance in foods and beverages and regulating your body's alkaline/acid chemistry through simple dietary changes can result in weight loss, increased energy, healing of ailments and disease, and a greater sense of well-being. Many of the foods and beverages we choose are acidic or turn acidic in our body, such as sweets, junk food, trans fats and oxidized oils, coffee, alcohol, meat, poultry, eggs, dairy, fish, most grains, and some fruit. The body must maintain a healthy pH balance—in the blood between 7.35 and 7.45. To deal with excess acid, the body will store it in fat cells. It will even make more fat cells in which to store acids to keep them from damaging delicate tissues and organs. The same is true of toxins, which are acidic. Many people have noticed that when they increase alkaline foods such as vegetables, sprouts, essential fats, and vegetable juices (all alkaline), their weight begins dropping off, pain from arthritis and fibromyalgia lessens, and ailments disappear. Choose whole, fresh, organic foods, with a high percentage being alkaline, as the foundation of your healthy diet—vegetables, vegetable juice, salads, sprouts, raw food dishes,

Alkaline Foods

Vegetables	Sesame seeds	Tahini
Vegetable juices	Flaxseed	Fats and Oils
Fruits	Buckwheat groats	• Flax
• Lemon	Spelt	• Hemp
• Lime	Lentils	• Avocado
• Avocado	Cumin seeds	• Virgin coconut
• Tomato	Any sprouted seed	• Palm
• Grapefruit	Sprouts (soy, alfalfa, mung	• Virgin olive
• Watermelon (neutral)	bean, wheat, radish,	• Evening primrose
• Rhubarb	chickpea, broccoli)	• Borage
Almonds	Bragg Liquid Aminos (soy	
Pumpkin seeds	sauce alternative)	
Sunflower seeds	Hummus	

dehydrated foods (dehydrated at 118°F. or below), and a little alkaline fruit, seeds, nuts, and good oils. Make the other 25 percent of your diet animal proteins, whole grains, and nuts (not on the alkaline list).

✻ Principle 3: Eat a high-fiber diet.

Fiber is important for good elimination, lowering cholesterol, and removing toxins. The recommended daily fiber intake is 20 to 35 grams daily. Choose complex carbohydrates—vegetables, fruit, legumes, and whole grains. These foods, which are abundant in insoluble and soluble fiber, should compose the largest portion of your food intake, 55 to 65 percent. Juice also contains soluble fiber. It is recommended that you limit the amount of grains; starchy vegetables such as potatoes, corn, and peas; and fruit to limit your sugar intake. This is especially important if you have diabetes, hypoglycemia, candidiasis, cancer, or metabolic syndrome, or are overweight. Protein should make up 15 to 20 percent of your diet, and fat should account for the remaining 15 to 25 percent. Although eating enough protein is important to overall health, there is evidence that too much protein can contribute to health problems.

✳ Principle 4: Choose healthy fats and avoid fats that contribute to disease.

Choose virgin coconut oil for cooking and virgin olive oil for salad dressings and other cold-food preparation. Eat more of the essential fatty acids (EFAs) found in cold-water fatty fish like salmon, mackerel, herring, trout, and sardines; fish oil such as cod-liver oil; flaxseed and hemp-seed oils and walnuts and walnut oil. Avoid as much as possible the unhealthy fats—saturated animal fat and processed fats such as margarine, trans fats, and hydrogenated oils. Be aware that the polyunsaturated vegetable oils such as corn, soy, safflower, sunflower, and canola oxidize easily. These fats are dominant in the omega-6 fats, and the American diet is too high in omega-6 fatty acids and too low in omega-3 fats. The unhealthy fats compromise immune-cell activity and contribute to a host of ailments and diseases.

✳ Principle 5: Avoid fast food, junk food, and commercially prepared foods.

Avoid sweets such as candy, chocolate, cookies, doughnuts, cakes, pies, ice cream, mochas, and refined-flour baked goods, such as pasta, pizza, rolls, bread and batter-coated fried foods. Most commercial foods are loaded with salt, sugar, preservatives, and additives. Too much salt causes sodium to be drawn into cells and potassium to be pulled out, which creates an imbalance in which cells are unable to efficiently absorb what they need or excrete wastes and unwanted materials. Consequently, they cease to effectively carry out vital metabolic processes. The foods listed above and toxins from the environment contribute to toxic-waste buildup inside the cells, and sludge accumulates outside the cells in tissue spaces. The symptoms of this "clogging up" and slowing down at the cellular level are fatigue, poor immune function, overweight, and, ultimately, disease. Preservatives and additives add to the body's toxic load and the decline of efficient organ function.

✳ The Health and Healing Food Categories

Following is a list of the food categories that make up the health and healing diet with recommended servings.

Vegetables: 6–11 servings per day

For this group, a single serving is one cup lettuce or other leafy greens; one-half cup chopped raw or cooked vegetables; one cup vegetable juice.

Recommended foods: all organically grown, fresh, raw or lightly cooked vegetables. Steamed or baked potatoes, new red potatoes, sweet potatoes, yams; baked squash. All vegetable juices.

Foods to avoid: canned vegetables, fried vegetables, canned or bottled vegetable juices. Frozen vegetables should be used only if fresh produce is not available.

Fruit: 2–3 servings per day

For this group, a single serving is one medium whole fruit; one-half cup chopped fruit; one cup fruit juice.

Recommended foods: all fresh, raw, organically grown fruits and freshly made fruit juices.

Foods to avoid: all canned fruits, and canned, bottled, or frozen juices. Frozen fruit should be used only if fresh produce is not available.

Grains: 1–3 servings per day (Choose only whole grains.)

For this group, one serving is equivalent to one slice of bread; one-half to one and one-quarter cups of dry cereal, depending on cereal type; one-half cup cooked brown rice, whole-grain pasta, or whole-grain cereal.

Recommended foods: all organically grown whole grains, such as rye, millet, buckwheat, whole wheat, corn, oats, brown rice, wheat germ, and bran. Dehydrated crackers are an excellent choice; they're usually made with sprouted seeds, vegetables, and sprouted grains. *Best bread choice:* sprouted whole-grain bread such as Ezekiel Bread; these breads can be found at most health food stores and should be refrigerated at all times. *Snacks:* air-popped popcorn.

Foods to avoid: white breads and crackers, refined-flour pasta and noodles, white rice, refined and sugared cereals, potato chips, corn chips, fried potatoes, buttered commercial popcorn, cakes, cookies, doughnuts, commercial muffins (high in sugar and fat).

Note: Be aware that brown-colored bread, muffins, bagels, and pasta doesn't mean those products are whole grain. Nor does a few whole grains thrown into the batter make it whole grain. Most brown bread is colored with something such as molasses. Only a few products are actually whole grain. See above.

Protein: 2–3 servings per day

For this group, one serving is four ounces cooked meat, poultry, or fish; one-half cup dried beans, lentils, or peas; one egg; two tablespoons nut butter; one-quarter cup nuts or seeds.

Recommended foods: eggs and skinless poultry (free-range and organically fed). Lean meat (free-range and no antibiotics or hormones); wild-caught fish and seafood, but especially fatty cold-water fish, chosen for its omega-3 fatty acids. All beans, lentils, and split peas, especially sprouted legumes such as bean, pea, and lentil sprouts (avoid soy products). All nuts (especially almonds, walnuts, and hazelnuts; soaked are the best), nut butters, seeds, and seed butters. Sprouted seeds such as sunflower and pumpkin.

Foods to avoid: luncheon or canned meats, hot dogs, bacon, sausage, salami, organ meat (which contains more toxins than does muscle meat), fatty meat, charbroiled meat, fried chicken, poultry skin, all deep-fried products. All meat and poultry not raised free-range or cage-free and raised with hormones, antibiotics, and other drugs. Peanut butter with added oil and sugar. Nuts roasted in oil and/or salted. Refried beans with lard.

Milk, Yogurt, Cheese (This is not a group of foods that I recommend.)

If you do choose to eat some dairy products, choose only organic dairy products and dairy alternatives. Growing numbers of people are allergic to or intolerant of dairy products. Dairy also tends to be quite mucus forming, which sets up a breeding ground for parasites, *Candida albicans,* and cancer cells. You can obtain calcium from dark leafy greens such as kale (very calcium rich); corn tortillas with lime added; seeds, especially sunflower and sesame; and nuts, especially almonds. For milk, you can substitute rice milk or almond milk. The best choices for cheese are pasture-fed sheep or goat cheese and plain yogurt. (Soymilk, soy ice cream, and soy cheese are not recommended because soy is high in phytoestrogens that can contribute to cancer in some people. Also, soy is a goitrogen, which means that it blocks iodine absorption and can contribute to low thyroid function and weight gain.)

Foods to avoid: nonorganic cheese, and especially cheese with yellow dye; nonorganic and non–pasture-fed milk, sweetened yogurt, ice cream, and sour cream.

Fats and oils: no more than 15 to 25 grams of fat daily; eat sparingly.

Recommended oils: virgin coconut oil, extra-virgin olive oil, hemp-seed oil; small amounts of sesame, almond, macadamia nut, and walnut oil.

You can also prepare dishes with any of these oils; however, olive and hemp-seed oils should not be heated. Virgin coconut oil is best for cooking since it has the least propensity to oxidize when heated. Purchase only pure, unrefined, organic oils; they can be found at health food stores. (Larger containers of coconut oil can be ordered, which offer good savings; see Sources, page 347.) For more information on the health benefits of coconut oil and more than seventy delicious recipes, see my book *The Coconut Diet.* Some fish oils are associated with clean arteries and freedom from fatty degeneration. The health secrets of these oils involve two omega-3 fatty acids: eicosapentaenoic acid (EPA) and docosahexaenoic acid (DHA). Essential fatty acids (EFAs) in hemp-seed and cod-liver oils provide the raw materials that allow our bodies to manufacture EPA and DHA. The richest sources of EPA and DHA are fatty cold-water fish such as salmon, herring, sardines, trout, halibut, cod, and mackerel. Fish oils are available in supplement form.

Americans eat too many unhealthy fats and not enough EFAs. Also, the American diet contains too many omega-6 fats and too few omega-3s. (The polyunsaturated oils—corn, canola, safflower, sunflower, and soy—are dominant in omega-6; they also oxidize easily and, therefore, are not recommended.) There are several oils rich in EFAs. They come in two types: omega-3 and omega-6 fatty acids. Hemp-seed oil is an example of oil that contains a good balance of omega-3 and omega-6 fatty acids, as well as gamma-linolenic acid (GLA). Extra-virgin olive oil contains small amounts of omega-3, and is good for cold-food preparation.

Your health will greatly benefit if you take one tablespoon of EFA-rich oil per day, such as cod-liver oil (also rich in vitamins A and D), evening primrose oil, borage oil, or unrefined hemp-seed oil, as a supplement. To help with taste, mix the oil with juice or "chase it" with juice.

Foods to avoid: margarine, shortening, partially hydrogenated oils (they contain trans-fatty acids), and fried and deep-fried foods—they contain toxic fatty-acid derivatives. The polyunsaturated oils—corn, canola, safflower, sunflower, and soy—oxidize easily. Trans-fatty acids and altered fatty-acid derivatives can have adverse effects on cell membranes and brain development in infants. In adults, they can damage the cardiovascular, liver, and immune systems.

Miscellaneous foods to avoid: coffee; soft drinks; fruit drinks; powdered drinks; alcohol; sweets; salt; anything with aspartame (NutraSweet), sucralose (Splenda), preservatives, dyes, additives, and fake fat; all food produced with pesticides and/or herbicides; and animal products grown with antibiotics and/or growth hormones, and not free-range or cage-free.

A SAMPLE MENU

To see how to put the diet guidelines to work in your everyday life, you can use this sample menu. Make adjustments to fit your lifestyle and specific needs.

Breakfast	✳	Juice, such as Morning Energizer (page 337) or Happy Morning (page 333) with protein powder, or Awesome Green Smoothie, (page 327) or toasted sprouted-grain bread (such as Ezekiel) with nut butter (organic almond is a great choice), or muesli with rice or almond milk, or soft-boiled egg with veggie patty
Midmorning Energy Snack	✳	Juice, such as The Ginger Hopper (page 332) or Icy Spicy Tomato (page 335), or vegetable sticks and/or one-quarter cup raw nuts or seeds
Lunch	✳	Green leafy salad with wild-caught salmon, or Cherie's Quick Energy Soup (page 330) and a dehydrated vegetable cracker
Midafternoon Energy Break	✳	Salsa in a Glass (page 340) or Afternoon Refresher (page 326), or two tablespoons sunflower or pumpkin seeds, or vegetable sticks
Dinner	✳	Main-course salad, such as Multigrain Salad Florentine or Chicken Curry Salad (see Two Main-Course Salads, below), or dinner salad and a cup of soup or baked squash or sweet potato, or stir-fry with lots of vegetables and a little organic tofu, chicken, meat, or seafood (optional) and brown rice
Evening Snack	✳	A piece of fresh fruit, or Sweet Dreams Nightcap (page 342)

Two Main-Course Salads

A main-course salad makes a great dinner. It's fast, healthy, and delicious. What you can put in a main-course salad is only limited by your tastes and imagination, but should always include a variety of natural, nutrient-packed ingredients. Here's a couple of ideas to help you get started.

Multigrain Salad Florentine

1 cup cooked or sprouted quinoa (optional)*
1 cup cooked or sprouted spelt berries (optional)*
½ cup cooked brown or wild rice, cooked or sprouted**
2 medium carrots, scrubbed and grated

1 bunch fresh spinach, washed, drained, and torn into bite-size pieces

½ cup chopped pecans, toasted (optional)

DRESSING:

1 lemon, juice and zest

2 to 3 tablespoons extra-virgin olive oil

2 tablespoons finely chopped fresh basil, or 2 teaspoons dried

1 large garlic clove, pressed

1 teaspoon honey or agave syrup

Pinch cayenne pepper

Pinch sea salt (optional)

*Quinoa and spelt are available at health food stores. If you do not use them, increase the amount of brown or wild rice used to 1 cup.

**Sprouted rice is rice that is soaked and sprouted, as seeds or nuts are sprouted.

1. In a large salad bowl, combine the quinoa and spelt (if using), brown or wild rice, and carrots. Add spinach and pecans.
2. In a small bowl, whisk together all of the dressing ingredients.
3. Pour dressing over salad ingredients and toss; serve within 30 minutes.

Serves 4

Chicken Curry Salad

2 cups cooked boneless, skinless chicken, cut into bite-size pieces

4 cups romaine or green leaf lettuce, washed, dried, and torn into bite-size pieces

1 cup baby field greens (or any other greens as desired), washed and dried

1 cup chopped cilantro

½ cup chopped red onion

½ cup chopped green onion

½ cup alfalfa sprouts (optional)

LEMON CURRY DRESSING:

3 tablespoons extra-virgin olive oil

3 tablespoons fresh lemon juice

3 tablespoons organic mayonnaise

2 teaspoons honey or agave syrup

1 to 2 teaspoons curry powder

2 tablespoons chopped fresh basil, or 1 to 2 teaspoons dried

¼ teaspoon sea salt (optional)

1. In a small bowl, whisk together the dressing ingredients, and set aside three-quarters of the dressing. Add the chicken to the remaining one-quarter dressing, and toss to coat. Chill until ready to serve.
2. In a large bowl, combine the remaining salad ingredients.
3. Just before serving, add the chicken and remaining dressing, toss to mix, and serve immediately.

   Serves 4

The Elimination Diet

M ANY PHYSICIANS BELIEVE THAT the best way to identify food allergies is with the "oral food challenge," in which potential food allergens are first eliminated from the diet and then gradually reintroduced. The elimination diet is designed to do just that. For the first seven days (the cleansing period), eat only the foods listed in the diet. (Read labels carefully to eliminate all other foods.) If your symptoms are related to food sensitivity, they will typically disappear by the end of the week. If they don't, it is possible that a reaction to a food in the elimination diet is responsible. In that case, go to an even more restricted diet. Lamb or sweet potato is usually at fault. After the diet period, you may introduce one food every two days. Keep a detailed record as to when the food was introduced and what symptoms appeared after it was eaten. Remember that some reactions are delayed up to forty-eight hours.

✳ Foods That Can Be Eaten During the Elimination Diet

- Beverage: water
- Cereal and grains: brown rice cereals, such as cream of brown rice; bread made with rice flour; rice cakes
- Condiments: Celtic sea salt or gray salt and white vinegar
- Fats: extra-virgin olive oil

- Fruit and juices: apricots, cranberries, peaches, pears, prunes (all juices should be freshly made, not bottled or canned)
- Meat: lamb
- Vegetables: sweet potatoes (boiled or baked), beetroot and beetroot greens (fresh), spinach (fresh or steamed). Vegetables can be steamed and seasoned with allowed condiments and fats.

SAMPLE ELIMINATION DIET MENU

Breakfast ✳ Stewed prunes or pear sauce

Brown rice cereal with pear juice or plain rice milk

Rice bread, toasted (no butter)

Lunch ✳ Pear juice

Baked sweet potato

Beetroot (with greens)

Broiled lamb chop

Rice cake

Peach

Dinner ✳ Steamed spinach

Baked sweet potato

Brown rice

Lamb roast

Pear

Or, you can follow the glutamate/aspartate restricted diet (GARD), which is also an elimination diet. It specifies the following foods (and food products/ingredients) that should be avoided:

- Gluten: commonly derived from wheat, rye, barley, and oats; avoid these grains
- Casein: protein found in cow's milk and most dairy products; avoid all dairy
- Soy: avoid all soy products; read labels to identify all soy, soybean oil, and textured vegetable protein
- Corn: including corn syrup and corn derivatives
- MSG (monosodium glutamate): a very common food ingredient in processed foods even though it is rarely clearly labeled as such; it's best to avoid all packaged and prepared foods. Make your food from scratch.
- Aspartame (NutraSweet): commonly used as a sugar substitute

The Cleansing Programs

JUST AS YOUR HOME needs a thorough cleaning occasionally, the interior of your physical house needs a thorough cleansing at least twice a year, if you want to achieve optimum health. The body was made to handle a certain amount of toxic substances, such as spoiled food or toxic plant substances, but not the kind of abuse we give it and are forced to encounter as a result of environmental toxicity. We are continually tempted to eat a host of unhealthy substances, such as fried foods; high-fat, preservative-laden snacks; refined foods; fake foods; and foods with additives and dyes. We are bombarded with pesticides, herbicides, chemical fertilizers, and other noxious stuff in our air, soil, and water. All these substances serve to weaken and congest our body.

Toxic and congestive substances can overwhelm the organs of elimination and build up within the body's tissues. Substances that are not broken down and excreted are generally stored in the intestines, gallbladder, kidneys, liver, fat cells, and skin. Therefore, cleansing our organs periodically helps promote health and healing. I've learned through personal experience this can only happen through specific plans designed to promote "housecleaning" in each specific organ or system.

Detoxifying the body is worth the effort because the benefits are astounding. You'll look more vibrant! Wrinkles will diminish, skin color will improve, dark circles under the eyes will eventually disappear, and hair and nails will grow better. Best of all, you'll enjoy health and vitality. You'll feel more energetic, and have greater mental clarity and a higher sense of well-being. If you have ailments, you'll give your body an opportunity to heal.

Freshly made fruit and vegetable juices from organically grown produce will help you no matter what else you do. But if your organs of elimination are congested, you'll get the best results for all your juicing efforts when you incorporate cleansing. Not cleaning your body is a bit like continuing to wax a linoleum floor that has a buildup of old wax and dirt. You'll achieve the clean, shiny floor you want after you strip off the old gunk and grime. Just like the floor, we all need to get rid of the "old gunk" that builds up inside our bodies.

What follows is the basic juice fast—a starting point for all internal cleansing. After the juice fast, you'll find the programs I've used for years to purify the intestines, gallbladder, liver, and kidneys. These programs work. If you use them periodically they can be one of the most important steps you take to improve your health, look younger, increase your energy and vitality, and prevent disease.

✳ The Juice Fast

No one has been able to explain why drinking only fresh juice for a period of a few days works such a miracle, but "miracle" is the right word. Wrinkles soften, the body firms, weight is lost, and the skin and hair look healthier. Blood pressure and cholesterol levels come down. Aches and pains diminish. Over time, disorders, illnesses, and diseases begin to heal, when people partake in periodic juice fasts.

Whenever you're sick, your body is sending you a signal. It needs rest from strenuous work and from foods that are toxic or difficult to digest. Vegetable-juice fasting gives the digestive system time out. It aids the immune system in clearing out dead, diseased, and damaged cells, and supports immune cells with an abundance of nutrients. Sludge that accumulates in spaces between the cells can be cleared away. There is also an opportunity to reduce amounts of lipofuscin—the brown material caused by fat degeneration that is responsible for age spots (also called sun spots or liver spots). Simply put—juice fasting clears out toxins right down to the cells.

Juice fasting is a safe, easy way to detoxify your internal organs, tissues, and cells. I don't recommend a water-only fast because it's hard on the body, and can cause internal damage. Many toxins are released when you fast, and without the addition of nutrients that neutralize and bind them, you can do yourself more harm than good. The antioxidants—vitamins C and E, beta-carotene, selenium, and various enzymes and phytochemicals—are found in large quantities in fresh juice; they bind to harmful toxins and carry them out of the body.

Anyone with hypoglycemia or diabetes should avoid fruit juice and dilute carrot juice and beetroot juice with an equal amount of purified water or green vegetable juices. Children under eighteen should not follow a strict juice fast unless recommended by a health professional, although fresh vegetable and small amounts of fruit juices are great supplements to a child's diet. Children can do a modified fast by adding lots of vegetables, fruit, juices, sprouts, seeds, nuts, and legumes to their diet and avoiding all other foods during the cleansing period.

On a personal note: For years my husband and I have made our annual pilgrimage to the Optimum Health Institute (OHI) in San Diego. We have been going there since 1991 for the cleansing benefits of their raw food and juice diet program. We call it our "tune-up." We lose weight. Facial lines fade. We both swear the program wipes away at least five years from our faces. We always leave feeling renewed and rejuvenated—and we never know the diseases we avoid because of our total body–cleansing weeks.

✳ Herbal Tea Recommendations for Fasting

Beneficial herbal teas include dandelion root and nettles, which help cleanse the liver and kidneys. If you purchase these herbs in bulk, steep one-half teaspoon of either herb in a pint of hot water for ten minutes, strain, and drink warm. Lemon may be added for flavor, but do not use any sweetener, with the exception of a little stevia.

✳ Fiber Recommendations

Bulking agents, such as psyllium husks, flax fiber, or pectin, can be added to fresh juice. (Psyllium can be drying for the colon. It's best mixed with other fiber.) These agents act as bulk laxatives. Mix two teaspoons to a glass of juice two to three times during the day. These high-fiber agents also help to curb appetite (see the Intestinal Cleanse, page 307).

✳ Juice Recommendations

Specific juices that are beneficial for cleansing include:

- Beetroot (especially good for the liver)
- Cabbage
- Wheatgrasss
- Sprouts (any kind)
- Lemon
- Lime
- Carrot
- Celery
- Green bell pepper
- Parsley
- Grapefruit
- Apple

Diuretic juices: Cucumber, parsley, watermelon, cantaloupe with the seeds, lemon, kiwifruit, and asparagus.

THE JUICE FAST SAMPLE MENU

The suggested menu is a guideline for the juice fast, and can be modified whenever necessary to meet your individual needs. The recipes are simply ideas; insert your favorites wherever you like. Keep the fast from one to three days. Make sure you drink at least two quarts of water each day in addition to the juice. These recipes are just suggestions. Choose the recipe you like from the recipe section.

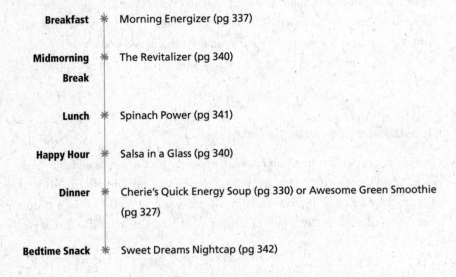

Breakfast ✳	Morning Energizer (pg 337)
Midmorning Break ✳	The Revitalizer (pg 340)
Lunch ✳	Spinach Power (pg 341)
Happy Hour ✳	Salsa in a Glass (pg 340)
Dinner ✳	Cherie's Quick Energy Soup (pg 330) or Awesome Green Smoothie (pg 327)
Bedtime Snack ✳	Sweet Dreams Nightcap (pg 342)

Breaking the Fast

Breaking the fast properly is as important as the fast itself. If the fast is broken with bad food choices, you could do more harm than good and possibly end up with a stomachache or worse. Make the day after a fast a strict vegan food day (no animal products), and eat the largest portion of your food raw—fresh fruits and vegetables. Make sure you also drink at least two quarts of water. A suggested menu for breaking the juice fast follows.

SAMPLE MENU

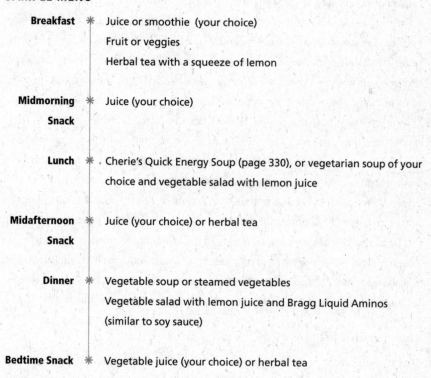

Breakfast	✳	Juice or smoothie (your choice)
		Fruit or veggies
		Herbal tea with a squeeze of lemon
Midmorning Snack	✳	Juice (your choice)
Lunch	✳	Cherie's Quick Energy Soup (page 330), or vegetarian soup of your choice and vegetable salad with lemon juice
Midafternoon Snack	✳	Juice (your choice) or herbal tea
Dinner	✳	Vegetable soup or steamed vegetables
		Vegetable salad with lemon juice and Bragg Liquid Aminos (similar to soy sauce)
Bedtime Snack	✳	Vegetable juice (your choice) or herbal tea

✳ The Intestinal Cleanse

The small intestine is made up of three segments: duodenum, jejunum, and ileum. Mineral absorption takes place in the duodenum, the first segment. Absorption of water-soluble vitamins, carbohydrates, and proteins occurs mostly in the jejunum, and the ileum, the last segment, is where fat-soluble vitamins, fat, cholesterol, and bile salts are absorbed. The large intestine (colon) also is made up of three segments: ascending, transverse, and descending. The large intestine is where the stool is formed. Although most of the water in the food is absorbed by the small intestine, more water is absorbed by the large intestine, as are electrolytes, which are mineral salts that help maintain the body's fluid balance.

Eating overly cooked food; fried food; junk food; spoiled food; or sweets like cookies, chocolate, and ice cream; drinking coffee or alcohol; or taking drugs (prescription or recreational) can stimulate mucus secretion throughout the entire alimentary canal. This is normal; it's the body's natural way of protecting itself against the occasional encounter with irritating food. When we ingest these substances every day, and for some people every meal, mucus and waste build up on the intestinal wall like crud builds up in bathroom pipes. Pancreatic juices help to digest food and cleanse mucus from the intestines. However, continual poor food choices lead to constant mucus secretion, and the digestive juices cannot keep up with this overload of waste. Mucus and waste buildup can interfere with nutrient absorption, provide a hiding place for *Candida albicans,* and contribute to poor elimination. This allows toxins to reenter the bloodstream.

As intestinal waste builds up, intestinal motion becomes less effective and material takes longer to pass through the digestive tract. This can contribute to constipation. Built-up mucus and waste also can be a breeding ground for parasites. I struggled with parasites for years, until I discovered the effectiveness of intestinal detoxification and parasite cleansing (for more information, see Parasitic Infections, page 238).

It's not hard to see why a clean intestinal tract is so important to good health. The following seven-day program will help you reduce waste buildup in the intestines and will allow for more efficient absorption of nutrients. If you have an intestinal disease, such as Crohn's disease or diverticulitis, check with your doctor before beginning.

The Intestinal Cleanse

Step 1: Drink three high-fiber shakes every day for seven days. Make these shakes with psyllium husk powder,* pectin, and/or flax fiber and betonite clay** (available at most health food stores). To make each shake, mix one tablespoon of betonite clay with eight to ten ounces of juice or water in a jar and shake. Add two teaspoons fiber and shake again. Drink immediately, as fiber gels quickly, and the mixture becomes very thick. If using water, you can add a little fresh lemon juice or cranberry juice concentrate to this mixture to make it more palatable.

Have a shake for breakfast, one for midmorning, and one midafternoon.

Enemas and Colonics

Though not a practice to rely on daily, enemas are very helpful during all the cleansing programs. The colon, kidneys, lungs, and skin can become overwhelmed with the release of toxins during a cleanse, and skin eruptions, rashes, headaches, and flu-like symptoms can result. Enemas assist the body in the elimination process, and help minimize symptoms. Many people are not familiar with enemas today; however, their therapeutic benefits have been known for centuries.

To prepare an enema, add two quarts of lukewarm water to an enema bag. To administer the enema, lie down on your right side, draw both knees toward the abdomen, and insert the nozzle into the anus. (It's a good idea to first lubricate the nozzle with vitamin E oil or a lubricant jelly.) Take a deep breath to facilitate drawing the greatest amount of fluid into the colon. Retain the fluid for between three and four minutes during a cleansing enema, if possible. Gently massage the lower abdomen while retaining the fluid.

After taking the enema, it is a good idea to replace lost minerals by drinking an eight-ounce glass of mixed carrot and celery juices. You also need to replace your beneficial intestinal flora by taking supplements of "friendly" probiotic bacteria—*Lactobacillus acidophilus* and *Bifidobacterium infantis*.

Colonics may be used for a more thorough cleansing. Colonics are administered higher in the bowel than is possible with standard enemas, and are performed by a trained technician using specialized equipment. See a certified colon therapist.

These shakes are very filling, and you probably won't be as hungry during the cleanse, which makes it easier to lose weight, if that is a goal.

Psyllium husk powder (also pectin and flax fiber) is a fibrous bulking agent that thickens and gels when mixed with juice or water. (It's best to choose or make a fiber blend that has more than just psyllium powder, since psyllium is quite drying to the intestinal tract.)

**Betonite clay* is absorbent clay used for centuries for internal purification. It draws out metals, drugs, toxins, waste, and mucus.

Step 2: Eat two meals a day; make the high-fiber shake and fresh vegetable juice your breakfast. (Choose from the recipes, pages 326–345.) The program works best if both meals are vegan (see the Juice Fast Sample Menu, page 306).

Step 3: Use colonics or cleansing enemas daily or at least every other day to remove excess waste that has accumulated. This will also help to relieve any adverse symptoms, such as headaches, fatigue, sleepiness, or aches and pains you may experience as toxins are released.

Diet Recommendations for the Intestinal Cleanse

Follow the high-alkaline diet. See principles 1 and 2 (pages 290–291).

Drink two to three glasses of fresh vegetable juice daily and juice-fast at least one day. (Short juice fasts from one to three days, which is drinking just vegetable juice, will greatly facilitate your intestinal cleanse.) Vegetables in particular are wise juice choices because they help immensely in alkalinizing your body. Minimize fruit juice because it contains fruit sugar; always dilute fruit juice by half with water or vegetable juices to dilute the sugar and prevent appetite stimulation. (Do not drink more than four ounces of fruit juice a day.)

✳ The Liver Cleanse

The liver is the largest internal organ of the body and one of the most important. Some of its major functions include carbohydrate, protein, and fat usage; metabolizing nutrients; and detoxification or excretion of hormones and chemical compounds, such as the breast cancer–promoting hormone 16-alphahydroxyestrone, drugs, and pesticides. The liver also filters more than one liter of blood each minute, and acts as a primary blood reservoir.

The liver creates and secretes bile. Bile acids are produced by liver cells and stored in the gallbladder until needed. They are critical to the digestion and absorption of fats. When fats enter the upper small bowel (which is composed of two sections, the duodenum and jejunum), the gallbladder releases bile acids that mix with the fats. This reaction forms a special chemical structure that can be further broken down by enzymes (lipases) to allow for better absorption. When bile stagnates in the gallbladder, gallstones can form, leading to possible bacteria growth. And liver congestion is nearly always present when a person has candidiasis.

To a great extent, your health and vitality depend on the healthy functioning of your liver. Many people have found that when they've completed a series of intestinal and liver cleanses, ailments and diseases have completely healed. Exposure to toxic chemicals, drugs, alcohol, or hepatitis, along with eating a typical Western diet, can lead to a sluggish or impaired liver. A liver that is even slightly sluggish can negatively impact your health, prevent weight loss, and affect your appearance by making you look older.

The liver is a prime place for the body to store toxins that can't be excreted. Highly toxic chemicals can pass through the liver, including residues from pesticides and herbicides. And it doesn't take a boatload of toxins or irritating substances to weaken the liver of some individuals. It can also be damaged by a variety of medications, alcohol, and viruses. One of the most common medications known to destroy liver cells is acetaminophen (as found in Tylenol). Even when taken in recommended amounts, this drug can do great harm to the liver.

Alcoholics are notorious for having bad livers because alcohol is a powerful liver toxin. Over time, heavy drinkers can develop severe scarring of the liver and loss of cells in that vital organ. Chronic heavy drinkers with damaged, poorly functioning livers are also at high risk of liver cancer. This is a result of the chronic scarring, inflammation, and exposure to toxins. But it may not be only heavy drinking that causes problems for some people. Researchers have found that even small amounts of alcohol can cause fat deposits in the livers of susceptible individuals.

As a consequence of our modern diet, many people have considerable congestion and even gallstones in their liver. This may be true even though a person has not had a history of gallstones. Gallstones in the liver are an impediment to acquiring and maintaining good health, youthfulness, and vitality. They are, indeed, one of the major reasons people become ill and have difficulty recuperating from illness or recovering from disease.

Liver congestion and stagnation are quite common, yet conventional medicine has no way to diagnose them. Relying on blood tests for diagnostic purposes concerning liver congestion is inadequate. Most people who have a physical ailment have perfectly normal liver enzymes in the blood, despite suffering liver congestion and stagnation. Liver enzymes become elevated in the blood only when there is advanced liver-cell destruction, as in hepatitis or liver inflammation. Liver cells contain large amounts of enzymes, and when they are ruptured, the enzymes enter the blood and signal liver abnormalities. By then, the damage has already occurred. It takes many years of congestion before such an event becomes possible. Therefore, cleansing the liver is an excellent preventive measure as well as a healing, restorative, and rejuvenating practice.

The symptoms of a sluggish liver are numerous and varied. They include abdominal discomfort, aches and pains, brown spots on the face and hands, dark circles under the eyes, anal itching, bad breath, body odor, sallow or jaundiced complexion, white or yellow tongue coating, digestive problems (belching and flatulence), dizziness, drowsiness after eating, fatigue, frequent urination at night, migraine headaches or headaches that involve a feeling of fullness or heaviness in the head, inability to tolerate heat or cold, sleeplessness (insomnia), irritability, loss of memory or inability to concentrate, loss of sexual desire, low back pain, malaise, menstrual problems, nervousness and anxiety, pain around the right shoulder blade and shoulder (also connected with gallbladder congestion), puffy eyes and/or face, red nose, small red spots on the skin (either smooth or raised and hard, known as cherry angiomas), and sinus problems. Allergies, candidiasis, constipation, hemorrhoids, cellulite, and premenstrual syndrome are also associated with a malfunctioning liver.

Optimizing liver function focuses on cleansing, protecting, and nourishing the liver. The following program does just that. **Note:** If you have a liver disease, consult your doctor first.

Benefits of Cleansing the Liver

- Complexion clears and brightens
- Dark circles disappear from under the eyes
- Some age spots may disappear
- Digestion improves
- Weight loss becomes easier; cellulite goes away
- Energy increases
- Sleep improves; need to urinate during the night improves
- Aches and pains disappear
- Headaches often cease
- Memory improves
- Mood is better
- Allergies go away
- Facial puffiness disappears
- Sinus problems clear

✳ The Seven-Day Liver Cleanse

You will follow this program for seven days. This program has a cumulative effect, and cheating or stopping midway stops the cleansing. If you miss a day or you cheat, you'll need to begin again.

Step 1: Start each day with lemon and hot water. Squeeze the juice of one-quarter lemon into eight to ten ounces of hot water and add a dash of cayenne pepper.

Step 2: Prepare the Gallbladder/Liver Flush Drink:

- Pour the juices of one lemon and one lime into your blender. If sweeter fruits do not adversely affect you, you can also add four ounces of freshly squeezed orange juice.
- Next, add one to five cloves of peeled garlic. Start with one clove on Day One and end with five cloves on Day Five. Each day increase by one garlic clove until you reach five. Continue with five garlic cloves on days Six and Seven.
- Add a one- to two-inch chunk of peeled fresh gingerroot.
- Add one to five tablespoons of extra-virgin olive oil. Start with one tablespoon on Day One and end with five tablespoons on Day Five. Each day increase by one tablespoon of olive oil until you reach five. Continue with five tablespoons for days Six and Seven.
- You may also add one tablespoon of virgin coconut oil each day (optional).
- Add four or five ice cubes.
- Add six to eight ounces of purified water.
- Blend until smooth and drink to your health!

Step 3: Drink the Gallbladder/Liver Cleansing Cocktail each day (see page 331).

Step 4: Eat a high-fiber, vegan diet that includes lots of vegetables, with at least 50 percent being raw. (Follow principles 1 and 2, pages 290–291.) Include several glasses of vegetable juice each day. Green smoothies are an excellent addition. You may also have fresh fruit, fruit smoothies, salads, sprouts, vegetable soup, vegetable broth, and brown rice. Avoid coffee, alcohol, tobacco, soft drinks, junk food, sweets, fried foods, wheat, and all animal products, including red meat, fish, poultry, eggs, dairy, and butter. It is best to finish your dinner by 6:30 p.m. if possible.

Step 5: Each day you'll eat one to two teaspoons of beetroot salad every other hour starting an hour after breakfast and ending with the last teaspoon(s) around 7:30 p.m. (see Beet Salad recipe, page 316).

Step 6: Each day drink one green drink (see page 317).

Step 7: Each day you'll eat one carrot salad (see recipe, page 316).

Liver-Friendly Vegetables

Eat an abundance of the following liver-friendly vegetables during the seven days of your detoxification program:

- Artichokes
- Beetroot
- Broccoli
- Brussels sprouts
- Cabbage
- Carrots
- Cauliflower
- Celery
- Chives

- Cucumber
- Eggplant
- Garlic
- Green beans
- Kale
- Kohlrabi
- Lettuce
- Mustard greens
- Okra

- Onion
- Parsley
- Parsnips
- Peas
- Pumpkin
- Spinach
- Squash
- Sweet potatoes or yams

Step 8: Drink one to two cups of vegetable broth each day (see recipe, page 317).

Step 9: Two times a day, take two liver-cleansing herbal supplements that contain milk thistle, artichoke, and turmeric. Three times a day, take one L-cysteine and one supplement containing vitamins, minerals, amino acids, and herbs. (For more information on these ingredients, see below; for products, see Sources, page 347.)

Step 10: Eat two teaspoons of fenugreek sprouts daily; they are very cleansing for the liver. (This is optional.) You can sprout fenugreek seeds easily. Just soak in purified water overnight and then place in a jar or colander, covered with a cloth or paper towel until they sprout. (They'll have little "tails" when sprouted.) Then refrigerate them. They should last about a week in the refrigerator.

Step 11: Either daily or every other day, use an enema to cleanse your colon (see Enemas and Colonics, page 309).

You may want to precede the Seven-Day Liver Cleanse with six weeks of a Chinese liver cleansing herbal formula, which is very helpful (see Sources for more information).

Liver Cleansing Supplements

(For a list of high-quality, effective liver supplements, see Sources.)

Milk thistle (Silymarin)

Silymarin, which is the most-studied active ingredient in milk thistle, enhances liver function and inhibits factors that cause hepatic damage. Because of its antioxidant properties, silymarin also helps prevent free-radical damage to the liver.

Artichoke

The chemical cyranin, which is found in the artichoke, gives this herb its pleasantly bitter taste and aids your liver during the detoxification process. This chemical, along with other compounds found in artichokes, helps increase the liver's production of bile and strengthens the bile duct so that it's better able to contract. The chemicals in artichokes also strengthen liver cell walls, protecting them from damage. They can also break up and mobilize fat stored in the liver, making them useful as well for lowering cholesterol.

Turmeric

Turmeric is known in Ayurvedic medicine as the king of spices. Its principal chemical component is curcumin. This spice helps cleanse the liver, purify the blood, and promote good digestion and elimination. It stimulates the gallbladder for bile production and scavenges free radicals.

N-Acetyl-L-Cysteine (NAC)

NAC is an antioxidant that helps increase glutathione synthesis, and has benefit during oxidative stress. NAC can help provide optimum antioxidant protection from free radicals caused by environmental pollution, cigarette smoke, and alcohol. Natural-health practitioners often prescribe it for patients with mercury or heavy metal toxicity (caused by environmental or dental amalgam fillings) because of its ability to bind to these toxins, allowing your body to excrete them.

L-methionine

L-methionine is an amino acid that the liver uses to create glutathione. It can help raise glutathione levels and thus improve the natural detoxification functions of the liver.

Beetroot Leaf and Black Radish

Beetroot leaf and black radish both work in conjunction with the liver's detoxification process and with carbohydrate and fat metabolism. Beetroot leaf may help to normalize the pH of the blood and stimulate bile flow. Black radish is rich in vitamins and bioflavonoids and may support heavy metal detoxification.

Dandelion

Dandelion has been used for centuries for general detox. Herbalists particularly recommend dandelion for the liver. It strengthens the liver by promoting bile secretion and provides a gentle cleansing action in the elimination of metabolic waste.

Recipes for the Liver Cleanse
Beet Salad with Lemon–Olive Oil Dressing

> 2 tablespoons extra-virgin, cold-pressed olive oil
>
> Juice of ½ lemon
>
> Dash of cinnamon (optional)
>
> 1 cup raw beetroot, finely grated or very finely chopped (or use the beetroot pulp from your juicer after making beetroot juice, which is the easiest)

Whisk the olive oil, lemon juice, and cinnamon (as desired) together and mix with the beetroot. Eat one to two teaspoons of this salad every other hour during the day for five days. You may get tired of eating beetroot all day, but remember how great it is for your liver. Eating a teaspoon or two of this salad every other hour is a small investment to help your precious liver. Don't be alarmed if your stools or urine are red from the beetroot.

Carrot Salad with Lemon–Olive Oil Dressing

> 1 cup raw carrots, finely grated or very finely chopped (or use the pulp from your juicer after making carrot juice, which is the easiest)
>
> 2 tablespoons extra-virgin, cold-pressed olive oil
>
> Juice of ½ lemon
>
> Dash of cinnamon (optional)

Place 1 cup of finely shredded carrots, or carrot pulp leftover from juicing, in a bowl. If you're shredding the carrots, they should be a mushy consistency; use a food processor or fine grater. (It's easiest to use carrot pulp.) Whisk the olive oil, lemon juice, and cinnamon (as desired) together. You may add more dressing, but not less. Pour the dressing over the shredded carrots (or carrot pulp) and mix well.

Green Drink

Preferably in the afternoon, drink ten ounces freshly juiced green vegetables—cucumber, parsley, spinach, kale, celery, or any other green herb or vegetable. Add fresh lemon juice and/or freshly juiced gingerroot to pep up the flavor. Fresh mint also makes a nice addition with cucumber and other milder-tasting greens.

Potassium-Rich Vegetable Broth

This vegetable broth provides important nutrients, especially minerals, that your body needs during the cleansing process. Drink one to two cups of the broth daily.

> 2 to 3 cups chopped fresh green beans (string beans) (frozen is acceptable when fresh is not available)
>
> 2 to 3 cups chopped zucchini
>
> 2 to 3 celery stalks
>
> Purified water, for steaming
>
> 1 to 3 tablespoons chopped parsley
>
> 1 tablespoon chopped garlic
>
> Seasonings and herbs, to taste
>
> Coconut oil on top (optional)

Steam the green beans, zucchini, and celery over purified water until soft, but still green and not mushy. Place the cooked vegetables, raw parsley, and garlic in a blender and puree until smooth. Add a bit of the steaming water, as needed, but keep the broth fairly thick. Season to taste with minced gingerroot, cayenne, vegetable seasoning, or herbs of your choice. Add coconut oil to the top of the broth, as desired.

> **Makes about 6 servings**

Gallbladder-Liver Cleansing Deluxe Cocktail

> 1 handful parsley, washed
>
> 4 medium carrots, scrubbed well, green tops removed, ends trimmed
>
> 1 small beetroot, with a few leaves

1 curly endive leaf

2 celery stalks with leaves, washed, ends trimmed

½ lemon, peeled

Bunch up the parsley and push it through the juicer feed tube with the carrots, beetroot, endive, celery, and lemon. Stir the juice and pour into a glass. Drink as soon as possible to maximize the nutritional value, or store in the refrigerator, covered, or take in a thermos.

Note: If you want a more substantial drink, you can pour the juice into a blender and add an avocado. Blend and serve in a glass or bowl, or you can make it thick like a soup with plenty of avocado and eat with a spoon.

Juice Therapy for Your Liver

Beetroot with leaves juice has been used for decades to cleanse and support the liver.

Curly endive has been traditionally used to promote the secretion of bile, which is helpful for the liver and gallbladder.

It's best to mix beetroot and endive, which are rather strong-tasting, with other juices that are milder in flavor, such as carrot, cucumber, lemon, or apple (see Gallbladder/Liver Cleansing Cocktail, page 317).

✳ Other Beneficial Juices

Juices that are beneficial for the liver include apricot, chervil, dandelion, gooseberry, papaya, radish, string bean, tomato, and wheatgrass. Many of these juices are used in the following recipes.

Liver Life Tonic *(pg 336)*   **Sinus Solution** *(pg 341)*   **Jack & the Bean** *(pg 335)*
Wheatgrass Light *(pg 345)*

✳ The Gallbladder Cleanse

The function of the gallbladder is to store and concentrate bile, which is made in the liver, until it is needed in the small intestine. The liver makes bile out of cholesterol, water, lecithin, mucin, bile acids, and other organic and inorganic substances. Bile acids are the check and balance of this system, designed to keep cholesterol soluble so it doesn't form stones. It is the typical Western diet of high-fat, fiber-depleted, refined foods that causes most gallstones. Symptoms can cause abdominal pain, nausea, and vomiting (for more information, see Gallstones and Liver—Gallbladder Congestion, page 164). When bile stagnates in the gallbladder, gallstones can form, leading to possible bacteria growth. This situation often triggers gallbladder attacks that spur severe cramping and pain, particularly if the gallstones block the bile duct—the tube connecting the gallbladder to the small intestine.

You can effectively prevent such attacks by regularly using curcumin, which stimulates the gallbladder to release its bile. Curcumin also has antibacterial and anti-inflammatory properties that help prevent infections and inflammation in this organ.

The cleansing program outlined here can help you purge the gallbladder of stones, "sand," or "mud," including the "silent stones" that don't cause symptoms.

On a personal note: I did a gallbladder flush for the first time when I was thirty because a reflexologist suggested it. I had experienced considerable pain when he worked on the reflex points on my feet that corresponded to the liver/gallbladder area. I was surprised by the purge and all the stones that were expelled. I've been a believer in this program ever since.

If you know that you have gallstones, suspect that you might, are over age forty, or have not used cleansing programs before, and if you've eaten a typical Western diet most of your life, it is advisable not to try the Advanced Seven-Day Gallbladder Flush until you've used several other cleansing programs, including the Liver Cleanse (page 310) and the Intestinal Cleanse (page 307). Use the Beginner's Seven-Day Gallbladder Cleanse first.

For several weeks beforehand, you should eat a low-fat, high-fiber diet that is mostly vegan, with the occasional addition of fish or chicken if you feel you need a little animal protein. It is especially important to follow this diet during the cleansing period.

This program is very similar to the Liver Cleanse. If you've completed the Liver Cleanse, you can go right into the Gallbladder Flush.

✳ The Beginner's Seven-Day Gallbladder Cleanse

Step 1: Start each day with lemon and hot water. Squeeze the juice of one-quarter lemon into eight to ten ounces of hot water and add a dash of cayenne pepper.

Step 2: Prepare the Gallbladder/Liver Flush Drink (see page 313).

Step 3: Drink at least two eight-ounce glasses of freshly made apple juice. Choose golden or red Delicious, Granny Smith, or pippin. Just make sure it's organic. If you have a blood-sugar disorder such as hypoglycemia or diabetes, choose only green apples (Granny Smith or pippin), and dilute the apple juice with at least four ounces of purified water. If apples don't agree with you, cranberry juice will also work. You can juice cranberries and add the juice to six to eight ounces of water, or you can use unsweetened cranberry juice concentrate mixed with water. (Unsweetened cranberry juice concentrate or concentrate sweetened with apple concentrate can be found at health food stores.) Also, drink one of the following juice combinations every day:

- Carrot, beetroot, and cucumber combined
- Carrot, celery, and endive combined

Step 4: Eat a low-fat, high-fiber diet that includes lots of vegetables, with at least 50 percent being raw. Include several glasses of vegetable juice each day. Green smoothies are also excellent. You may have fresh fruit, fruit smoothies, salads, sprouts, vegetable soup, vegetable broth, and brown rice. Avoid coffee, alcohol, soft drinks, junk food, sweets, red meat, fried foods, dairy, and wheat.

Step 5: Either daily or every other day, use an enema to gently cleanse your colon (see Enemas and Colonics, page 309).

Step 6: Use a lipotropic supplement formula that includes choline, methionine, betaine, folic acid, and vitamin B_{12}. The lipotropic formula helps remove fat from the liver and increases bile solubility. Also, use an herbal formula that includes milk thistle, artichoke, and turmeric (see Sources for product recommendations). The herbal formula also increases bile solubility.

Step 7: Use a gel-forming fiber, such as psyllium husk, prune fiber, apple pectin, and/or flax fiber, daily. Mix two teaspoons in eight ounces of fresh juice or water, two or three times a day. (For fiber recommendations, see Sources.)

✳ The Advanced Seven-Day Gallbladder Flush

Days One through Five

Step 1: Start each day with lemon and hot water. Squeeze the juice of one-quarter lemon into eight to ten ounces of hot water and add a dash of cayenne pepper.

Step 2: Prepare the Gallbladder/Liver Flush Drink (see page 313).

Step 3: Drink at least two eight-ounce glasses of freshly made apple juice or cranberry juice. Choose any kind of apple you wish such as golden or red Delicious, Granny Smith, or pippin. Just make sure they're organic. If you have a blood-sugar disorder such as hypoglycemia or diabetes, choose only green apples (Granny Smith or pippins) and dilute the apple juice with at least four ounces of purified water. If apples don't agree with your cranberry juice will also work. You can juice cranberries and add six to eight ounces of water, or you can use unsweetened cranberry juice concentrate (or a cranberry concentrate sweetened with apple concentrate) mixed with water. (Unsweetened cranberry juice concentrate or concentrate sweetened with apple concentrate can be found at health food stores.)

Step 4: Eat a low-fat, high-fiber diet that includes lots of vegetables, with at least 50 percent being raw. Include several glasses of vegetable juice each day. Green smoothies are also excellent. You may have fresh fruit, fruit smoothies, salads, sprouts, vegetable soup, vegetable broth, and brown rice. Avoid coffee, alcohol, soft drinks, junk food, sweets, red meat, dairy, and wheat.

Step 5: Either daily or every other day, use an enema to gently cleanse your colon (see Enemas and Colonics, page 309).

Day Six

Drink only freshly made vegetable and fruit juice and eat no solid food (see the Juice Fast Sample Menu, page 306). In the evening before retiring, drink four ounces of gently warmed extra-virgin, cold-pressed olive oil mixed with four ounces of freshly made grapefruit, lemon, or apple juice. Shake them in a jar to combine, and drink it all at one time. You can sip through a straw. This will not taste pleasant. Immediately after drinking the mixture, go to bed and lie down on your right side. Stay on your right side as long as you can; hopefully you'll go right to sleep. (This is a very important step. Actually, it's so important that some people prefer to sip the olive oil–juice mixture by the bed and then immediately lie down.)

Day Seven

On the morning of the seventh day, drink eight ounces of prune juice. (You will want to be at home during this process.) Dilute the prune juice with four ounces of purified water if you have a sugar-metabolism challenge. Wait an hour before you eat. You should have only vegetable juice, vegetable broth, or lightly steamed vegetables with nothing on them except lemon juice and herbs for the rest of the day. (Eat no meat, eggs, dairy, grains, or fat.) Within a few hours, the gallbladder should purge.

What should you expect? Your body ought to expel stones that can range in size from that of orange seeds to dimes, or you may expel a thick liquid (hence the reference to sand or mud), if the stones have been softened by the juices. Colors can range from light to dark green to turquoise. If you pass stones, sand, or mud, it's a sign that you should do another gallbladder cleanse because the gallbladder or liver will empty what is least embedded. As you continue to cleanse, your body will clear out the liver. You should continue to cleanse, allowing three or four weeks in between, until there is no more sign of congestion. Then it's a good idea to cleanse the liver and gallbladder at least once, or preferably twice, a year.

✳ The Kidney Cleanse

The kidneys perform many important functions, including:

- Elimination of wastes; excretion of urine
- Regulation of blood pressure
- Balancing of pH—acid/alkaline balance
- Balancing of fluids and electrolytes

Poor dietary habits such as eating refined carbohydrates (sweets and white-flour baked goods), drinking too much alcohol, eating large amounts of animal protein and fat, consuming mucus-forming foods like dairy products, and eating too much salt, along with prescription drugs, pesticides, and environmental toxins, overload the kidneys, making them less effective. This reduced effectiveness contributes to more congestion, kidney stone development, and other kidney ailments.

Symptoms of possible kidney congestion or other problems include burning or pain during urination, cloudy urine, a cold sensation in the lower half of the body, dark circles under the eyes, frequent urination (especially at night), foul-smelling or dark urine, incontinence, pain in the eyes, and blood in the urine. (If you suspect kidney stones or have a urinary tract infection, see your doctor immediately.)

As you cleanse and support your kidney and urinary health, you will also expel toxins and wastes from your kidneys. The following kidney cleanse program can reduce the toxic load on the kidneys, which allows them in turn to do their job of clearing toxins from the bloodstream. If you have a kidney disease, consult your health-care provider first.

✳ The Five-Day Kidney Cleanse Program

Throughout the day, drink a minimum of ten eight-ounce glasses (2¼ quarts) of purified water. The kidneys need water to cleanse efficiently, so make sure you drink enough water.

UPON RISING

Drink 1 cup of herbal tea such as nettle, agrimony, marshmallow, juniper, or buchu. (These can be found at health food stores.) These diuretic herbs will help rid the body of excess water and benefit the urinary tract as well. Drink fresh juice chosen from the list below or cranberry water (see page 325).

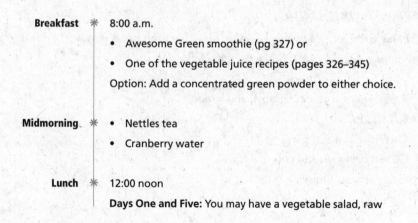

Breakfast ✳ 8:00 a.m.
- Awesome Green smoothie (pg 327) or
- One of the vegetable juice recipes (pages 326–345)

Option: Add a concentrated green powder to either choice.

Midmorning ✳
- Nettles tea
- Cranberry water

Lunch ✳ 12:00 noon

Days One and Five: You may have a vegetable salad, raw

vegetable sticks, or lightly steamed vegetables like broccoli or cooked artichoke. Or choose from any of the juice, smoothie, or raw soup recipes. For salad dressing, choose from olive oil, lemon juice, avocado, garlic, and any spices or herbs.

Days Two through Four: Choose any juice, smoothie, or raw soup recipes from the recipe section. You will not be consuming any solid food on these days.

Midafternoon: ✳ Cranberry water (and kidney herbal supplement, as desired)

Dinner ✳ 5:00 to 6:00 p.m.*

Days One and Five: You may have a vegetable salad, raw vegetable sticks, or lightly steamed vegetables like broccoli or cooked artichoke. Or choose from any of the juice, smoothie, or raw soup recipes. For salad dressing, choose from olive oil, lemon juice, avocado, garlic, or any spices or herbs.

Days Two through Four: Choose any juice, smoothie, or raw soup recipes from the recipe section, or have one cup Potassium-Rich Vegetable Broth (see page 317). You will not be consuming any solid food on these days.

Evening ✳ Herbal tea (and herbal supplement, as desired)

* Avoid eating after 7:00 p.m. to give your kidneys a chance to do their work of detoxing while you sleep.

Kidney-Cleansing Recipes and Products

Each day, drink one to two eight-ounce glasses of fresh juices that help to cleanse and support the kidneys. Choose from the following:

- Asparagus, tomato, cucumber, and lemon
- Cantaloupe with seed
- Carrot, celery, and parsley
- Carrot, beetroot, and coconut
- Cucumber and mint

- Watermelon
- Nettles, cucumber, and lemon

Good diuretics include cucumber, watermelon, cantaloupe, asparagus, lemon, kiwifruit, and parsley juices.

Cranberry Water

Mix one to two teaspoons unsweetened cranberry juice concentrate in eight to ten ounces water. (Unsweetened cranberry juice concentrate or cranberry sweetened with apple concentrate can be purchased at health food stores.) Add a little stevia, if desired. (Do not use any artificial sweeteners, including Splenda.)

Nettles Tea

The herb nettles is used traditionally for kidney cleansing and support; it helps eliminate uric acid. Drink one cup of this tea each day.

Beneficial Herbs
- Buchu
- Sarsaparilla root
- Hydrangea root
- Gingerroot
- Barberry
- Fenugreek

If you have a urinary tract infection, drink cranberry juice every day. (For more information, see Bladder Infections, page 59.)

Juice Recipes

Afternoon Refresher

  1 medium to large organic cucumber, scrubbed well if organic, or peeled if not
    organic
  ½ small or medium lemon, peeled

Cut the produce to fit your juicer's feed tube. Juice the ingredients and stir. Pour into a
glass and drink as soon as possible.

  Serves 1

Allergy Relief

  1 small bunch parsley
  ¼ to ½ small or medium lemon, washed, or peeled if not organic
  2 celery stalks with leaves
  2 to 3 large carrots, scrubbed well, green tops removed, and ends trimmed

Cut the produce to fit your juicer's feed tube. Bunch up the parsley and add to the
juicer before turning it on. Then add the lemon and place the plunger in place. Juice
the remaining ingredients and stir. Pour into a glass and drink as soon as possible.

  Serves 1

Antiulcer Cabbage Cocktail

¼ small head green cabbage

3 carrots, scrubbed well, tops removed, and ends trimmed

4 celery stalks, with leaves if desired

Cut the produce to fit your juicer's feed tube. Juice the ingredients and stir. Pour into a glass and drink as soon as possible.

Serves 1

NOTE: Scientific research has proven that cabbage juice is an effective treatment for stomach ulcers.

Antiviral Cocktail

1 green apple

1 large garlic clove with peel

1 turnip, scrubbed well

1 handful watercress, rinsed

5 carrots, scrubbed well, green tops removed, and ends trimmed

Cut the produce to fit your juicer's feed tube. Juice the ingredients and stir. Pour into a glass and drink as soon as possible.

Serves 1–2

Awesome Green Smoothie

½ cucumber, peeled and cut in chunks

1 avocado, peeled, seeded, and cut in quarters

1 cup raw spinach

½ cup coconut milk

Juice of 1 lime

1 tablespoon green powder of choice (optional)

2 to 3 tablespoons ground almonds (optional)

Combine all ingredients except almonds in a blender and blend well. Sprinkle ground almonds on top, as desired.

Serves 1–2

Beautiful-Bone Solution

1 green apple

1 to 2 kale leaves

1 handful parsley

1 organic celery stalk

$1/4$ small or medium lemon, peeled

$1/2$- to 1-inch piece gingerroot, peeled

Cut the apple into sections to fit your juicer's feed tube. Bunch up the kale and parsley, and push through the feed tube with the apple, celery, lemon, and gingerroot. Stir the juice, and pour into a glass. Serve at room temperature or chilled, as desired.

Serves 1

Beautiful-Skin Cocktail

1 cucumber, peeled

1 parsnip, peeled

2 to 3 carrots, scrubbed well, tops removed, and ends trimmed

$1/2$ lemon, peeled

$1/4$ green bell pepper, seeded

Cut the produce to fit your juicer's feed tube. Juice the ingredients and stir. Pour into a glass and drink as soon as possible.

Serves 1–2

NOTE: Cucumber and bell pepper are good sources of the trace mineral silicon, which is recommended to strengthen skin, hair, and fingernails along with bones. In studies, silicon has been shown to reduce signs of aging by improving thickness of skin and reducing wrinkles.

Beet-Cucumber Cleansing Cocktail

1 cucumber, peeled

3 carrots, scrubbed well, tops removed, and ends trimmed

1 beetroot with stem and leaves, scrubbed well

2 celery stalks

1 handful parsley

1- to 2-inch piece gingerroot, scrubbed or peeled if old

$\frac{1}{2}$ lemon, peeled

Cut the produce to fit your juicer's feed tube. Juice the ingredients and stir. Pour into a glass and drink as soon as possible.

> **Serves 1–2**

Bladder Tonic

1 medium vine-ripened tomato

1 organic cucumber, peeled if not organic

8 asparagus stems

$\frac{1}{2}$ medium lemon, washed, or peeled if not organic

Dash hot sauce

Cut the produce to fit your juicer's feed tube. Juice the ingredients except hot sauce. Pour into a glass, stir in hot sauce, and drink as soon as possible.

> **Serves 1–2**

Cabbage Patch Cocktail

3 to 4 pounds green cabbage (spring or summer cabbage is best)

1 tomato or 1 lemon, peeled

1 pound organic celery with leaves

Cut the produce to fit your juicer's feed tube. Juice the ingredients and stir. Pour into a glass and drink as soon as possible.

> **Serves 1**

Calcium-Rich Cocktail

1 cucumber, peeled

1 to 2 medium-large kale leaves

1 handful parsley

1 celery stalk

$\frac{1}{2}$ lemon, peeled

1-inch piece gingerroot, scrubbed or peeled if old

Cut the produce to fit your juicer's feed tube. Juice the ingredients and stir. Pour into a glass and drink as soon as possible.

Serves 1–2

Cherie's Green Smoothie

½ cucumber, peeled and cut into chunks

1 avocado, peeled, seeded, and cut into quarters

1 cup raw spinach

Juice of 1 lime

1 tablespoon green powder of choice (optional)

2 to 3 tablespoons ground almonds (optional)

Combine all ingredients except almonds in a blender and blend well. Sprinkle ground almonds on top, as desired.

Serves 2

Cherie's Quick Energy Soup

1¼ cups fresh carrot juice (5 to 7 medium, or approximately 1 pound, yield about 1 cup)

1 avocado, peeled and seeded

½ teaspoon ground cumin

Juice the carrots and pour the juice into a blender. Add the avocado and cumin and blend until smooth. Serve chilled.

Serves 1

Colon Cleanser

2 green apples

½ medium lemon

1 bunch spinach

1 handful parsley

Cut the produce to fit your juicer's feed tube. Juice the ingredients and stir. Pour into a glass and drink as soon as possible.

Serves 1

Cranberry-Apple Cocktail

2 organic green apples

1/4 to 1/2 cup fresh or frozen (thawed) cranberries

1/4 small or medium lemon, washed, or peeled if not organic

1/2 cup purified water (optional)

Cut the produce to fit your juicer's feed tube. Juice one apple first. Turn off the machine, add the cranberries, and put the plunger in, then turn the machine on and juice. Follow with the lemon and second apple, and stir. Pour into a glass and drink as soon as possible.

Serves 1

Gallbladder-Liver Cleansing Cocktail

1/2 organic cucumber, scrubbed

1/2 medium lemon, peeled

5 carrots, scrubbed well, green tops removed, and ends trimmed

1/2 small to medium beetroot with leaves and stems, scrubbed well

Cut the produce to fit your juicer's feed tube. Juice the ingredients and stir. Pour into a glass and drink as soon as possible.

Serves 1

Gallbladder Rejuvenator

1/4 purple cabbage

3 to 4 carrots, scrubbed well, green tops removed, and ends trimmed

1/2 beetroot with leaves and stems, scrubbed well

1/2 lemon, peeled

1/2 green apple

1-inch piece gingerroot, scrubbed or peeled if old

Cut the produce to fit your juicer's feed tube. Juice the ingredients and stir. Pour into a glass and drink as soon as possible.

Serves 1–2

Garlic Surprise

1 handful parsley

1 lettuce leaf

1/2 medium cucumber, peeled

1 garlic clove

3 carrots, scrubbed well, green tops removed, and ends trimmed

2 celery stalks

Roll the parsley in the lettuce leaf. Juice the cucumber and the parsley rolled in the lettuce leaf. Add the garlic and push through the juicer with the carrots, followed by the celery. Stir and pour into a glass.

Serves 1–2

The Ginger Hopper

1/2 green apple

1/2- to 1-inch piece gingerroot, peeled

5 medium carrots, scrubbed well, green tops removed, and ends trimmed

Cut the produce to fit your juicer's feed tube. Juice the ingredients and stir. Pour into a glass and drink as soon as possible.

Serves 1

Ginger Twist

1 handful parsley

1/2 lemon, peeled

4 carrots, scrubbed well, green tops removed, and ends trimmed

1-inch piece gingerroot, peeled

Cut the produce to fit your juicer's feed tube. Juice the ingredients and stir. Pour into a glass and drink as soon as possible.

Serves 1

Gout-Fighting Tonic

1 green apple

1 cup strawberries or ½ pound organic cherries, pits removed

2 celery stalks

½ lemon, peeled

Cut the produce to fit your juicer's feed tube. Juice the ingredients and stir. Pour into a glass and drink as soon as possible.

Serves 1

Happy Morning

½ green apple

4 to 5 carrots, well scrubbed, green tops removed, and ends trimmed

3 fennel stalks; include leaves and flowers

½ cucumber, peeled

1 handful spinach

1-inch piece gingerroot, peeled

Cut the produce to fit your juicer's feed tube. Juice the apple first and follow with the other ingredients. Stir and pour into a glass; drink as soon as possible.

Serves 1

NOTE: Fennel juice has been used as a traditional tonic to help the body release endorphins, the feel-good peptides, from the brain into the bloodstream. Endorphins help diminish anxiety and fear, and generate a mood of euphoria.

Healthy Lungs

1 handful watercress

1 small turnip, scrubbed well, tops removed, and ends trimmed

2-inch piece of jicama, scrubbed well or peeled

2 to 3 carrots, scrubbed well, tops removed, and ends trimmed

1 garlic clove

½ lemon, peeled

Bunch up the watercress. Cut the produce to fit your juicer's feed tube. Tuck the watercress in the feed tube and push through with the turnip. Juice the remaining ingredients, finishing with a carrot. Stir the juice, pour into a glass, and drink as soon as possible.

Serves 1

NOTE: Turnip juice has traditionally been used a remedy to strengthen lung tissue.

Healthy-Sinus Solution

2 vine-ripened tomatoes
½ cucumber, peeled
6 radishes, scrubbed
½ lime, peeled

Cut the produce to fit your juicer's feed tube. Juice the ingredients and stir. Pour into a glass and drink as soon as possible.

Serves 1

NOTE: Radish juice is a traditional remedy to open up the sinuses and support the mucous membranes.

Hot Ginger-Lemon Tea

2-inch piece gingerroot
Dash ground cardamom
½ small or medium lemon, washed, or peeled if not organic
2 cups pure water
1 tablespoon loose licorice tea, or 1 tea bag (optional)
1 stick cinnamon, broken
4 to 5 whole cloves
Dash ground nutmeg

Place all ingredients in a saucepan and simmer for 10 minutes. Strain and drink immediately.

Serves 2

Icy Spicy Tomato

2 medium vine-ripened tomatoes

2 dark green lettuce leaves

2 radishes, scrubbed

4 sprigs parsley

$\frac{1}{2}$ lime or lemon, peeled

Cut the produce to fit your juicer's feed tube. Juice the ingredients and stir. Pour into a glass and drink as soon as possible.

Serves 1

Immune Builder

1 handful watercress

1 turnip, scrubbed, tops removed, and ends trimmed

3 carrots, scrubbed well, tops removed, and ends trimmed

1 to 2 garlic cloves

$\frac{1}{2}$ green apple such as Granny Smith or pippin

Bunch up the watercress. Cut the produce to fit your juicer's feed tube. Tuck the watercress in the feed tube and push through with the turnip. Juice the remaining ingredients, finishing with a carrot. Stir the juice, pour into a glass, and drink as soon as possible.

Serves 1

NOTE: Studies show that garlic has a compound that has a natural antibiotic-like effect. It is antibacterial, antifungal, antiparasitic, and antiviral, but it must be consumed raw to have this effect.

Jack & the Bean

1 large vine-ripened tomato

2 romaine lettuce leaves

8 organic string beans

3 Brussels sprouts

$\frac{1}{2}$ small or medium lemon, peeled

Cut the produce to fit your juicer's feed tube. Juice the ingredients and stir. Pour into a glass and drink as soon as possible.

Serves 1

Liver Life Tonic

1 handful dandelion greens
3 to 4 carrots, scrubbed well, tops removed, and ends trimmed
½ cucumber, peeled
½ lemon, peeled

Bunch up the dandelion greens. Cut the produce to fit your juicer's feed tube. Tuck the dandelion greens in the feed tube and push through with the carrots. Juice the remaining ingredients, finishing with a carrot. Stir the juice, pour into a glass, and drink as soon as possible.

Serves 1

NOTE: Dandelion juice is a traditional remedy for cleansing the liver.

Magnesium-Rich Cocktail

3 to 4 carrots, scrubbed well, tops removed, and ends trimmed
2 celery stalks, with leaves as desired
½ small beetroot, scrubbed well
2 to 3 broccoli florets
½ lemon, peeled

Cut the produce to fit your juicer's feed tube. Juice the ingredients and stir. Pour into a glass and drink as soon as possible.

Serves 1

Memory Mender

2 medium vine-ripened tomatoes
½ small or medium lemon, washed, or peeled if not organic
¼ small head iceberg lettuce
4 cauliflower florets, washed

Cut the produce to fit your juicer's feed tube. Juice the ingredients and stir. Pour into a glass and drink as soon as possible.

Serves 1–2

Mint Refresher

2 stalks fennel with leaves

$1/2$ cucumber, peeled

$1/2$ green apple such as Granny Smith or pippin

1 small handful mint

1-inch piece gingerroot, scrubbed or peeled if old

Cut the produce to fit your juicer's feed tube. Juice the ingredients and stir. Pour into a glass and drink as soon as possible.

Serves 1–2

Mood Mender

3 fennel stalks; include leaves and flowers

3 carrots, scrubbed well, tops removed, and ends trimmed

2 celery stalks

$1/2$ pear

$1/2$-inch piece gingerroot, scrubbed or peeled if old

Cut the produce to fit your juicer's feed tube. Juice the ingredients and stir. Pour into a glass and drink as soon as possible.

Serves 1–2

NOTE: Fennel juice has long been used as a tonic to help the body release endorphins, the feel-good peptides, from the brain into the bloodstream. Endorphins help diminish anxiety and fear, and generate a mood of euphoria.

Morning Energizer

3 to 4 carrots, scrubbed well, tops removed, and ends trimmed

1 cucumber, peeled

$1/2$ beetroot, scrubbed well (may include stem and 1 to 2 leaves)

½ lemon, peeled

1-inch piece gingerroot, scrubbed or peeled if old

Cut the produce to fit your juicer's feed tube. Juice the ingredients and stir. Pour into a glass and drink as soon as possible.

Serves 1–2

Natural Diuretic Cocktail

1 medium vine-ripened tomato

½ small or medium lemon, washed, or peeled if not organic

1 small handful parsley, rinsed

1 organic cucumber, scrubbed well

4 asparagus stems, washed

Cut the produce to fit your juicer's feed tube. Juice the tomato and lemon. Turn off the juicer and add the parsley, followed by half the cucumber. Put in the plunger and turn the machine on. Juice the remaining ingredients and stir. Pour into a glass and drink as soon as possible.

Serves 1

NOTE: Lemon, parsley, cucumber, and asparagus all act as diuretics.

Orient Express

2 to 3 carrots, scrubbed well, tops removed, and ends trimmed

1 daikon radish, trimmed and scrubbed

1-inch piece gingerroot, scrubbed or peeled if old

Cut the produce to fit your juicer's feed tube. Juice the ingredients and stir. Pour into a glass and drink as soon as possible.

Serves 1

Pancreas Helper

2 romaine lettuce leaves

½ cucumber, peeled

1 large vine-ripened tomato

8 to 10 string beans

2 Brussels sprouts

½ lemon, peeled

Bunch up the lettuce leaves. Cut the produce to fit your juicer's feed tube. Tuck the lettuce in the feed tube and push through with the cucumber. Juice the remaining ingredients, finishing with some tomato. Pour into a glass and drink as soon as possible.

Serves 1

NOTE: Brussels sprouts and string bean juice are traditional remedies to help strengthen and support the pancreas. Drink before a meal. (If this drink is too strong, dilute with a little water.) For best pancreas support, also avoid refined carbohydrates such as white-flour products, sugars of all types, soda, and all sweets.

Peppy Parsley

1 bunch parsley

2 celery stalks

1 to 2 carrots, scrubbed well, tops removed, and ends trimmed

½ cucumber, peeled

½ lemon, peeled

Cut the produce to fit your juicer's feed tube. Juice the ingredients and stir. Pour into a glass and drink as soon as possible.

Serves 1

The Pink Onion

1 large yellow onion

1-inch piece gingerroot, washed

1 large pink grapefruit, peeled, or enough to make 2 cups juice

1 small or medium lemon, washed, or peeled if not organic

Cut the produce to fit your juicer's feed tube. Juice the ingredients and stir. Pour into a glass and drink as soon as possible.

Serves 1

Pure Green Sprout Drink

1 organic cucumber, scrubbed well

1 small handful clover sprouts

1 large handful sunflower sprouts

1 small handful buckwheat sprouts

Cut the produce to fit your juicer's feed tube. Juice the ingredients and stir. Pour into a glass and drink as soon as possible.

Serves 1

Radish Care

5 carrots, scrubbed well, green tops removed, and ends trimmed

5 to 6 radishes (green tops removed), washed well

$1/2$ small or medium lemon, washed, or peeled if not organic

Cut the produce to fit your juicer's feed tube. Juice the ingredients and stir. Pour into a glass. Serve at room temperature or chilled, as desired.

Serves 1

The Revitalizer

2 tomatoes

$1/2$ cucumber, peeled

6 to 8 string beans

$1/2$ lemon or lime, peeled

Dash hot sauce

Cut the produce to fit your juicer's feed tube. Juice the ingredients and stir. Pour into a glass and drink as soon as possible.

Serves 1

Salsa in a Glass

1 medium vine-ripened tomato

$1/2$ cucumber, peeled

1 small handful cilantro

½ lime, peeled

Dash hot sauce (optional)

Cut the produce to fit your juicer's feed tube. Juice the ingredients and stir. Pour into a glass and drink as soon as possible.

Serves 1

Sinus Solution

2 medium vine-ripened tomatoes

4 radishes with green tops, washed

½ small or medium lime or lemon, peeled

Cut the produce to fit your juicer's feed tube. Juice the ingredients and stir. Pour into a glass and drink as soon as possible.

Serves 1

Sleep Mender

2 romaine lettuce leaves

½ lemon, peeled

5 medium carrots, scrubbed well, green tops removed, and ends trimmed

4 cauliflower florets, washed

Cut the produce to fit your juicer's feed tube. Juice the ingredients and stir. Pour into a glass and drink as soon as possible.

Serves 1

Spinach Power

½ cucumber, peeled

3 carrots, scrubbed well, tops removed, and ends trimmed

2 celery stalks, with leaves as desired

½ beetroot, scrubbed well (may include stem and 1 to 2 leaves)

1 small handful parsley

½ lemon, peeled

Cut the produce to fit your juicer's feed tube. Juice the ingredients and stir. Pour into a glass and drink as soon as possible.

Serves 1–2

Spring Tonic

1 vine-ripened tomato

1 cucumber, peeled

8 asparagus stems

$\frac{1}{2}$ lemon, peeled

Cut the produce to fit your juicer's feed tube. Juice the ingredients and stir. Pour into a glass and drink as soon as possible.

Serves 1–2

NOTE: Asparagus is a natural diuretic, which helps flush toxins from the body and promotes kidney cleansing.

Sweet Dreams Nightcap

1 small handful parsley

2 romaine lettuce leaves

$\frac{1}{2}$ cucumber, peeled

3 carrots, scrubbed well, tops removed, and ends trimmed

$\frac{1}{2}$ cucumber, peeled

1 celery stalk

Bunch up the parsley and roll in a romaine leaf. Juice the cucumber and turn off the juicer. Add the romaine and parsley to the feed tube, turn the machine back on, and tap them through with a carrot. Juice the remaining ingredients and stir. Pour into a glass and drink as soon as possible.

Serves 1

Super Green Sprout Drink

1 cucumber, peeled

1 large handful sunflower sprouts

1 small handful buckwheat sprouts

1 small handful clover sprouts

1 large handful spinach

Cut the cucumber to fit your juicer's feed tube. Juice part of the cucumber first. Bunch up the sprouts and wrap in spinach leaves, turn off the machine, and add them to the feed tube. Turn the machine back on and tap with the rest of the cucumber to gently push the sprouts and spinach through, and then juice the remaining part of the cucumber. Stir the ingredients, pour into a glass, and drink as soon as possible.

Serves 1

Sweet & Regular

1 pear, washed

1 organic apple, any kind, washed

Cut the produce to fit your juicer's feed tube. Juice the ingredients and stir. Pour into a glass and drink as soon as possible.

Serves 1

Thyroid Tonic

5 carrots, scrubbed well, green tops removed, and ends trimmed

$\frac{1}{2}$ medium lemon, peeled

5 to 6 radishes with green tops

Cut the produce to fit your juicer's feed tube. Juice the ingredients and stir. Pour into a glass and drink as soon as possible.

Serves 1

NOTE: Radishes are a traditional remedy for the thyroid.

Tomato Florentine

2 vine-ripened tomatoes

4 to 5 sprigs basil

1 large handful spinach

$\frac{1}{2}$ lemon, peeled

Juice one tomato. Wrap the basil in several spinach leaves. Turn off the juicer and add the spinach and basil. Turn the juicer back on and gently tap to juice them. Juice the remaining tomato and the lemon, and stir. Pour in a glass, and drink as soon as possible.

Serves 1

Triple C

   ¼ small head green cabbage

   4 organic celery stalks with leaves

   4 carrots, scrubbed well, green tops removed, and ends trimmed

Cut the produce to fit your juicer's feed tube. Juice the ingredients and stir. Pour into a glass and drink as soon as possible.

Serves 1–2

Turnip Time

   1 turnip, scrubbed well

   ½ small or medium lemon, peeled

   2-inch piece jicama, scrubbed, or peeled if not organic

   1 handful watercress

   4 carrots, scrubbed well, green tops removed, and ends trimmed

   1 garlic clove with peel, washed (optional)

Cut the produce to fit your juicer's feed tube. Juice the ingredients and stir. Pour into a glass and drink as soon as possible.

Serves 1–2

Veggie Delight

   1 cucumber, peeled

   2 to 3 celery stalks (leaves can be included)

   ½ lemon, with peel, seeded (use only organic)

   1-inch piece gingerroot

Cut the produce to fit your juicer's feed tube. Juice the ingredients and stir. Pour into a glass and drink as soon as possible.

Serves 1–2

Waldorf Twist

1 green apple

3 organic celery stalks with leaves

$\frac{1}{2}$ lemon, peeled

Cut the produce to fit your juicer's feed tube. Juice the ingredients and stir. Pour into a glass and drink as soon as possible.

Serves 1

Weight-Loss Buddy

1 small Jerusalem artichoke, scrubbed well

3 to 4 carrots, scrubbed well, tops removed, and ends trimmed

$\frac{1}{2}$ small beetroot, scrubbed well

$\frac{1}{2}$ cucumber

$\frac{1}{2}$ lemon

Cut the produce to fit your juicer's feed tube. Juice the ingredients and stir. Pour into a glass and drink as soon as possible.

Serves 1

NOTE: Jerusalem artichoke juice combined with carrot and beetroot juices is a traditional remedy for satisfying cravings for sweets and junk food. The key is to sip it slowly when you get a craving for high-fat or high-carb foods.

Wheatgrass Light

1 green apple, washed

1 handful wheatgrass, rinsed

2 to 3 sprigs mint, rinsed (optional)

$\frac{1}{2}$ small or medium lemon, washed, or peeled if not organic

Cut the produce to fit your juicer's feed tube. Starting with the apple, juice all the ingredients and stir. Pour into a glass and drink as soon as possible.

Serves 1

Sources

Web Sites for Cherie and John Calbom

www.juicebookinfo.com

www.sleepawaythepounds.com: information about the Sleep Away the Pounds Program and products

www.gococonuts.com: information about the coconut diet and coconut oil

www.wrinklecleanse.com: information about the wrinkle cleanse

www.ultimatesmoothie.com: information about *The Ultimate Smoothie Book* and healthy smoothies

www.cancercleanse.net: information about *The Complete Cancer Cleanse*

www.cheriecalbom.com: information about the authors and their books and other Web sites

Other Books by Cherie and John Calbom

Note: All these books can be ordered at any of the Web sites noted above or by calling 866-843-8935.

Juicing, Fasting, and Detoxing for Life (Grand Central Wellness)

Sleep Away the Pounds (Warner Wellness)

The Wrinkle Cleanse (Avery)

The Coconut Diet (Warner)

The Complete Cancer Cleanse (Warner)

The Ultimate Smoothie Book (Warner)

Juicers

To learn which juicers are recommended by Cherie, call 866-8-GET-WEL (866-843-8935) or see the Web site www.juicebookinfo.com

Lymphasizer

866-8-GET-WEL (866-843-8935) or see the Web site www.juicebookinfo.com

Food Products

Virgin coconut oil: call 866-843-8935 or see the Web site www.juicebookinfo.com to order virgin coconut oil. (Larger quantities, such as quarts and gallons, represent the most savings.)

Cleanse Products

General Cleanse

Silver Creek Labs Creation's Cleanse (800-493-1146)

Colon Cleanse Products

Cherie's fiber recommendation: Medibulk by Thorne (Psyllium powder, prune powder, apple pectin; 866-843-8935)

Dr. Schultz Colon Cleanse Products Formula I & II (877-832-2463)

Silver Creek Labs Colon Cleanser Complete (800-493-1146)

Liver/Gallbladder Cleanse Products and Liver Support

Cherie recommends: S.A.T. by Thorne (milk thistle, artichoke, turmeric) along with Cysteplus (N-Acetyl-L-Cysteine) and Lipotropein (vitamins, minerals, L-methionine, and herbs including dandelion, beetroot leaf, and black radish root; 866-843-8935) and/or Chinese herbal tinctures (4-part kit) to use with Cherie's Liver Detox Program (866-843-8935)

Candida albicans Cleanse Products

Fungal Defense Garden of Life (www.gardenoflifeusa.com; 800-622-8986)

Yeast Max Advanced Naturals (health food stores)

Silver Creek Labs Candida Cleanse (800-493-1146)

Parasite Cleanse Products

Worm Squirm I and II Arise & Shine (866-843-8935)

Silver Creek Labs ParaCease & ParaAssist (800-493-1146)

Kidney Cleanse Herbs

Arise & Shine Kidney Life (888-557-4463)

Dr. Schultz's Kidney Cleanse Detox Kit (877-832-2463)

Heavy Metal and Toxic Compounds Cleanse Products

For all these products, call 866-843-8935.

Captomer by Thorne (Succinic acid from 100 mg DMSA); chelates heavy metals.

Heavy Metal Support by Thorne (replaces important minerals and other nutrients lost during metal chelating)

Toxic Relief Booster by Thorne (nutrients designed to aid in metabolizing the increased amount of fat-stored toxins released into the bloodstream during a cleanse

Formaldehyde Relief by Thorne (provides nutrients necessary for detoxification of formaldehyde from new carpet and furniture out-gassing, as well as compounds produced by *Candida albicans* or by alcohol metabolism)

Solvent Remover by Thorne (contains amino acids specific to solvent detoxification in the liver, as well as nutrients that help protect nerves from solvent damage)

Pesticide Protector by Thorne (aids in detoxification of chlorinated pesticides, organophosphates, carbamates, and pyrethrins)

Information and Products for Specific Disorders

Alzheimer's Disease

Amino Acids: Neurotransmitter testing is the best way to quantify depletion in brain chemicals. Testing can be completed whether you are taking medications or not. For more information regarding how to get tested, please check my Web site www.juicebookinfo.com or call 866-848-8935.

Anxiety and Panic Attacks

Amino Acids: Neurotransmitter testing is the best way to quantify depletion in brain chemicals. Testing can be completed whether you are taking medications or not. For more information regarding how to get tested, please check my Web site www.juicebookinfo.com or call 866-848-8935.

ADD/ADHD

Amino Acids: Neurotransmitter testing is the best way to quantify depletion in brain chemicals. Testing can be completed whether you are taking medications or not. For more information regarding how to get tested, please check my Web site www.juicebookinfo.com or call 866-848-8935.

Attention Deficit Disorder

Is This Your Child? by Doris Rapp (New York: William Morrow, 1991)

Is This Your Child's World? by Doris Rapp (New York: Bantam Books, 1996)

Cancer

Center for Alternative Cancer Research
412 G Street N.E.
Washington, DC 20069

People Against Cancer
P.O. Box 10
Otho, IA 50569
515-972-4444 or fax 515-972-4415

Third Opinion by John M. Fink (Garden City Park, NY: Avery Publishing Group, 1997), 800-548-5757

Depression

Amino Acids: Neurotransmitter testing is the best way to quantify depletion in brain chemicals. Testing can be completed whether you are taking medications or not. For more information regarding how to get tested, please check my Web site www.juicebookinfo.com or call 866-848-8935.

Diverticulitis and Diverticulosis

Ness Formula Enzymes 866-843-8935

Eczema

Ness Formula Enzymes 866-843-8935

Epilepsy and Seizures

Amino Acids: Neurotransmitter testing is the best way to quantify depletion in brain chemicals. Testing can be completed whether you are taking medications or not. For more information regarding how to get tested, please check my Web site www.juicebookinfo.com or call 866-848-8935.

Virgin coconut oil: 866-843-8935

The Epilepsy Diet Treatment: An Introduction to the Ketogenic Diet by John Freeman (New York: Demos Publications, 1994)

Eye Disorders

Amino Acids: Neurotransmitter testing is the best way to quantify depletion in brain chemicals. Testing can be completed whether you are taking medications or not. For more information regarding how to get tested, please check my Web site www.juicebookinfo.com or call 866-848-8935.

Fibromyalgia

Amino Acids: Neurotransmitter testing is the best way to quantify depletion in brain chemicals. Testing can be completed whether you are taking medications or not. For more information regarding how to get tested, please check my Web site www.juicebookinfo.com or call 866-848-8935.

Insomnia and Jet Lag

Amino Acids: Neurotransmitter testing is the best way to quantify depletion in brain chemicals. Testing can be completed whether you are taking medications or not. For more information regarding how to get tested, please check my Web site www.juicebookinfo.com or call 866-848-8935.

Migraines

Amino Acids: Neurotransmitter testing is the best way to quantify depletion in brain chemicals. Testing can be completed whether you are taking medications or not. For more information regarding how to get tested, please check my Web site www.juicebookinfo.com or call 866-848-8935.

Stress

Amino Acids: Neurotransmitter testing is the best way to quantify depletion in brain chemicals. Testing can be completed whether you are taking medications or not. For more information regarding how to get tested, please check my Web site www.juicebookinfo.com or call 866-848-8935.

Organic Produce—Information

Campaign for Sustainable Agriculture
12 North Church Street
Goshen, NY 10924
914-294-0633

Environmental Working Group
Suite 600
1718 Connecticut Avenue NW
Washington, DC 20009
202-667-6982

Mothers & Others for a Livable Planet
40 West 20th Street
New York, NY 10011
212-242-0010

The Organic Food Alliance
Suite 531
2111 Wilson Boulevard
Arlington, VA 22201
703-276-9498

Organic Foods Production of North America
P.O. Box 1078
Greenfield, MA 01302

Organic Produce—Mail Order

Diamond Organics
P.O. Box 2159
Freedom, CA 95019
800-922-2396

Walnut Acres Organic Farms
Penn Creek, PA 17862
800-433-3998

Health Centers Utilizing Juice and Raw Foods Cleanse Programs

The following centers offer a raw-foods and/or juice-detoxification program. You will find nutritional classes or other health classes that address the emotional, mental, and spiritual aspects of health and renewal. Most of the centers also provide massage and colonics. It is best to contact the various centers to find out which one best fits your needs.

Cedar Springs Renewal Center
Michael Mahaffey and Nan Monk, Directors
31459 Barben Road
Sedro Woolley, WA 98284
360-826-3599
Fax: 360-422-1524
www.cedarsprings.org

Creative Health Institute
112 West Union City Road
Union City, MI 49094
800-426-1213
Fax: 517-278-5837
www.creativehealthinstitute.com

HealthQuarters Ministries
David Frahm, N.D., Director
3620 W. Colorado Avenue
Colorado Springs, CO 80904
719-593-8694
Fax: 719-531-7884
e-mail: healthqu@healthquarters.org
www.healthquarters.org

Hippocrates Institute
Brian and Anna Maria Clement, Directors
1443 Palmdale Court
West Palm Beach, FL 33411
800-842-2125

Fax: 561-471-9464

e-mail: hippocrates@worldnet.att.net

www.hippocratesinstitute.org

Optimum Health Institute of Austin

Route 1, Box 339 J

Cedar Creek, TX 78612

512-303-4817

Fax: 512-303-1239

e-mail: austin@optimumhealth.org

www.optimumhealth.org

Optimum Health Institute of San Diego

6970 Central Avenue

Lemon Grove, CA 91945-2198

800-993-4325

Fax: 619-589-4098

e-mail: optimum@optimumhealth.org

www.optimumhealth.org

Sanoviv Medical Institute

Dr. Myron Wentz, Director

Playa de Rosarito, Km 39

Baja California, Mexico

800-726-6848

Fax: 801-954-7477

www.sanoviv.com

We Care

Susana and Susan Lombardi, Directors

18000 Long Canyon Road

Desert Hot Springs, CA 92241

800-888-2523

Fax: 760-251-5399

e-mail: info@wecarespa.com

www.wecarespa.com

Appendix

Body Mass Index (BMI) Chart

There are a lot of ways to determine your ideal weight, but one of the most accurate and easiest to use is the Body Mass Index (BMI) system. BMI is calculated from height and weight; basically the more you weigh, the higher your BMI will be. Overweight is defined as having a BMI of 25.0 to 29.9 and obesity as having a BMI of 30.0 and above. To use the following chart, simply find your height, look across to find your weight, and then go to the top of the chart to find your BMI.

BMI	20	21	22	23	24	25	26	27	28	29	30	31	32	33	34
HEIGHT							WEIGHT IN POUNDS								
4'10"	96	100	105	110	115	119	124	129	134	138	143	148	153	158	162
4'11"	99	104	190	114	119	124	128	133	138	143	148	153	158	163	168
5'0"	102	107	112	117	122	127	132	138	143	148	153	158	163	168	174
5'1"	106	111	116	122	127	132	138	143	148	153	158	164	169	174	180
5'2"	109	115	120	126	131	136	142	147	153	158	163	169	175	180	186
5'3"	113	118	124	130	135	141	146	152	158	164	164	169	175	180	186
5'4"	116	122	128	134	140	145	151	157	163	169	175	180	186	192	197
5'5"	120	126	132	138	144	150	156	162	168	174	180	186	192	198	204
5'6"	124	130	136	142	148	155	161	167	173	179	186	192	198	204	210
5'7"	127	134	140	147	153	159	166	172	178	185	191	198	204	211	217
5'8"	132	139	145	152	158	165	172	178	185	191	197	203	210	216	223
5'9"	135	142	149	155	162	169	176	182	189	196	203	209	216	223	230
5'10"	140	147	154	161	168	175	182	189	196	202	209	216	222	229	236

BMI	20	21	22	23	24	25	26	27	28	29	30	31	32	33	34
HEIGHT							**WEIGHT IN POUNDS**								
5'11"	143	150	157	164	171	179	186	193	200	208	215	222	229	236	243
6'0"	147	155	162	170	177	185	192	199	207	214	221	228	235	242	250
6'1"	151	158	166	174	181	189	196	204	211	219	227	235	242	250	257
6'2"	155	164	171	179	187	195	203	210	218	225	233	241	249	256	264
6'3"	160	168	176	184	192	200	207	216	224	232	240	248	256	264	272
6'4"	164	172	181	189	197	205	214	222	230	238	246	254	263	271	279

Clinical guidelines on the identification, evaluation and treatment of overweight and obesity in adults. National Institutes of Health; National Heart, Lung and Blood Institute (1998).

If your height or weight is not listed you can determine your own BMI by using the following formula:

$$\frac{\text{Weight (pounds)}}{\text{Height (inches)}^2} \times 705 = \text{BMI}$$

To use this formula, just follow these steps. Let's assume, for the sake of this example, that you are 5 feet, 4 inches tall, and weigh 121 pounds.

1. First, calculate your height in inches, and square it—in other words, multiply the number by itself. In our example, your height is 64 inches. So:

$$64 \times 64 = 4,096$$

2. Now, write down your weight in pounds. In our example, your weight is 121 pounds.

3. Divide the smaller number (in this case, 121) by the larger number (4,096), rounding off your answer to the nearest hundredth:

$$121 \div 4,096 = .03$$

4. Multiply your final number (.03) by 705.

$$.03 \times 705 = 21$$

In this example, your BMI is 21.

It is important to remember that if you are very muscular you can have a higher-than-recommended BMI and not be overweight. You should also note that if you have been overweight for many years the recommended BMI for your height may not be a realistic goal. Don't be discouraged—any weight loss is better than no loss at all.

References

Using Juices for Healing

Nutritional Content of Organic Food organic.lovetoknow.com/Nutritional_Content_of_Organic_Food

Organics www.well.blogs.nytimes.com/2007/10/22/five-easy-ways-to-go-organic

Allergies

"Allergies." Herbs2000.com. http://www.herbs2000.com/disorders/allergies.htm.

"Allergies: How to Avoid Them." Natural Ways to Health. http://www.naturalways.com/alergy1.htm.

"Allergies" RX Insider.com. http://rxinsider.com/monographs/allergies.htm.

Barnett, R. A. *Tonics.* (New York: HarperCollins, 1997).

Damjanov, I. *Pathology for the Health-Related Professional.* (Philadelphia: W. B. Saunders, 1996).

"Diet and Disease: Food Allergies." USDA National Agriculture Library. Food and Nutrition Information Center. http://fnic.nal.usda.gov.

"Eczema and Hay Fever May Be in Decline, but Food Allergies Are Soaring." *Science Daily.* Source: BMJ Specialty Journals, August 31, 2006, http://www.sciencedaily.com/releases/2006/08/060830215643 .htm.

The Environmental Working Group. "Shopper's Guide," 5th ed. [No date given; data is from the USFDA between 2000–2005]. http://www.foodnews.org/index.php.

"Food Allergy." MedlinePlus. NIH. National Institute of Allergy and Infectious Diseases, http://www .niaid.nih.gov/healthscience/healthtopics/foodAllergy/default.htm.

"Food Allergy." MedlinePlus. NIH. National Institute of Allergy and Infectious Diseases, http://www .nlm.nih.gov/medlineplus/foodallergy.html.

Heinerman, J. *Heinerman's Encyclopedia of Healing Juices.* (Englewood Cliffs, NJ: Prentice Hall, 1994).

Keegan, L. *Healing Nutrition.* (Albany, NY: Delmar Publications, 1996).

Kenton, L., and S. Kenton. *Raw Energy.* (London: Century Publishing, 1985).

Lust, J. B. *Raw Juice Therapy.* (London: Thorsons Publishers Limited, 1958).

Murray, M. T. *The Healing Power of Foods* (Rocklin, CA: Prima Publishing, 1993).

Murray, M.T., and J. Pizzorno. *The Encyclopedia of Natural Medicine,* 2nd ed. (Rocklin, CA: Prima Publishing, 1998).

"Pollen, Fruits, Veggies Help Trigger Oral Allergy Syndrome." MedicineNet.com. http://www .medicinenet.com/script/main/art.asp?articlekey=83564. Source: American Academy of Allergy, Asthma and Immunology, news release, August 2007.

Polunin, M. *Healing Foods*. (New York: DK Publishing, 1997).

Smith, J. M. "Genetically Modified Foods May Cause Rising Food Allergies," Institute for Responsible Technology: Spilling the Beans (June 2007). http://www.seedsofdeception.com/utility/showArticle/objectID=1264.

Squires, S. "When Food Is a Danger," July 10, 2007. WashingtonPost.com. www.washingtonpost.com.

"Understanding Food Allergy." International Food Information Council. http://www.ific.org/publications/brochures/allergybroch.cfm (May 2007).

Alzheimer's Disease and Dementia

Alzheimer's and Dementia journal, reported in *USA Today*, August 2005. http://www.usatoday.com-news/health/2005-08-14-alzheimers-folate_x.htm.

"Alzheimer's Disease." Alzheimer's Association. http://www.alz.org.

"Alzheimer's Epidemic to Be Larger Than Estimated." Mercola.com. http://www.mercola.com/2005/apr/9/alzheimers_epidemic.htm.

"Aspartame's toxic effects." http://www.health-report.co.uk/aspartame-toxic-effects.htm.

Blaylock, R. "Aspartame and Pilots." http://www.aspartame.com/blalockpilot.htm.

———. "Excitotoxins, the Taste That Kills." http://www.aspartame.com/ram/mpr060398.ram.

———. "Food Additives and Brain Damage." http://www.aspartame.com/ram/blaylocknoha.ram.

———. "Not Just Another Scare: Toxin Additives in Your Food and Drink." http://www.aspartame.com/blayart1.htm.

Behl, C., et al. "Vitamin E Protects Nerve Cells from Amyloid Protein Toxicity," *Biochemical and Biophysical Research Communications* 944–950, July 1992.

Copestake, P. "Aluminum and Alzheimer's Disease—An Update." *Food and Chemical Toxicology* 31:670–685, 1993.

Dai, Q., et al. "Fruit and Vegetable Juices and Alzheimer's Disease: The Kame Project." *American Journal of Medicine* 119 (9): 751–759, 2006.

Damjanov, I. *Pathology for the Health-Related Professional* (Philadelphia: W. B. Saunders, 1996).

"Folate May Lower Alzheimer's Risk," CBS news, reporting from WebMD. http://www.cbsnews.com/stories/2005/08/15/health/webmd/main779484.shtml.

"Fluoridated Water Implicated as Contributing Factor in AD." Fluoride Action Network. http://www.fluorideaction.net/.

Giselle, P. et al. "The Curry Spice Curcumin Reduces Oxidative Damage and Amyloid Pathology in an Alzheimer Transgenic Mouse." *Journal of Neuroscience* 21 (4): 8370–8377, 2001.

"How to Easily and Inexpensively Blow Away Alzheimer's Disease." Mercola.com. http://www.mercola.com/2005/jan/26/alzheimers.htm.

Johnson-Marcel, T. Revolution Health Group. "Folic Acid Found to Slow Cognitive Decline in Older Adults," June 13, 2007. Revolution Health online: www.revolutionhealth.com/news/?id=article.2007-01-23.2300236381.

Joseph, J., et al. "Fruit Extracts Antagonize Abeta- or DA-induced Deficits in Ca2+ Flux in M1-transfected COS-7 Cells." *Journal of Alzheimer's Disease* 6 (4): 403–411; discussion 443–449, 2004.

Le Bars, P. L. "A Placebo-controlled, Double-blind, Randomized Trial of an Extract of Ginkgo biloba for Dementia." *Journal of the American Medical Association* (October 22/29, 1997).

Lim, W., et al. "Omega 3 Fatty Acid for the Prevention of Dementia." Cochrane Database of Systematic Reviews (online): CD005379. January 2006.

Lyketsos, C., et al. "Position Statement of the American Association for Geriatric Psychiatry (AAGP) Regarding Principles of Care for Patients with Dementia Resulting from Alzheimer's Disease." *American Journal of Geriatric Psychiatry* 14 (7): 561–572, 2006.

Mercola, J. "Alzheimer's Disease Will Become 'Enormous' Public Health Burden in US." http://www.mercola.com/1998/archive/alzheimers_disease.htm. *American Journal of Public Health* 1998;88:1337–1342.

———. "Curry Ingredient Helps Treat Alzheimer's." Mercola.com. http://www.mercola.com/2005/jan/15/curry_alzheimers.htm.

———. "Vegetarian Diet Increases Alzheimer's Risk." Mercola.com. http://www.mercola.com/2001/may/19/alzheimers.htm.

Morris, M., et al. "Fish Consumption and Cognitive Decline with Age in a Large Community Study." *Archives of Neurology* 62 (12): 1849–1853, December 2005.

Morris, M., et al. "Thoughts on B-vitamins and Dementia." *Journal of Alzheimer's Disease* 9 (4): 429–433, 2006.

Murray, M. T. *The Healing Power of Foods* (Rocklin, CA: Prima Publishing, 1993).

Murray, M. T., and J. Pizzorno. *The Encyclopedia of Natural Medicine,* 2nd ed. (Rocklin, CA: Prima Publishing, 1998).

National Institutes of Health. "Folic Acid Possibly a Key Factor in Alzheimer's Disease Prevention," March 2002. http://www.nih.gov/news/pr/mar2002/nia-01.htm.

Newman, P. E. "Could Diet Be One of the Causal Factors of Alzheimer's Disease?" *Medical Hypotheses* 39:123–126, October 1992.

Petersen, R., et al. "Vitamin E and Donepezil for the Treatment of Mild Cognitive Impairment." *New England Journal of Medicine* 352 (23): 2379–2388, 2005.

Riley M. E., et al. "Evaluation of a New Nutritional Supplement for Patients with Alzheimer's Disease." *Journal of the American Dietetic Association* 90:433–435, March 1990.

Rister, Robert. *Japanese Herbal Medicine: The Healing Art of Kampo* (Garden City Park, NY: Avery Publishing Group, 1999).

Roberts, H. J. "Allopathic Specific Condition Review: Alzheimer's Disease." *Protocol Journal of Botanical Medicine* 2(1):94, 1997.

Rondeau, V., et al. "Aluminum in Drinking Water and Cognitive Decline in Elderly Subjects: The Paquid Cohort." *Journal of Epidemiology.* 1543: 288–290, 2001. http://aje.oxfordjournals.org/cgi/content/full/154/3/288-a.

Scarmeas, N., et al. "Mediterranean Diet, Alzheimer's Disease, and Vascular Mediation." *Archives of Neurology* 63 (12): 1709–1717, 2006.

Young, R. Article on sugar and Alzheimer's disease. *"Are You Losing Your Mind?"* www.articlesofhealth.blogspot.com.

Zandi, P., et al. "Reduced Risk of Alzheimer's Disease in Users of Antioxidant Vitamin Supplements: The Cache County Study," *Archives of Neurology* 61 (1): 82–88, 2004.

Anemia

"Anemia." Wikipedia. http://en.wikipedia.org/wiki/Anemia.

Centers for Disease Control and Prevention (CDC). "Iron Deficiency." http://www.cdc.gov/nccdphp/dnpa/nutrition/nutrition_for_everyone/iron_deficiency/index.htm.

el-Shobaki F. A., and Z. A. Saleh. "[The Effect of Some Beverage Extracts on Intestinal Iron Absorption]," *Zeitschrift fur Ernahrungswissenchaft* 29(4):264–269, 1990 [in German].

"Folic Acid." MedlinePlus, NIH. http://www.nlm.nih.gov/medlineplus/folicacid.html.

Gleerup, A. et al. "Iron Absorption from the Whole Diet: Comparison of the Effect of Two Different Distributions of Daily Calcium Intake," *American Journal of Clinical Nutrition* 61(1):97–104, 1995.

Haas, E. M. *Staying Healthy with Nutrition* (Berkeley, CA: Celestial Arts, 1992).

Hallberg, L., et al. "Calcium Effect of Different Amounts on Nonheme- and Heme-Iron Absorption in Humans," *American Journal of Clinical Nutrition* 53(1):112–119, 1991.

Healthcastle.com. "Anemia Diet: Iron Deficiency Anemia." http://www.healthcastle.com/iron-anemia-diet.shtml.

"Herbs." MotherNature.com. http://www.mothernature.com/Library/Bookshelf/Books/15/58.cfm.

Herbs 2000.com. http://www.herbs2000.com/disorders/anemia.htm.

Hoffmann, D. *The Herbal Handbook: A User's Guide to Medical Herbalism.* (Rochester, NY: The Healing Arts Press, 1988).

Holistic Online.com. "Herbal Medicine—Anemia," http://www.holisticonline.com/remedies/anemia.htm.

JAMA. http://jama.ama-assn.org/cgi/content/full/296/22/2758.

Kappor, R., and U. Mehta. "Iron Status and Growth of Rats Fed Different Dietary Iron Sources." *Plant Foods for Human Nutrition* L44(1):29–34, 1993.

Layrisse, M., and M. N. Garcia-Casal. "Strategies for the Prevention of Iron Deficiency Through Foods in the Household." *Nutrition Reviews* 55(6):233–239, 1997.

Layrisse, M., et al. "The Role of Vitamin A on the Inhibitors of Nonheme Iron Absorption: Preliminary Results." *Nutritional Biochemistry* 8:61–67, 1997.

Lieberman, S., and N. Bruning. *The Real Vitamin & Mineral Book,* 4th ed. (New York: Avery, 2007).

Lynch, S. R., et al. "Inhibitory Effect of Soybean Protein-Related Moiety on Iron Absorption in Humans." *American Journal of Clinical Nutrition* 60(4):567–572, 1994.

Mercola, J. "How to Know If You Are Anemic." Mercola.com. http://v.mercola.com/blogs/public_blog/How-do-You-Know-if-You-Are-Anemic—23885.aspx.

———. "The Plague of High-Fructose Corn Syrup in Processed Foods." Mercola.com. http://v.mercola.com/blogs/public_blog/The-Plague-of-High-Fructose-Corn-Syrup-in-Processed-Foods-4192.aspx.

———. "Too Much Zinc Can Cause Anemia." Mercola.com. http://www.mercola.com/2003/aug/6/zinc_anemia.htm.

Murray, M. T., and J. Pizzorno. *The Encyclopedia of Natural Medicine,* 2nd ed. (Rocklin, CA: Prima Publishing, 1998).

Office of Dietary Supplements, NIH Clinical Center, National Institutes of Health. http://ods.od.nih.gov/factsheets/iron.asp.

"Recommendations to Prevent and Control Iron Deficiency in the United States." *Morbidity and Mortality Weekly Report* 1998; 47 (No. RR-3), p. 5.

Siegenber, D., et al. "Ascorbic Acid Prevents the Dose-Dependent Inhibitory Effects of Polyphenols and Phytates on Nonheme-Iron Absorption." *American Journal of Clinical Nutrition* 53:537–541, 1991.

Whiting, S. J. "The Inhibitory Effect of Dietary Calcium on Iron Availability: A Cause for Concern?" *Nutrition Reviews* 53(3):77–80, 1995.

Anxiety and Panic Attacks

Alschuler, L. "Botanical Medicine I, II, III, IV" (lectures). Seattle: Bastyr University, 1998.

Benjamin, J., et al. "Inositol Treatment in Psychiatry." *Psychopharmacology Bulletin* 31:167–175, 1995.

Boulenger J. P., and T. W. Uhde. "Caffeine Consumption and Anxiety: Preliminary Results of a Survey Comparing Patients with Anxiety Disorders with Normal Controls." *Psychopharmacology Bulletin* 18:53, 1982.

Bruce, M., et al. "Anxiogenic Effects of Caffeine in Patients with Anxiety Disorders." *Archives of General Psychiatry* 49: 867–869, 1992.

Charney D. S., et al. "Increased Anxiogenic Effects of Caffeine in Patients with Panic Disorders." *Archives of General Psychiatry* 43:233, 1985.

Dean, C. "The Miracle of Magnesium." http://www.mercola.com/2004/aug/7/miracle_magnesium.htm.

DePrietas, E. T., et al. "Effects of Caffeine in Chronic Psychiatry Patients." *American Journal of Psychiatry* 136:1337–1338, 1979.

Gorman, J. M., et al. "Hypoglycemia and Panic Attacks." *American Journal of Psychiatry* 141:101, 1984.

Grogg, J. L., et al. *Advanced Nutrition and Human Metabolism,* 2nd ed. (New York: West Publishing Co., 1995).

Haas, E. M. *Staying Healthy with Nutrition.* (Berkeley, CA: Celestial Arts, 1992).

HealthyPlace.com, Anxiety Community. "Nutrition Therapy for Anxiety Disorders." http://www.healthyplace.com/Communities/Anxiety/treatment/nutrition_therapy.asp.

"Java, Vino, Chocolate, and Cigars" (lecture). Seattle: Thorne Research Seminar, November 15, 1997.

Kahn, R. S., and H. G. M. Westenberg. "L-5-Hydroxytryptophan in the Treatment of Anxiety Disorders." *Journal of Affective Disorders* 8:197–200, 1985.

Kirschmann, G. J., and J. D. Kirschmann. *Nutrition Almanac,* 4th ed. (New York: McGraw-Hill, 1996).

Leznoff, A. "Preventative Challenges to Patients with Multiple Chemical Sensitivity." *Journal of Allergy and Clinical Immunology* 99(4):438–442, 1997.

Mercola, J. "Panic Attacks, Depression Harm Your Mind and Body." http://www.mercola.com. October 13, 2005.

Mohler, H., et al. "Nicotinamide Is a Brain Constituent with Benzodiazepine Actions." *Nature* 278:563, 1979.

"Panic Disorder." http://panicdisorder.about.com/od/herbsandmore/Herbs_Vitamins_and_Supplements .htm.

Rowe, K. S., et al. "Synthetic Food Coloring and Behavior: A Dose Response Effect in a Double-Blind, Placebo-Controlled, Repeated-Measures Study." *Pediatrics* 125: 691–698, 1994.

Smith, Claire. "Too Much Coffee Lands Sleepy Teenager in Hospital with Caffeine Overdose." News .Scotsman.com. http://news.scotsman.com/uk.cfm?id=1280372007 August 14, 2007.

Volz, H. P., and M. Kieser. "Kava-Kava Extract WS 1490 Versus Placebo in Anxiety Disorders—A Randomized Placebo-Controlled 25-Week Outpatient Trial." *Pharmacopsychiatry* 30:1–5, 1997.

Voocovi, P. P., et al. "Nicotinic Acid Effectiveness in the Treatment of Benzadiazepine Withdrawal." *Current Therapy Research* 41:1017, 1987.

White, H. L., et al. "Extracts of Ginkgo Biloba Leaves Inhibit Monoamine Oxidase." *Life Sciences* 58(16):1315–1321, 1996.

Wilson, Reid. "Panic Attacks." Anxieties.com. http://www.anxieties.com/panic-step1f.php.

Asthma

"Allergy." MedicineNet.com. http://www.medicinenet.com/asthma/page6.htm.

Barnett, R. A. *Tonics* (New York: HarperCollins, 1997).

Britton, J. "Dietary Magnesium, Lung Function, Wheezing, and Airway Hyperreactivity in a Random Adult Population Sample." *Lancet* 344:357–362, 1994.

Chatzi, L., et al. "Protective Effect of Fruits, Vegetables and the Mediterranean Diet on Asthma and Allergies Among Children in Crete." *Thorax* 62(8):677–683 August 2007.

Damjanov, I. *Pathology for the Health-Related Professions.* (Philadelphia: W. B. Saunders, 1996).

Dry, J., and D. Vincent. "Effect of Fish Oil Diet on Asthma: Results of a 1-Year Double-Blind Study." *International Archive of Allergy and Applied Immunology* 95:156–157, 1991.

Forastiere, F., et al. "Consumption of Fresh Fruit Rich in Vitamin C and Wheezing Symptoms in Children." *Thorax* 55(4):283–288, April 2000.

Gursche, S. *Healing with Herbal Juices.* (Burnaby, BC, Canada: Alive Books, 1993).

Hatch, G. E. "Asthma, Inhaled Oxidants and Dietary Antioxidants." *American Journal of Clinical Nutrition* 61(Suppl.): 625S–630S, 1995.

Litonjua, A. A., et al. "Maternal Antioxidant Intake in Pregnancy and Wheezing Illnesses in Children at 2 Years of Age." *American Journal of Clinical Nutrition* 84(4):903–911, October 2006.

Monteleone, C. A., and A. R. Sherman. "Nutrition and Asthma." *Archives of Internal Medicine* 157:23–34, January 1997.

Murray, M. T., and J. Pizzorno. *The Encyclopedia of Natural Medicine,* 2nd ed. (Rocklin CA: Prima Publishing, 1998).

Nariman, H., et al. "Diet and Childhood Asthma in a Society in Transition: A Study in Urban and Rural Saudi Arabia." *Thorax* online. http://thorax.bmj.com/cgi/content/abstract/55/9/775. *Thorax* 55:775–779, September 2000.

National Heart, Lung, and Blood Institute. *Diseases and Conditions Index.* http://www.nhlbi.nih .gov/health/dci/Diseases/Asthma/Asthma_Causes.html.

Soutar, A., et al. "Bronchial Reactivity and Dietary Antioxidants." *Thorax* 52:166–170, February 1997.

Tabak, C., et al. "Diet and Asthma in Dutch School Children." *Thorax* 61(12):1048–1053, December 2006. E-pub October 21, 2005.

Troisi, R. J. "A Prospective Study of Diet and Adult-Onset Asthma." *American Respiratory and Critical Care Medicine* 151: 1401–1408, 1995.

Willers, S., et al. "Maternal Food Consumption During Pregnancy and Asthma, Respiratory and Atopic Symptoms in 5-Year-old Children." *Thorax* online, http://thorax.bmj.com/cgi/content/abstract/thx .2006.074187vi.

ADD (Attention Deficit Disorder) and ADHD (Attention Deficit Hyperactivity Disorder)

Antalis, C. J., et al. (2006). "Omega-3 Fatty Acid Status in Attention-Deficit/Hyperactivity Disorder." *Prostaglandins Leukot. Essent. Fatty Acids* 75 (4–5): 299–308, October–November 2006.

Arnold, L. E., and R. A. DiSilvestro. "Zinc in Attention-Deficit/Hyperactivity Disorder." *Journal of Child and Adolescent Psychopharmacology* 15 (4): 619–627, August 2005.

"Attention Deficit Disorder (ADD) Can Respond to a Diet Change." www.homeschoolmath.net/teaching/add-adhd-diet.php.

"Attention Deficit/Hyperactivity Disorder." Centers for Disease Control and Prevention (CDC). http://www.cdc.gov/ncbddd/adhd/.

Barkley, R. A. "Attention-Deficit/Hyperactivity Disorder: Nature, Course, Outcomes, and Comorbidity." ContinuedEdCourse.net. Retrieved on December 8, 2007, from Wikipedia http://en.wikipedia.org/wiki/Attention-deficit_hyperactivity_disorder.

Boris, M., et al. "Foods and Additives Are Common Causes of the Attention Deficit Hyperactive Disorder in Children." *Annals of Allergy* 72:462–468, 1994.

Braun, J. M., et al. "Exposures to Environmental Toxicants and Attention Deficit Hyperactivity Disorder in U.S. Children." *Environmental Health Perspectives* 114 (12): 1904–1909, December 2006, from Wikipedia, "ADHD." http://en.wikipedia.org.

"Frequently Asked Questions." Attention Disorder Deficit Association (ADDA): http://www.add.org/help/faqs.html#1.

Rosenthal, E. "Study Links Food Additives and Hyperactivity." *International Herald Tribune*, September 10, 2007. http://www.boston.com.

Bladder Infections

Alschuler, L. "Botanical Medicine I, II, III, IV" (lectures). Seattle: Bastyr University, 1998.

Avorn, J., et al. "Reduction of Bacteriuria and Pyuria After Ingestion of Cranberry Juice." *Journal of the American Medical Association* 271(10):751–754, 9 March 1994.

Bernstein, J., et al. "Depression of Lymphocyte Transformation Following Oral Glucose Ingestion." *American Journal of Clinical Nutrition* 30:613, 1977.

Bodel, P. T., et al. "Cranberry Juice and the Antimicrobial Action of Hippuric Acid." *Journal of Laboratory and Clinical Medicine* 54:881–888, 1959.

"Cranberry Juice Tannins Can Defeat E. Coli Bacteria." ScientistLive.com. http://www.scientistlive.com.

Fleet, J. C. "New Support for a Folk Remedy: Cranberry Juice Reduces Bacteriuria and Pyuria in Elderly Women." *Nutrition Reviews* 52(5):168–170, May 1994.

Foxman, B., et al. "First-time Urinary Tract Infection and Sexual Behavior." *Epidemiology* 6(2):162–168, March 1995.

Gaby, A. "Therapeutic Nutrition I, II" (lectures). Seattle: Bastyr University, 1998.

Girodon, F., et al. "Effect of Micronutrient Supplementation on Infection in Institutionalized Elderly Subjects: A Controlled Trial." *Annals of Nutrition and Metabolism* 41(2):98–107, 1997.

Goldhar, J. "Anti-Escherichia coli Adhesion Activity of Cranberry and Blueberry Juices." *Advances in Experimental Medicine and Biology* 15:179–183, 1996.

Grimble, R. F. "Effects of Antioxidative Vitamins on Immune Function with Clinical Applications." *International Journal for Vitamin and Nutrition Research* 67(5):312–320, 1997.

Jepson, R., et al. "Cranberries for Preventing Urinary Tract Infections." Cochrane Database of Systematic Reviews: CD001321, 2004.

Kuzminski, L. N. "Cranberry Juice and Urinary Tract Infections: Is There a Beneficial Relationship?" *Nutrition Reviews* 1996;54(11 pt 2):S87–S90.

Levy, R., et al. "Vitamin C for the Treatment of Recurrent Furunculosis in Patients with Impaired Neutrophil Functions." *Journal of Infectious Disease* 173(6):1502–1505, June 1996.

Lundberg, J. O., et al. "Urinary Nitrite: More Than a Marker of Infection." *Urology* 50(2):189–191, August 1997.

Naganawa, R., et al. "Inhibition of Microbial Growth by Ajoene, a Sulfur-Containing Compound Derived from Garlic." *Applied and Environmental Microbiology* 62(11):4238–4242, November 1996.

"Natural Remedies: Bladder Infections." Health Ninjas.com. http://www.healthninjas.com/remedies/bladder_infections.shtml.

Ofek, I., et al. "Anti-Escherichia Coli Adhesion Activity of Cranberry and Blueberry Juices" [letter]. *New England Journal of Medicine* 324:1599, 1991.

Okie, S. "New E. Coli Strain Drug-Resistant Urinary Tract Infections." http://www.mercola.com/2001/oct/17/e_coli.htm (excerpted from *Washington Post,* October 4, 2001; page A03).

Pitchford, P. *Healing with Whole Foods: Oriental Traditions and Modern Nutrition.* (Berkeley, CA: North Atlantic Books, 1993).

Rees, L. P., et al. "A Quantitative Assessment of the Antimicrobial Activity of Garlic." *World Journal of Microbiology and Biotechnology* 9:303–307, 1993.

Sanchez, A., et al. "Role of Sugars in Human Neutrophilic Phagocytosis." *American Journal of Clinical Nutrition* 26(11): 1180–1184, November 1973.

"Urinary Tract Infection." MedLinePlus. NIH. http://www.nlm.nih.gov/medlineplus/ency/article/000521.htm#Treatment.

"Urinary Tract Infection in Adults (UTI in Adults)." MedicineNet.com. http://www.medicinenet.com-urine_infection/article.htm.

Walker, E. B., et al. "Cranberry Concentrate: UTI Prophylaxis." *Journal of Family Practice* 45:167–168, 1997.

"What Is a Bladder Infection?" Cool Nurse.com. http://www.coolnurse.com/bladder.htm.

Zafriri, D., et al. "Inhibitory Activity of Cranberry Juice on Adherence of Type 1 and Type P Fimbriated Escherichia coli to Eukaryotic Cells." *Antimicrobial Agents and Chemotherapy* 33(1): 92–98, January 1989.

Bruises

Beckham, N. *Family Guide to Natural Therapies* (New Canaan, CT: Keats Publishing, 1996).

"Bruise Remedies." Organic Nutrition. http://www.organicnutrition.co.uk/articles/bruises.htm.

"Bruises and Blood Spots Under the Skin." WebMD. http://www.webmd.com/a-to-z-guides/Bruises-and-Blood-Spots-Under-the-Skin-Home-Treatment.

"Bruises: Self-treatment." eMedicine Health. http://www.emedicinehealth.com/bruises/page6_em.htm. Reference: *Harrison's Principles of Internal Medicine.* (McGraw-Hill, edited by Eugene Braunwald. et al., 2001).

Haas, E. M. *Staying Healthy with Nutrition.* (Berkeley, CA: Celestial Arts, 1992).

Hoffmann, D. *The Herbal Handbook: A User's Guide to Medical Herbalism.* (Rochester, NY: Healing Arts Press, 1988).

———. *The New Holistic Herbal,* 3rd ed. (Rockport, MA: Element Books, 1992).

Moore, M. *Medicinal Plants of the Pacific West.* (Santa Fe: Red Crane Books, 1993).

Murray, M. T., and J. Pizzorno. *Encyclopedia of Nutritional Supplements,* 2nd ed. (Rocklin, CA: Prima Publishing, 1998).

Pitchford, P. *Healing with Whole Foods: Oriental Traditions and Modern Nutrition.* (Berkeley, CA: North Atlantic Books, 1993).

"Remedies to Speed Bruise Healing." Mercola.com. May 24, 2007. http://v.mercola.com/blogs/public_blog/Eight-Natural-Remedies-to-Speed-Bruise-Healing-17487.aspx.

Thomas, C. L. *Taber's Cyclopedic Medical Dictionary,* 17th ed. (Philadelphia: F. A. Davis, 1993).

Bursitis and Tendinitis

Arora, R. et al. "Anti-inflammatory Studies on *Curcuma longa* (Turmeric)." *Indian Journal of Medical Research* 59:1289–1295, 1971.

"Bursitis." Mayo Clinic.com. http://www.mayoclinic.com/health/bursitis/DS00032/DSECTION=3.

"Bursitis." MedicineNet.com. http://www.medicinenet.com/bursitis/article.htm.

Murray M. T., and J. Pizzorno. *Encyclopedia of Natural Medicine,* 2nd ed. (Rocklin, CA: Prima Publishing, 1998).

Taussig, S. "The Mechanism of the Physiological Action of Bromelain." *Medical Hypotheses* 6:9–14, 1980.

Weil A. *Vitamins and Minerals.* (New York: Ivy Books, 1997).

Yoshimoto, T., et al. "Flavonoids: Potent Inhibitors of Arachidonate 5-Lipoxygonase." *Biochemistry and Biophysical Research Communications* 116: 612–618, 1983.

Cancer

Albrecht, M., et al. "Pomegranate Extracts Potently Suppress Proliferation, Xenograft Growth, and Invasion of Human Prostate Cancer cells." *Journal of Medicinal Food* 7(3):274–283, Fall 2004.

Belman, S. "Onion and Garlic Oil Inhibit Tumor Growth." *Carcinogenesis* 4(8):1063–1065, 1983.

Bendich, A. "Vitamin C and Immune Response." *Food Technology* 41:112–114, 1987.

Cameron, E., and L. Pauling. *Proceedings of the National Academy of Sciences* 73(10): 3685–3689 (October 1976). In: Lieberman S., and N. Bruning. *The Real Vitamin and Mineral Book,* 4th ed. (New York: Avery, 2007).

Craig, W. J. "Phytochemicals: Guardians of Our Health." *Journal of the American Dietetic Association* 97(10 Suppl2):S199–S204, October 1997.

Digirolamo, M. *Diet and Cancer: Markers, Prevention and Treatment.* (New York: Plenum Press; 1994), p. 203.

Dowd, P., et al. "Single-Nutrient Effects of Immunologic Functions." *Journal of the American Medical Association* 245:53–58, 1981.

Egner, P. A., et al. "Chemoprevention with Chlorophyllin in Individuals Exposed to Dietary Aflatoxin." *Mutation Research* 523–524:209–16, February–March 2003.

Gerster, H. "Anticarcinogenic Effect of the Common Carotenoids." *International Journal for Vitamin and Nutrition Research* 63:93–121, 1993.

"The Hidden Dangers of Soy Allergens." www.nexusmagazine.com/articles/Soy%20Allergens.html.

Hoffer, A., and L. Pauling. *Journal of Orthomolecular Medicine* 5(3):143–154, 1990. In: Lieberman, S., and N. Bruning. *The Real Vitamin and Mineral Book,* 4th ed. (New York: Avery, 2007).

Jeune, M. A., et al. "Anticancer Activities of Pomegranate Extracts and Genistein in Human Breast Cancer Cells." *Journal of Medicinal Food* 8(4):469–475, Winter 2005.

Kage, B. "Soda Warning: High Sugar Intake Linked to Pancreatic Cancer." November 9, 2006, www.newstarget.com/021031.html.

Khan, N., et al. "Pomegranate Fruit Extract Inhibits Prosurvival Pathways in Human A549 Lung Carcinoma Cells and Tumor Growth in Athymic Nude Mice." *Carcinogenesis* 28(1):163–173, January 2007. E-pub August 18, 2006.

Kuhnau, J. "The Flavonoids: A Class of Semi-Essential Food Components: Their Role in Human Nutrition." *World Review of Nutrition and Diet* 24:117–191, 1976.

Kumar, S. S., et al. "Effect of Chlorophyllin Against Oxidative Stress in Splenic Lymphocytes in Vitro and in Vivo." *Biochimica et Biophysica Acta* 1672(2):100–111, May 3, 2004.

Lai, C. N., et al. "Anti-mutagenic Activities of Common Vegetables and Their Chlorophyll Content," *Mutation Research* 77: 245–250, 1980. In: Kenton, L., and S. Kenton. *Raw Energy* (London: Century Publishing, 1985).

Lai, C. N., et al. "Chlorophyll: The Active Factor in Wheat Sprout Extract Inhibiting the Metabolic Activation of Carcinogens in Vitro." *Nutrition and Cancer* 1(3):19–21, 1978. In: Wigmore, A. *The Wheatgrass Book* (Garden City Park, NY: Avery Publishing Group, 1985).

Leeper, D. B., et al. "Effect of I.V. Glucose versus Combined I.V. Plus Oral Glucose on Human Tumor Extracellular pH for Potential Sensitization to Thermoradiotherapy." *International Journal of Hyperthermia* 14(3):257–269, May–June 1998.

Malik, A., et al. "Pomegranate Fruit Juice for Chemoprevention and Chemotherapy of Prostate Cancer." *Proceedings of the National Academy of Sciences* 102; published online before print as 10.1073/pnas .0505870102.

McEligot, A. J., et al. "Comparison of Serum Carotenoid Responses Between Women Consuming Vegetable Juice and Women Consuming Raw or Cooked Vegetables" *Epidemiology Biomarkers & Prevention* 8:227–231, March 1999. Online at American Association for Cancer Research: cebp.aacrjournals .org/cgi/content/full/8/3/227.

Ogawa, K., et al. "Beneficial Effects of the Vegetable Juice Aojiru on Cellular Immunity in Japanese Young Women." *Nutrition Research Journal* 24(8):613–620, August 2004. www.nrjournal.com/article/PIIS0271531704000442/abstract.

Ornish, D., et al. "Intensive Lifestyle Changes May Affect the Progression of Prostate Cancer. *Journal of Urology* 2005; 274:1065–1069.

Park, K. K., et al. "Inhibitory Effects of Chlorophyllin, Hemin and Tetrakis (4-benzoic acid) Porphyrin on Oxidative DNA Damage and Mouse Skin Inflammation Induced by 12-O-tetradecanoylphorbol-13-acetate as a Possible Anti-tumor Promoting Mechanism." *Mutation Research* 542(1–2):89–97WY, December 9, 2003.

Pierce, J. P., et al. "Greater Survival After Breast Cancer in Physically Active Women with High Vegetable-Fruit Intake Regardless of Obesity." *Journal of Clinical Oncology* 25:2345–2351, 2007.

Pierce, J. P., et al. "Influence of a Diet Very High in Vegetables, Fruit, and Fiber and Low in Fat on Prognosis Following Treatment for Breast Cancer: The Women's Healthy Eating and Living (WHEL) Randomized Trial." *JAMA* 298:289–298, 2007.

Pizzorno, J. *Total Wellness.* (Rocklin, CA: Prima Publishing, 1996).

Rock, C. L., et al. "Plasma Carotenoids and Recurrence-free Survival in Women with a History of Breast Cancer." *Journal of Clinical Oncology* 23:6631–6638, 2005.

Seeram, N. P., et al. "In Vitro Antiproliferative, Apoptotic and Antioxidant Activities of Punicalagin, Ellagic Acid and a Total Pomegranate Tannin Extract Are Enhanced in Combination with Other Polyphenols as Found in Pomegranate Juice." *Journal of Nutritional Biochemistry* 16(6):360–367, June 2005.

Semba, R. D. "Vitamin A, Immunity and Infection." *Clinical Infectious Diseases* 19:489–499, 1994.

Steinmetz, K., and J. D. Potter. "Vegetables, Fruit and Cancer, I: Epidemiology." *Cancer Causes Control* 2:325–357, 1991.

———. "Vegetables, Fruit and Cancer, II: Mechanisms," *Cancer Causes Control* 2:427–442, 1991.

"Study Links High Carbohydrate Diet to Increased Breast Cancer Risk." www.sciencedaily.com/releases/2004/08/040806094822.htm.

Talska, G., et al. "Genetically Based n-Acetyltransferase Metabolic Polymorphism and Low-Level Environmental Exposure in Carcinogens," *Nature* 369: 154–156, 1994. In: Murray, M. T., and J. Pizzorno. *Encyclopedia of Natural Medicine,* 2nd ed. (Rocklin, CA: Prima Publishing, 1998).

"The Truth About Soy." www.soyonlineservice.co.nz.

Volk, T. et al. "PH in Human Tumor Xenografts: Effect of Intravenous Administration of Glucose." *British Journal of Cancer* 68(3):492–500, September 1993.

Warburg, O. "On the Origin of Cancer Cells." *Science* 123:309–314, February 1956.

Watson, R. R., et al. "Selenium and Vitamins A, E, and C: Nutrients with Cancer Prevention Properties." *Journal of the American Dietetic Association* 86(4): 505–510, 1986.

Weil, A. *Vitamins and Minerals.* (New York: Ivy Books, 1997).

Weissman, G., et al. "Polyphenols Stop Cancer, Heart Disease, Depending on the Dose," October 31, 2007, www.news-medical.net/?id=31953.

Candidiasis

Alchemical Medicine Research and Teaching Association. "Condition: Vaginitis/leukorrhea. Body System: Reproductive System." IBIS: Integrative BodyMind Information System, Version 1.2, 1994. Gaia Multimedia, Inc.

Babu, U., and M. L. Failla. "Respiratory Burst and Candidacidal Activity of Peritoneal Macrophages Are Impaired in Copper-Deficient Rats." *Journal of Nutrition* 120(12): 1692–1699, December 1990.

Boyne, R., and J. R. Arthur. "The Response of Selenium-Dependent Mice to Candida albicans Infection." *Journal of Nutrition* 116: 816–822, May 1986.

The Burton Goldberg Group (J. Strohecker, exec. ed.). *Alternative Medicine: The Definitive Guide* (Puyallup, WA: Future Medicine Publishing, 1994), pp. 587–593.

"Candida Albicans and Foods Containing Yeast." Seattle: Bastyr University Nutrition Clinic, 1998.

De Schepper, L. *Candida.* Online publication of American College of Physicians. 1986, pp. 28–32.

Drutz, D. J. "Lactobacillus Prophylaxis for Candida Vaginitis." Comment in *Annals of Internal Medicine* 116(5):419–420, March 1992.

Edman, J., et al. "Zinc Status in Women with Recurrent Vulvovaginal Candidiasis." *American Journal of Obstetrics and Gynecology* 155:1082–1085, 1986.

Hilton, E., et al. "Ingestion of Yogurt Containing Lactobacillus Acidophilus as Prophylaxis for Candidal Vaginitis." *Annals of Internal Medicine* 116(5):353–357, March 1992.

Horowitz, B. J., et al. "Sugar Chromatography Studies in Recurrent Candida Vulvovaginitis." *The Journal of Reproductive Medicine* 29(7):441–443, July 1984.

Kennedy, M. J., et al. "Mechanisms of Association of *Candida albicans* with Intestinal Mucosa." *Journal of Medical Microbiology* 24(4):333–341, December 1987.

MacDonald, T. M., et al. "The Risks of Symptomatic Vaginal Candidiasis After Oral Antibiotic Therapy," *Quarterly Journal of Medicine* 86(7):419–424, July 1993.

Olkowski, A. A., et al. "Effects of Diets of High Sulphur Content and Varied Concentrations of Copper, Molybdenum, and Thiamin on In Vitro Phagocytic and Candidacidal Activity of Neutrophils in Sheep." *Research in Veterinary Science* 48(1):82–86, January 1990.

Pizzorno, J., and M. T. Murray. *The Textbook of Natural Medicine* (Seattle: Bastyr University Publications, 1992).

Reed, B. D., et al. "The Association Between Dietary Intake and Reported History of Candida Vulvovaginitis." *The Family Practice* 29(5):509–515, 1989.

Rochilitz, S. *Allergies and Candida with the Physicist's Rapid Solution,* 2nd ed. (Setauket, NY: Human Ecology Balancing Sciences, Inc.) 1989, pp. 69–91.

Canker Sores

Balch, P., and J. Balch. *Prescription for Nutritional Healing,* 4th ed. (New York: Avery, 2006).

Hay, K. D., et al. "The Use of an Elimination Diet in the Treatment of Recurrent Aphthous Ulceration of the Oral Cavity." *Oral Surgery* 57:504–507, 1984.

Murray, M. T., and J. Pizzorno. *Encyclopedia of Nutritional Supplements.* (Rocklin, CA: Prima Publishing, 1996).

Wray, D., et al. "Recurrent Aphthae Treatment With Vitamin B_{12}, Folic Acid, and Iron." *British Medical Journal* 2:490–493, 1975.

Cardiovascular Disease

Anderson, J. W., et al. "Meta Analysis of the Effects of Soy Protein Intake on Serum Lipids." *New England Journal of Medicine* 333:276–282, 1995.

————. "Oat Bran Cereal Lowers Serum Total and LDL Cholesterol in Hypercholesterolemic Men," *American Journal of Clinical Nutrition* 52:495–499, 1990.

Aronov, D. M., et al. "Clinical Trial of Wax-Matrix Sustained Release Niacin in a Russian Population with Hypercholesteremia." *Archives of Family Medicine* 5:567–575, 1996.

Ascherio, A., et al. "Trans Fatty Acids Intake and Risk of Myocardial Infarction," *Circulation* 89:94–101, 1994.

Baggesen, J. R. High Tech Health. www.richmond.com/health-fitness/article/23476.

Bakalar, N. "Symptoms: Metabolic Syndrome Is Tied to Diet Soda." *The New York Times,* February 5, 2008.

Berkow, R. (ed.). *The Merck Manual, 16th ed.* (Rahway, NJ: Merck Research Laboratories, 1992).

Bianchi, C., et al. "Alcohol Consumption and the Risk of Acute Myocardial Infarction in Women." *Journal of Epidemiology and Community Health* 47:308–311, 1993.

Block, G., and L. Langseth. "Antioxidant Vitamins and Disease Prevention." *Food Technology* 80–84, July 1994.

Breithaupt-Grogler, K., et al. "Protective Effect of Chronic Garlic Intake on Elastic Properties of Aorta in the Elderly," *Circulation* 96:2649–2655, 1997.

Camargo, C. A., et al. "Prospective Study of Moderate Alcohol Consumption and Risk of Peripheral Arterial Disease in U.S. Male Physicians." *Circulation* 95:577–580, 1997.

Cappuccio, F. P., and G. A. MacGregor. "Does Potassium Supplementation Lower Blood Pressure? A Meta-Analysis of Published Trials." *Journal of Hypertension* 9:465–473, 1991.

Carbonneau, M. A., et al. "Supplementation with Wine Phenolic Compounds Increases the Antioxidant Capacity of Plasma and Vitamin E of Low-Density Lipoprotein Without Changing the Lipoprotein Copper Ion Oxidability: Possible Explanation by Phenolic Location." *European Journal of Clinical Nutrition* 51: 682–690, 1997.

Carper, Jean. "Your Big New Threat: Inflammation." www.usaweekend.com/03_issues/030309/030309eatsmart.html.

Cerda, J. J., et al. "The Effects of Grapefruit Pectin on Patients at Risk for Coronary Heart Disease Without Altering Diet or Lifestyle." *Clinical Cardiology* 11:589–594, 1988.

Chisholm, A., et al. "Effect on Lipoprotein Profile of Replacing Butter with Margarine in a Low Fat Diet: Randomized Study with Hypercholesteremic Subjects." *British Medical Journal* 312:931–934, 1996.

Cotran, R. S., et al. *Robbins Pathologic Basis of Disease,* 5th ed. (Philadelphia: W. B. Saunders, 1994).

Crestanello, J. A., et al. "Elucidation of a Tripartite Mechanism Underlying the Improvement in Cardiac Tolerance to Ischemia by Coenzyme Q10 Pretreatment." *Journal of Thoracic and Cardiovascular Surgery* 111:443–450, 1996.

Croft, K. D., et al. "Oxidative Susceptibility of Low-Density Lipoproteins—Influence of Regular Alcohol Use." *Alcoholism and Clinical Experimental Research* 20:980–984, 1996.

Davini, P., et al. "Controlled Study on L-carnitine Therapeutic Efficacy in Post-Infarction." *Drugs Under Experimental Clinical Research* 18:355–365, 1992.

Frankel, E. N., et al. "Inhibition of Oxidation of Human Low-Density Lipoprotein by Phenolic Substances in Red Wine." *Lancet* 341:454–457, 1993.

Gatto, L. M., et al. "Ascorbic Acid Induces a Favourable Lipoprotein Profile in Women." *Journal of the American College of Nutrition* 15:154–158, 1996.

Geleijnse, J. M., et al. "Dietary Electrolyte Intake and Blood Pressure in Older Subjects: The Rotterdam Study." *Journal of Hypertension* 14:737–741, 1996.

Gey, K. F. "Cardiovascular Disease and Vitamins. Concurrent Correction of Suboptimal Plasma Antioxidant Levels May, as Important Part of Optimal Nutrition, Help to Prevent Early Stages of Cardiovascular Disease and Cancer, Respectively." *Bibliotheca Nutritio et Dieta* 52:75–91, 1995.

Gillman, M. W., et al. "Protective Effect of Fruits and Vegetables on Development of Stroke in Men." *Journal of the American Medical Association* 273:1113–1117, 1995.

Graham, I. M., et al. "Plasma Homocysteine as a Risk Factor for Vascular Disease. The European Concerted Action Project." *Journal of the American Medical Association* 277:1775–1781, 1997.

Imai, K., and K. Nakachi. "Cross Sectional Study of Effects of Drinking Green Tea on Cardiovascular and Liver Diseases." *British Medical Journal* 310:693–696, 1995.

Jenkins, D. J., et al. "Effect of Diet High in Vegetables, Fruit, and Nuts on Serum Lipids." *Metabolism* 46:530–537, 1997.

Kurowska, E. M., et al. "Effects of Substituting Dietary Soybean Protein and Oil for Milk Protein and Fat in Subjects with Hypercholesteremia." *Clinical and Investigative Medicine* 20:162–170, 1997.

Lark, S. M. *Women's Health Companion.* (Berkeley, CA: Celestial Arts, 1995).

Lovegren, Stefan. "Pomegranate Juice Fights Heart Disease, Study Says." *National Geographic News,* March 22, 2005. news.nationalgeographic.com/news/2005/03/0322_050322_pomegranates.html.

McCarron, D. A. "Role of Adequate Dietary Calcium Intake in the Prevention and Management of Salt-Sensitive Hypertension." *American Journal of Clinical Nutrition* 65:712S–716S, 1997.

Miura, S., et al. "Effects of Various Natural Antioxidants on the Copper Ion Mediated Oxidative Modification of Low Density Lipoprotein." *Biological and Pharmaceutical Bulletin* 18:1–4, 1995.

Mizushima, S., et al. "Fish Intake and Cardiovascular Risk Among Middle-Aged Japanese in Japan and Brazil." *Journal of Cardiovascular Risk* 4:191–199, 1997.

Mori, T. A., et al. "Interactions Between Dietary Fat, Fish and Fish Oils and Their Effects on Platelet Function in Men at Risk of Cardiovascular Disease." *Artheriosclerosis, Thrombosis, and Vascular Biology* 17:279–286, 1997.

Morrison, H. I., et al. "Serum Folate and Risk of Fatal Coronary Heart Disease." *Journal of the American Medical Association* 275:1893–1896, 1996.

Murray, M. T. *The Complete Book of Juicing.* (Rocklin, CA: Prima Publishing, 1992).

———. *The Healing Power of Herbs,* 2nd ed. (Rocklin, CA: Prima Publishing, 1995).

Murray, M. T., and J. Pizzorno. *The Encyclopedia of Natural Medicine,* 2nd ed. (Rocklin, CA: Prima Publishing, 1998).

Ness, A. R., and J. W. Powles. "Fruits and Vegetables, and Cardiovascular Disease: A Review." *International Journal of Epidemiology* 26:1–13, 1997.

Ness, A. R., et al. "Vitamin C Status and Blood Pressure." *Journal of Hypertension* 14:503–508, 1996.

Oliver, M. F. "It Is More Important to Increase the Intake of Unsaturated Fats Than to Decrease the Intake of Saturated Fats: Evidence from Clinical Trials Relating to Ischemic Heart Disease." *American Journal of Clinical Nutrition* 66:980S–986S, 1997.

Olson, B. H., et al. "Psyllium Enriched Cereals Lower Blood Total Cholesterol and LDL Cholesterol but Not HDL Cholesterol in Hypercholesterolemic Adults: Results of Meta-Analysis." *Journal of Nutrition* 127:1973–1980, 1997.

Orekhov, A. N., and V. V. Tertov. "In Vitro Effect of Garlic Powder Extract on Lipid Content in Normal and Atherosclerotic Human Aortic Cells." *Lipids* 32:1055–1060, 1997.

Ornish, D., et al. "Can Lifestyle Changes Reverse Coronary Heart Disease? The Lifestyle Heart Trial." *Lancet* 336:129–133, 1990.

Palmer, J. R., et al. "Coffee Consumption and Myocardial Infarction in Women." *American Journal of Epidemiology* 141: 724–731, 1995.

Pucciarelli, G., et al. "The Clinical and Hemodynamic Effects of Propionyl-L-Carnitine in the Treatment of Congestive Heart Failure." *Clinica Terapeutica* 141: 379–384, 1992.

Rifier, V. A., and A. K. Khachadurian. "Effects of Vitamin C and E Supplementation on the Copper Mediated Oxidation of HDL and on HDL Mediated Cholesterol Efflux." *Atherosclerosis* 127:19–26, 1996.

Robbers, J., et al. *Pharmacognosy and Pharmacobiotechnology.* (Baltimore: Williams & Wilkins, 1996).

Robertson, D., et al. "Tolerance to the Humoral and Hemodynamic Effects of Caffeine in Man." *Journal of Clinical Investigation* 67:1111–1117, 1981.

Robertson, J., et al. "The Effect of Raw Carrots on Serum Lipids and Colon Function." *American Journal of Clinical Nutrition* 32:1889–1892, 1979.

Robinson, K., et al. "Low Circulating Folate and Vitamin B_6 Concentrations: Risk Factors for Stroke, Peripheral Vascular Disease, and Coronary Artery Disease, European COMAC Group." *Circulation* 97:437–443, 1998.

Salonen, J. T., et al. "Effects of Antioxidant Supplementation on Platelet Function: A Randomized Pair-Matched Placebo-Controlled Double-Blind Trial in Men with Low Antioxidant Status." *American Journal of Clinical Nutrition* 53:1222–1229, 1991.

Santos, M. J., et al. "Influence of Dietary Supplementation with Fish on Plasma Fatty Acid Composition in Coronary Heart Disease Patients." *Annals of Nutrition and Metabolism* 39:52–62, 1995.

Schneider, J., et al. "Alcohol Lipid Metabolism and Coronary Heart Disease." *Herz* 21:217–226, 1996.

"Science News Study Provides New Evidence That Cranberry Juice May Help Fight Heart Disease," *ScienceDaily* March 26, 2003. www.sciencedaily.com/releases/2003/03/030326074425.htm

"Science News UC Davis Study Finds Heart Benefits from Apples and Juice," *ScienceDaily,* February 26, 2001. www.sciencedaily.com/releases/2001/02/010223081211.htm

Science and Nutrition. "Fruit and Vegetables Cut Heart Disease Risk, Says Study." www.food-decisions.com/news/ng.asp?id=70841-fruit-vegetables-chd.

Skrabal F., et al. "Low Sodium/High Potassium Diet for Prevention of Hypertension: Probable Mechanisms of Action." *Lancet* 2:895–900, 1981.

Soja, A. M., and S. A. Mortensen. "Treatment of Chronic Cardiac Insufficiency with Coenzyme Q10, Results of Meta-Analysis in Controlled Clinical Trials." *Ugeskr Laeger* 159:7302–7308, 1997.

Takamatsu, S., et al. "Effects on Health of Dietary Supplementation with 100 mg d-Alpha Tocopheryl Acetate Daily for 6 Years." *Journal of International Medical Research* 23:342–357, 1995.

Tavani, A., et al. "Beta Carotene Intake and Risk of Nonfatal Acute Myocardial Infarction in Women." *European Journal of Epidemiology* 13:631–637, 1997.

Troisi, R., et al. "Trans Fatty Acid Intake in Relation to Serum Lipid Concentrations in Adult Men." *American Journal of Clinical Nutrition* 56:1019–1024, 1992.

Weber, C., et al. "The Coenzyme Q10 Content of the Average Danish Diet." *International Journal for Vitamin and Nutrition Research* 67:123–129, 1997.

Werbach, M. *Healing with Food* (New York: HarperCollins, 1993).

Willett, W. C., et al. "Intake of Trans Fatty Acids and Risk of Coronary Heart Disease Among Women." *Lancet* 341:581–585, 1993.

Wise, K. J., et al. "Interactions Between Dietary Calcium and Caffeine Consumption on Calcium Metabolism in Hypertensive Humans." *American Journal of Hypertension* 9:223–229, 1996.

Carpal Tunnel Syndrome

Alchemical Medicine Research and Teaching Association. "Condition: Carpal Tunnel Syndrome." IBIS: Integrative BodyMind Information System, Version 1.2, 1994. Gaia Multimedia, Inc. http://www.alternative-medicine-and-health.com/conditions/carpal.htm.

Bernstein, A. L., and J. S. Dinesen. "Brief Communication: Effect of Pharmacologic Doses of Vitamin B_6 on Carpal Tunnel Syndrome, Electroencephalographic Results in Pain." *Journal of the American College of Nutrition* 12(1):73–76, February 1993.

Folkers, K., and J. Ellis. "Successful Therapy with Vitamin B_6 and Vitamin B_2 of the Carpal Tunnel Syndrome and Need for Determination of the RDAs for Vitamin B_6 and B_2 Disease States." *Annals of the New York Academy of Sciences* 585:295–301, 1990.

Fuhr, J. E., et al. "Vitamin B_6 Levels in Patients with Carpal Tunnel Syndrome." *Archives of Surgery* 124:1329–1330, 1989.

Gaby, A., and J. Wright. *Nutritional Therapy in Medical Practice.* (Seattle: Gaby/Wright Seminars, 1996), p. 18.

Gould, J. S., and H. A. Wissinger. "Carpal Tunnel Syndrome in Pregnancy." *Southern Medical Journal* 71:144, 1978.

Haas, E. M. *Staying Healthy with Nutrition* (Berkeley, CA: Celestial Arts, 1992), p. 22.

"Natural Carpal Tunnel Syndrome Treatments." altmedicine.about.com/od/carpaltunnelsyndrome/a/carpal_tunnel.htm.

Ombregt, L., et al. *A System of Orthopedic Medicine.* (Philadelphia: W. B. Saunders, 1995), pp. 393–399.

Pizzorno, J., and M. T. Murray. *Textbook of Natural Medicine.* (Seattle: Bastyr University Publications, 1992).

Roe, D. *Drug-Induced Nutritional Deficiencies.* (Westport, CT: AVI, 1976), pp. 166–167.

Werbach, M. *Nutritional Influences on Illness.* (New Canaan, CT: Keats Publishing, 1988), pp. 192–193.

Chronic Fatigue Syndrome

Barnes, C. L., et al. "Chronic Fatigue Syndrome: What Are the Facts?" *The Journal of Practical Nursing* 24–31, September 1993.

The Burton Goldberg Group (J. Strohecker, exec. ed.). *Alternative Medicine: The Definitive Guide.* (Puyallup, WA: Future Medicine Publishing, 1994), pp. 616–624.

Carter, R. E. "Chronic Intestinal Candidiasis as a Possible Etiological Factor in the Chronic Fatigue Syndrome." *Medical Hypotheses* June 44(6):507–515, 1995.

Cox, I. M., et al. "Red Blood Cell Magnesium and Chronic Fatigue Syndrome." *Lancet* 337:757–760, 1991.

Douglass, J. "Nutrition, Nonthermally Prepared Food and Nature's Message to Man." *Journal of the International Academy of Preventative Medicine* VII(2). July 1982. In: Kenton, L. and S. Kenton, *Raw Energy.* (London: Century Publishing Co.) 1984.

Galland, L. and M. Leem. "*Giardia lamblia* Infection as a Cause of Chronic Fatigue." *Journal of Nutrition and Medicine* 1:27, 1990.

Haas, E. M. *Staying Healthy with Nutrition.* (Berkeley, CA: Celestial Arts, 1992).

Hoffmann, D. *The Herbal Handbook: A User's Guide to Medical Herbalism* (Rochester, NY: Healing Arts Press, 1988).

Hoffmann, D. *The New Holistic Herbal.* 3rd ed. (Rockport, MA: Element Books, 1992).

Jacobson, W., et al. "Serum Folate and Chronic Fatigue Syndrome." *Neuropsychobiology* 35(1):16–23, 1997.

Murray, M. T., and J. Pizzorno. *The Encyclopedia of Natural Medicine,* 2nd ed. (Rocklin, CA: Prima Publishing, 1998).

Pitchford, P. *Healing with Whole Foods: Oriental Traditions and Modern Nutrition.* (Berkeley, CA: North Atlantic Books, 1993).

Pizzorno, J., and M. T. Murray. *The Textbook of Natural Medicine* (Seattle: Bastyr University Publications, 1992), Mono Ch-1.

Pliophys, A. V. and S. Pliophys. "Amantadine and L-Carnitine Treatment of Chronic Fatigue Syndrome." *Lancet* 337:757–760, 1991.

———. "Serum Levels of Carnitine in Chronic Fatigue Syndrome: Clinical Correlates." *Neuropsychobiology* 32(3):132–138, 1995.

Pompei, R., et al. "Antiviral Activity of Glycyrrhizic Acid." *Experientia* 36(3):304–305, 1980.

Straus, S. E., et al. "Allergy and the Chronic Fatigue Syndrome." *Journal of Allergy and Clinical Immunology* 81(5):791–795, 1988.

Colds

Abbas, A. K., A. H. Lichtman, et al. *Cellular and Molecular Immunology.* (Philadelphia: W. B. Saunders, 1994), pp. 328, 396.

Balch, P., and J. Balch. *Prescription for Nutritional Healing,* 4th ed. (New York: Avery, 2006).

Baurn, M. K., et al. "HIV-1 Infection in Women Is Associated with Severe Nutritional Deficiencies." *Journal of Acquired Immune Deficiency Syndromes and Human Retrovirology* 16(4):272–278, 1997.

Cowgill, U. M. "The Distribution of Selenium and Mortality Owing to Acquired Immune Deficiency Syndrome in the Continental US." *Biological Trace Element Research* 56(1):43–61, 1997.

Garland, M. I., and K. O. Hagneyer. "The Role of Zinc Lozenges in Treatment of the Common Cold." *Annals of Pharmacotherapy* 32(1):63–69, 1998.

Glasziou, P. P., and D. E. M. MacKerras. "Vitamin A Supplementation in Infectious Diseases: A Meta Analysis." *British Medical Journal* 306:366–370, 1993.

Haas, E. *Staying Healthy with Nutrition: The Complete Guide to Diet and Nutritional Medicine.* (Berkeley, CA: Celestial Arts Publishing, 1992), pp. 96, 213.

Hemil, A. H. "Vitamin C and Common Cold Incidence: A Review of Studies with Subjects Under Heavy Physical Stress." *International Journal of Sports Medicine* 17(5):379–383, 1996.

———. "Vitamin C Intake and Susceptibility to the Common Cold." *British Journal of Nutrition* 77(1):59–72, 1997.

———. "Vitamin C, the Placebo Effect, and the Common Cold: A Case Study of How Preconceptions Influence the Analysis of Results." *Journal of Clinical Epidemiology* 49(10):1079–1084, October 1996.

Hunt, C., et al. "The Clinical Effects of Vitamin C Supplementation in Elderly Hospitalized Patients with Acute Respiratory Infections." *International Journal for Vitamin and Nutrition Research* 64(3):212–219, 1994.

Kiremidjian-Schumacher, L., et al. "Supplementation with Selenium and Human Immune Cell Functions II: Effect on Cytotoxic Lymphocytes and Natural Killer Cells." *Biological Trace Element Research* 41(1–2):115–127, 1994.

Makowska-Zwierz, W., et al. "The Effect of Vitamin E on Granulocyte Function in Patients with Recurrent Infections." *Archivm Immunologiae et Therapiae Experimentalis* (Warz) 39(1–2):109–115, 1991.

Mossad S. B., et al. "Zinc Gluconate Lozenges for Treating the Common Cold: A Randomized Double-Blind, Placebo-Controlled Study." *Annals of Internal Medicine* 125(2):81–88, 1996.

Murray, M. T. *The Complete Book of Juicing.* (Rocklin, CA: Prima Publishing, 1992), pp. 71, 136, 157, 209–210, 214.

———. *The Healing Power of Herbs,* 2nd ed. (Rocklin, CA: Prima Publishing, 1992), pp. 102, 124, 355.

Murray M. T., and J. Pizzorno. *The Encyclopedia of Natural Medicine,* 2nd ed. (Rocklin, CA: Prima Publishing, 1998), pp. 148–157, 371–376.

Novick, S. G., et al. "Zinc Induced Suppression of Inflammation in the Respiratory Tract, Caused by Infection with Human Rhinovirus and Other Irritants." *Medical Hypotheses* 49(4):347–357, 1997.

"Nutrition for Colds and Flu." www.fooddemocracy.wordpress.com/2007/11/29/nutrition-for-colds-and-flu.

Peretz, A. "Lymphocyte Response Is Enhanced by Supplementation of Elderly Subjects with Selenium-Enriched Yeast." *American Journal of Clinical Nutrition* 53(5):1323–1328, 1991.

Price, S., and L. Price. *Aromatherapy for Health Professionals*. (New York: Churchill Livingstone, 1995), pp. 249, 253.

See, D. M., et al. "In Vitro Effects of Echinacea and Ginseng on Natural Killer and Antibody-Dependent Cell Cytotoxicity in Healthy Subjects and Chronic Fatigue Syndrome or Acquired Immunodeficiency Syndrome Patients." *Immunopharmacology* 35(3):229–235, 1997.

Werbach, M. *Healing with Food*. (New York: HarperCollins, 1993), pp. 77, 201.

Colitis, IBS, and Other Bowel Diseases

Bartels, M. et al. "What Is the Role of Nutrition in Ulcerative Colitis? A Contribution to the Current Status of Diet Therapy in Treatment of Inflammatory Bowel Disease." *Langenbecks Arch fur Chirurgie* 380(1):4–11, 1995.

Belluzzi, A., et al. "Effect of an Enteric-Coated Fish-Oil Preparation on Relapses in Crohn's Disease." *New England Journal of Medicine* 34:1557–1560, June 13, 1996.

Burke, A., et al. "Nutrition and Ulcerative Colitis." *Baillieres Clinical Gastroenterology* 11(1):153–174, March 1997.

"Dietary and Other Risk Factors of Ulcerative Colitis: A Case-Controlled Study in Japan." *Journal of Clinical Gastroenterology* 19(2):166–171, September 1994.

Heaton, K., et al. "Treatment of Crohn's Disease with an Unrefined-Carbohydrate, Fibre-Rich Diet." *British Medical Journal* 2:764–766, September 1979.

Hoffmann, D. *The New Holistic Herbal*. (Rockport, MA: Element, Inc. 1990).

Hyde, A. C. "An Herbal Practitioner's Approach to Irritable Bowel Syndrome." *The European Journal of Herbal Medicine* 1(2):44–47, Summer 1994.

Jarrett, M., et al. "Comparison of Diet Composition in Women with and without Functional Bowel Disorder." *Gastroenterology Nursing* 16(6):253–258, June 1994.

Jones, V., et al. "Crohn's Disease: Maintenance of Remission by Diet." *Lancet* 1:177–180, July 1985.

Meier, R. "Chronic Inflammatory Bowel Disease and Nutrition." *Schweizerische Medizinische Wochenschrift Supplement* 79:14S–24S, 1996.

Murray, M. T., and J. Pizzorno. *Encyclopedia of Natural Medicine*, 2nd ed. (Rocklin, CA: Prima Publishing, 1998).

Peck, P. "Glutamine Should Be Figured into IBD Formulation." *Family Practice News* 22, June 1, 1994.

Raif, S., et al. "Pre-illness Dietary Factors in Inflammatory Bowel Disease." *Gut* 40(6):754–760, June 1997.

Reichert, R. "Treatment of Ulcerative Colitis with *Boswellia Serrata*." *Quarterly Review of Natural Medicine* 175–176, Fall 1997.

Rhodes, J. M. "Unifying Hypothesis for Inflammatory Bowel Disease and Associated Colon Cancer: Sticking the Pieces Together with Sugar." *Lancet* 346:40–44, 6 January 1996.

Sandler, R. S. "Epidemiology of Irritable Bowel Syndrome in the United States." *Gastroenterology* 99(2):409–415, August 1990.

Shoda, R., et al. "Epidemiologic Analysis of Crohn's Disease in Japan: Increased Dietary Intake of n-6 Polyunsaturated Fatty Acids and Animal Protein Relates to the Increased Incidence of Crohn's Disease in Japan." *American Journal of Clinical Nutrition* 63:741–745, 1996.

Sonnerville, K., et al. "Delayed Release Peppermint Oil Capsules (Colpermin) for the Spastic Colon Syndrome: A Pharmacokinetic Study." *British Journal of Clinical Pharmacology* 18:638–640, 1984. In: Murray, M. T., and J. Pizzorno. *The Encyclopedia of Natural Medicine*. (Rocklin, CA: Prima Publishing, 1990), p. 399.

Thornton J., et al. "Diet and Crohn's Disease: Characteristics of the Pre-Illness Diet." *British Medical Journal*, 762–764, September 2, 1979.

Tragnone, A., et al. "Dietary Habits as Risk Factors for Inflammatory Bowel Disease." *European Journal of Gastroenterology* 7(1):47–51, January 1995.

Vernia, P., et al. "Lactose Malabsorption and Irritable Bowel Syndrome. Effect of a Long-Term Lactose-Free Diet." *Italian Journal of Gastroenterology* 27(3):117–121, April 1995.

Walker, A. R. "Diet and Bowel Diseases—Past History and Future Prospects." *South African Medical Journal* 68(3):148–152, 3 August 1985.

Constipation

Banaszkiewicz, A., and H. Szajewska. "Ineffectiveness of Lactobacillus GG as an Adjunct to Lactulose for the Treatment of Constipation in Children: A Double-Blind, Placebo-Controlled Randomized Trial." *Journal of Pediatrics* 146.3: 364–369, 2005, from www.altmedicine.about.com/od/constipation/a/constipation_2.htm.

"Help for When You're Constipated." *Family Practice Recertification* 17(4):54, April 1995.

Lupton J. R., et al. "Barley Bran Flour Accelerates Gastrointestinal Transit Time." *Journal of the American Dietetic Association* 93:881–885, 1993.

"Nonorganic Constipation: A Double-Blind Controlled Trial," *Digestive Diseases and Sciences* 40(2): 349–356, February 1995.

Voderholzer, W. A., et al. "Dietary Fiber in the Treatment of Constipation." *Nutrition Research Newsletter*, March, 1997. www.findarticles.com.

Cravings

Barnett, R. A. *Tonics* (New York: HarperCollins, 1997).

Blundell, J. E, et al. "Mechanisms of Appetite Control and Their Abnormalities in Obese Patients." *Hormone Research* 39:72–76, 1993.

Burton, B. T., and W. R. Foster. *Human Nutrition* (New York: McGraw-Hill, 1998).

Carper, J. *Food: Your Miracle Medicine.* (New York: HarperCollins, 1993).

Christensen, L., and S. Somers. "Comparison of Nutrient Intake Among Depressed and Nondepressed Individuals." *International Journal of Eating Disorders* 20:105–109, July 1996.

Douglass, J. M., et al. "Effects of a Raw Food Diet on Hypertension and Obesity." *South Medical Journal* 78(7):841–844, July 1985.

Dye, L., and J. E. Blundell. "Menstrual Cycle and Appetite Control: Implications for Weight Regulation." *Human Reproduction* 12:1142–1151, June 1997.

Haas, E. M. *Staying Healthy with Nutrition.* (Berkeley, CA: Celestial Arts, 1992).

Hart, C. *Secrets of Serotonin.* (New York: St. Martin's Press, 1996).

Heller, R. F. "Hyperinsulinemic Obesity and Carbohydrate Addiction: The Missing Link Is the Carbohydrate Frequency Factor." *Medical Hypotheses* 42:307–312, May 1994.

Hunt, D. *No More Cravings.* (New York: Warner Books, 1987).

Kenton, L., and S. Kenton. *Raw Energy* (London: Century Publishing, 1985).

Mercer, M. E. "Food Cravings, Endogenous Opioid Peptides, and Food Intake: A Review." *Appetite* 29:3225–3252, December 1997.

Monte, T. *World Medicine: The East West Guide to Healing Your Body.* (New York: Jeremy P. Tarcher, 1993), p. 216.

Plesman, J. "The Serotonin Connection." Online at The Hypoglycemic Health Association of Australia: www.hypoglycemia.asn.au/articles/serotonin_connection.html.

Sayegh, R., et al. "The Effect of a Carbohydrate-Rich Beverage on Mood, Appetite, and Cognitive Function in Women with Premenstrual Syndrome." *Obstetrics and Gynecology* 86:520–528, October 1995.

Wallach, J. D., and M. Lan. *Rare Earth's Forbidden Cures* (Bonita, CA: Double Happiness Publishing, 1994).

Depression

Alpert, J. E., and M. Fava. "Nutrition and Depression: The Role of Folate." *Nutrition Reviews* 55:145–149, 1997.

Anada, R. F., et al. "Depression and the Dynamics of Smoking. A National Perspective." *Journal of the American Medical Association* 264:1583–1584, 1990.

Balch P., and J. Balch. *Prescription for Nutritional Healing,* 4th ed. (New York: Avery, 2006).

Bell, J. R., et al. "Brief Communication. Vitamin B_1, B_2, and B_6 Augmentation of Tricyclic Antidepressant Treatment in Geriatric Depression with Cognitive Dysfunction." *Journal of the American College of Nutrition* 11:159–163, 1992.

Bell, J. R., et al. "Symptom and Personality Profiles of Young Adults from College Student Population with Self-Reported Illness from Foods and Chemicals." *Journal of the American College of Nutrition* 12:693–702, 1993.

Birmaher, B., et al. "Cellular Immunity in Depressed, Conduct Disorder, and Normal Adolescents: Role of Adverse Life Events." *Journal of the American Academy of Child and Adolescent Psychiatry* 33:671–678, 1994.

Bottiglieri, T. "Folate, Vitamin B_{12}, and Neuropsychiatric Disorders." *Nutrition Review* 54:382–390, 1996.

Bucco, G. "Fading the Winter Blues." *Herbs for Health* 1:34–37, 1998.

Christensen, L., and S. Somers. "Adequacy of the Dietary Intake of Depressed Individuals." *Journal of the American College of Nutrition* 13:597–600, 1994.

Ellenbogen, M. A., et al. "Mood Response to Acute Tryptophan Depletion in Healthy Volunteers: Sex Differences and Temporal Stability." *Neuropsychopharmacology* 15:465–474, 1996.

Fetrow, C. W., and J. R. Avila. "Efficacy of the Dietary Supplement S-Adenosyl-L-Methionine." *Annals of Pharmacotherapy* 35(11):1414–1425.

Freyre, A. V., and J. C. Flichman. "Spasmophilia Caused by Magnesium Deficit." *Psychosomatics* 11:500–502, 1970.

Frizel, D., et al. "Plasma Magnesium and Calcium in Depression." *British Journal of Psychiatry* 115:1375–1377, 1969.

Hibben, J. R., and N. Salem. "Dietary Polyunsaturated Fatty Acids and Depression: When Cholesterol Does Not Satisfy." *Journal of the American College of Nutrition* 62:1–9, 1995.

Irwin, M., et al. "Depression and Reduced Natural Killer Cytoxicity: A Longitudinal Study of Depressed Patients and Control Subjects." *Psychological Medicine* 22:1045–1050, 1992.

Maes, M. "A Review of the Acute Phase Response in Major Depression." *Reviews in the Neurosciences* 4:407–416, 1993.

Murray, M. T., and J. Pizzorno. *Encyclopedia of Natural Medicine,* 2nd ed. (Rocklin, CA: Prima Publishing, 1998).

Pancheri, P., et al. "A Double-Blind, Randomized Parallel-Group, Efficacy and Safety Study of Intramuscular S-adenosyl-L-methionine 1,4-Butanedisulphonate (SAMe) versus Imipramine in Patients with Major Depressive Disorder. *International Journal of Neuropsychopharmacology* (4) 2002 Dec;5:287–294.

Van Straten, M. *Healing Foods.* (New York: Barnes & Noble, 1997).

Werbach, M. R. *Nutritional Influences on Illness.* (New Canaan, CT: Keats, 1990).

Wong, Cathy. "SAMe." www.altmedicine.about.com.

Young, S. N. "Use of Tryptophan in Combination with Other Antidepressant Treatments: A Review." *Journal of Psychiatry and Neuroscience* 16:241–246, 1991.

Diabetes Mellitus

Alschuler, L. "Botanical Medicine I, II, III, IV" (lectures). Seattle: Bastyr University, 1998.

Bantle, J. P., et al. (2006). "Nutrition Recommendations and Interventions for Diabetes—2006: A Position Statement of the American Diabetes Association." *Diabetes Care* 29 (9): 2140–2157, 2006. http://care.diabetesjournals.org/cgi/content/full/29/9/2140.

Borkman, M., et al. "The Relation Between Insulin Sensitivity and the Fatty-Acid Composition of Skeletal-Muscle Phospholipids." *New England Journal of Medicine* 328:238, 1993. In: Rudin D., and C. Felix, *Omega 3 Oils* (Garden City Park, NY: Avery Publishing Group, 1996), pp. 63–64.

Chandalia, M., et al. "Beneficial Effects of High Dietary Fiber Intake in Patients with Type 2 Diabetes Mellitus, *New England Journal of Medicine* 342:1392–1398, 2000.

Cunningham, J. J. "Micronutrients as Nutriceutical Interventions in Diabetes Mellitus." *Journal of the American College of Nutrition* 17:7–10, 1998.

"Diabetes." MedlinePlus. NIH. National Institute of Diabetes and Digestive and Kidney Diseases. www.nlm.nih.gov/medlineplus/diabetes.html.

Gaby, A. "Therapeutic Nutrition I, II" (lectures). Seattle: Bastyr University, 1998.

Geil, P. B., and J. W. Anderson. "Nutrition and Health Implications of Dry Beans: Review." *Journal of the American College of Nutrition* 13:549–558, 1994.

Grogg, J. L., Gropper, S. S., Hunt, S. M. *Advanced Nutrition and Human Metabolism,* 2nd ed. (New York: West Publishing Co., 1995).

Haas, E. M. *Staying Healthy with Nutrition.* (Berkeley, CA: Celestial Arts, 1992).

He, K. et al. "Magnesium Intake and the Metabolic Syndrome: Epidemiologic Evidence to Date." *Journal of the CardioMetabolic Syndrome* 1(5):356–357, Fall 2006.

Heinerman, J. *Heinerman's Encyclopedia of Healing Juices.* (Englewood Cliffs, NJ: Prentice Hall, 1994).

Jovanovic-Peterson, L. and C. M. Peterson. "Review of Gestational Diabetes Mellitus and Low-Calorie Diet and Physical Exercise as Therapy." *Diabetes/Metabolism Reviews* 12: 287–308, 1996.

———. "Vitamin and Mineral Deficiencies Which May Predispose to Glucose Intolerance of Pregnancy." *Journal of the American College of Nutrition* 15:14–20, 1996.

Kenton, L. and S. Kenton. *Raw Energy.* (London: Century Publishing, 1985).

Kirschmann, G. J., and J. D. Kirschmann. *Nutrition Almanac,* 4th ed. (New York: McGraw-Hill, 1996).

Mann, J. I. "The Role of Nutritional Modifications in the Prevention of Macrovascular Complications of Diabetes." *Diabetes* 46(2):S125–S130, 1997.

McCarron, D. A., et al. "Nutritional Management of Cardiovascular Risk Factors: A Randomized Clinical Trial." *Archives of Internal Medicine* 157:169–177, 1997.

Mertz, W. "A Balanced Approach to Nutrition for Health: The Need for Biologically Essential Minerals and Vitamins" (see comments). *Journal of the American Dietetic Association* 94:1259–1262, 1994.

Moffat, D., "What to Juice and Why: Vegetable Juices." HOME:Health-and-Fitness/Nutrition. www.ezinearticles.com/?What-to-Juice-and-Why:-Vegetable-Juices&id=417420.

Mooradian, A. D., et al. "Selected Vitamins and Minerals in Diabetes." *Diabetes Care* 17:464–479, 1994.

"Natural Remedies to Treat Diabetes and Related Conditions." Earth Clinic. www.earthclinic.com/CURES/diabetes.html

"Nutrition Recommendations and Principles for People with Diabetes Mellitus." *Journal of the American Dietetic Association* 504–506, 1994.

Rayssiguier, Y., et al. "High Fructose Consumption Combined with Low Dietary Magnesium Intake May Increase the Incidence of the Metabolic Syndrome by Inducing Inflammation." *Magnesium Research* 19(4):237–243, December 2006.

Rosedale, R. "Diabetes Is Not a Disease of Blood Sugar!" Mereola.com. http://www.mercola.com/article/diabetes/index.htm.

Toeller, M. "Diet and Diabetes." *Diabetes/Metabolism Reviews* 9:93–108, 1993.

Wong, K. "Natural Treatments for Type 2 Diabetes," About.com, Alternative Medicine. http://altmedicine.about.com/cs/conditionsatod/a/Diabetes.htm.

Diverticulosis and Diverticulitis

Aldoori, W. H., et al. "A Prospective Study of Dietary Fiber Types and Symptomatic Diverticular Disease in Men." *Journal of Nutrition* 128:714–719, 1998.

Balch, P., and J. Balch. *Prescription for Nutritional Healing,* 4th ed. (New York: Avery, 2006).

Burton, B. T. *Human Nutrition.* (New York: McGraw-Hill, 1988).

Dean, R., et al. "Preventing Diverticulosis." *Canadian Nurse* 86:35–36, September 1990.

Diverticulitis Diet: www.mayoclinic.com/health/diverticulitis-diet.

Malbey, R. *The New Age Herbalist.* (New York: McMillan, 1988).

O'Keefe, S. "Nutrition and Gastrointestinal Disease." *Scandinavian Journal of Gastroenterology Supplement* 220:52–58, 1996.

Pitchford, P. *Healing with Whole Foods: Oriental Traditions and Modern Nutrition*. (Berkeley, CA: North Atlantic Books, 1993).

Silverman, H. M. "Therapeutic Fiber: Its Role in Disease Treatment and Prevention." *The Journal of Practical Nursing* 40:18–26, June 1990.

Tursi, A. "Acute Diverticulitis of the Colon—Current Medical Therapeutic Management." *Expert Opinion on Pharmacotherapy* 5(1): 55–59, 2004.

Weiss, R. F. *Herbal Medicine* (Beaconsfield, UK: Beaconsfield Publishers, 1988).

Eczema (Atopic Dermatitis)

Anderson, J. A. "Milk, Eggs and Peanuts: Food Allergies in Children." *American Family Physician* 56(5):1365–1374, October 1997.

Bindslev-Jensen, C., et al. "Atopic Dermatitis." *Ugeeskr-Laeger* 159(42):6199–6204, October 1997.

Borrek, S., et al. "Gamma-Linolenic Acid-Rich Borage Seed Oil Capsules in Children with Atopic Dermatitis. A Placebo-Controlled Double-Blind Study." *Klinisch Padiatrie* 209(3):100–104, May 1997.

Businco, L., et al. "Breast Milk from Mothers of Children with Newly Developed Atopic Eczema Has Low Levels of Long Chain Polyunsaturated Fatty Acids." *Journal of Allergy and Clinical Immunology* 91(6):1134–1139, June 1993.

Cotterill, J. A. "Psychophysiological Aspects of Eczema." *Seminars in Dermatology* 3:216–219, 9 September 1990.

Di-Gioacchino, M., et al. "Allergic Contact Dermatitis to Nickel: Modification of Receptor Expression on Peripheral Lymphocytes of Woman After Oral Provocation Tests." *Giornale Italiano di Medicina del Lavoro ed Ergonomia* 19(1):56–58, January-March 1997.

Dotterud, L. K. "Role of Food in Atopic Eczema," *Tidsskrift Norske Laegeforening* 116(28):3335–3340, November 1996.

Eberlein-Konig, B., et al. "Change of Skin Roughness Due to Lowering Air Humidity in Climate Chamber." *Acta Dermatologica Venerologica* 76(6):447–449, November 1996.

Flyvholm, M. A., et al. "Nickel Content of Food and Estimation of Dietary Intake." *Zitschrift fur Lebensum Unters Forsch* 179(6):427–431, December 1984.

Gmoshinski, I. V., et al. "Disordered Permeability of the Gastrointestinal Tract Barrier for Macromolecules and the Possibilities for Its Experimental Dietetic Correction." *Fiziolohichnyi Zhurnal I. M. Sechenova* 79(6):115–127, June 1993.

Hosynek, J. J. "Gold: An Allergen of Growing Significance." *Food and Chemical Toxicology* 35(8):839–844, August 1997.

Leung, D. Y. "Atopic Dermatitis: Immunobiology and Treatment with Immune Modulators." *Clinical and Experimental Immunology* 7(1):25–30, January 10, 1997.

Majamaa, H., et al. "Intestinal Inflammation in Children with Atopic Eczema; Faecal Eosinophil Cationic Protein and Tumor Necrosis Factor-Alpha as Non-Invasive Indicators of Food Allergy." *Clinical and Experimental Allergy* 26(2):181–187, February 1996.

———. "Probiotics: A Novel Approach in the Management of Food Allergy," *Journal of Allergy and Clinical Immunology* 99(2):179–185, February 1997.

"Metabolic Pathways of Essential Fatty Acids." *Protocol Journal of Botanical Medicine* 1(1):18–19, Summer 1995.

Morse, P. F. et al. "Meta Analysis of Placebo Controlled Studies of the Efficacy of Epogam in the Treatment of Atopic Eczema. Relationship Between Plasma Essential Fatty Acid Changes and Clinical Response." *British Journal of Dermatology* 121(1):75–90, July 1989.

Murray, M., *Understanding Fats and Oils: Your Guide to Healing with Essential Fatty Acids*. (Encinitas, CA: Progressive Health Publishing, 1996).

Murray, M. T., and J. Pizzorno. *The Encyclopedia of Natural Medicine*, 2nd ed. (Rocklin, CA: Prima Publishing, 1998).

Ockenfels, H. M., et al. "Contact Allergy in Patients with Periorbital Eczema: An Analysis of Allergens. Data Recorded by the Information Network of the Department of Dermatology," *Dermatology* 195(2):119–124, 1997.

Ring, J., et al. "Atopic Eczema, Langerhans Cells and Allergy." *International Archives of Allergy and Applied Immunology* 94(1–4): 194–201, 1991.

Skin problems. www.greenpeople.co.uk/info_features_skinproblems.

Wollenberg, A., et al. "Immunomorphological and Ultrastructural Characterization of Langerhans Cells and a Novel, Inflammatory Dendritic Epidermal Cell (IDEC) Population in Lesional Skin of Atopic Eczema." *Journal of Investigative Dermatology* 106(3):446–453, March 1996.

Wong, C. "Natural Treatments for Eczema." www.altmedicine.about.com.

Wright, S., and T. A. Sanders. "Adipose Tissue Essential Fatty Acid Composition in Patients with Atopic Eczema." *European Journal of Clinical Nutrition* 45(10):501–505, October 1991.

Zajic, L. J. "Raw Food Diet Study: An Investigation of Over 500 People Who Have Eaten a Raw Food Diet for Over 2 Years." www.iowasource.com.

Epilepsy and Seizures

Barnett, L. "Magnesium, the Nutrient That Could Change Your Life." www.mgwater.com/rod07.shtml.

Burhanoglin, M. "Hypozincemia in Febrile Convulsions." *European Journal of Pediatrics* 155:498–501, 1996.

Bykowski, M. "Unhealthy Liquids May Promote Obesity." *Family Practice News* 61, March 1, 1997.

"Dietary Therapies." Epilepsy.com. http://www.epilepsy.com/epilepsy/dietary_therapies.

"Epilepsy." Life Extension. Updated: 04/25/2006. http://search.lef.org/cgi-src-bin/MsmGo.exe?grab_id=0&page_id=592&query=seizures&hiword=SEIZURE%20seizures%20

"Glutamate Aspartate Restricted Diet (GARD)." Coping with Epilepsy. http://www.coping-with-epilepsy.com/index.php?p=glutamate-aspartate-gard

Gobbi, G., et al. "Celiac Disease, Epilepsy and Cerebral Calcifications." *Lancet* 340: 439–442, August 22, 1992.

Hardin, P. "FDA Pivotal Safety Study: Aspartame Caused Brain Seizures." www.mercola.com/article/aspartame/fda_safety_study.htm.

Kiviranta, T., and E. M. Airaksinen. "Low Sodium Levels in Serum Are Associated with Subsequent Febrile Seizures." *Acta Pediatrics* 84:1372–1374, 1995.

Krahn, L. E. "Use of Caffeine in Medically Refractory Seizure Patients." *Neuropsychiatry, Neuropsychology and Behavioral Neurology* 7(2):136, 1994.

Maltz, G. "Ketogenic Diet Can Control Seizures in Epileptic Children." *Family Practice News* 23, December 15, 1994.

"The MCT Diet." Epilepsy.com. www.epilepsy.com/epilepsy/keto_news_august07.

Mercola, J. "Low-Grain Diet Great for Seizures." Mercola.com. www.mercola.com/2003/dec/27/seizure_diet.htm.

Murray, M. *The Encyclopedia of Nutritional Supplements.* (Rocklin, CA: Prima Publishing, 1996).

Nakagawa, E., et al. "Efficacy of Pyridoxal Phosphate in Treating an Adult with Intractable Status Epilepticus." *Neurology* 48:1468–1469, May 1997.

National Institute of Neurological Disorders and Stroke. "Seizures and Epilepsy: Hope Through Research." www.ninds.nih.gov/disorders/epilepsy/detail_epilepsy.htm#107313109.

Newell, G. W., et al. "Effect of Administering Agenized Amino Acids and Wheat Gluten to Dogs." *American Journal of Physiology* 152 (3):637–644, 1948.

"Non-Drug Therapies." Epilepsy.com. www.epilepsy.com/epilepsy/alternative_therapies.

Pfeifer, H. H. "The Low Glycemic Index Treatment and the Ketogenic Diet." Epilepsy.com. www.epilepsy.com/epilepsy/keto_news_may07.

Prasad, A. N., et al. "Alternative Epilepsy Therapies: The Ketogenic Diet, Immunoglobulins, and Steroids." *Epilepsia* 37 (Suppl. 1):S81–S95, 1996.

Ramaekers, V., et al. "Selenium Deficiency Triggering Intractable Seizures." *Neurological Pediatrics* 25:216–223, 1994.

Spinella, M. "Herbal Medicines and Epilepsy: The Potential for Benefit and Adverse Effects." *Epilepsy & Behavior* 2(6):524–532, 2001.

Stoddard, M. N. Conversations between Mary Nash Stoddard of the Aspartame Consumer Safety Network and Mark D. Gold, 1995. www.health-report.co.uk/aspartame-toxic-effects.htm#misdiagnosed.

Torbi, D., et al. "Free Radical Generation in the Brain Precedes Hyperbaric Oxygen-Induced Convulsions." *Free Radical Biology in Medicine* 13:101–106, 1992.

"Vitamin/Mineral Supplementation." Coping with Epilepsy. www.coping-with-epilepsy.com/index.php?p=vitamins-minerals.

"What Is Epilepsy?" Epilepsy Foundation. www.epilepsyfoundation.org/about/faq/index.cfm.

Eye Disorders

Ahirot-Westerlund, B., and A. Norrby. "Cataracts, Vitamin E and Selenomethionine." *Acta Ophthalmologica Scandinavica* 237–238, April 1988.

Awasthi, S., et al. "Curcumin Protects Against 4-Hydroxy-2-Trans-Nonenal-Induced Cataract Formation in Rat Lenses." *American Journal of Clinical Nutrition* 64:761–766, 1996.

Bunce, G. E. "Nutrition and Eye Diseases of the Elderly." *Journal of Nutritional Biochemistry* 5:66–76, February 1994.

Daniels, S. "Omega-3 Eyed for Retina Protection," 6/25/2007, www.mediomega.com.

Harding, J. "Cigarettes and Cataract: Cadmium or a Lack of Vitamin C?" *British Journal of Ophthalmology* 70:199–201, 1995.

Karakucuk, S., et al. "Selenium Concentrations in Serum, Lens, and Aqueous Humor of Patients with Senile Cataracts." *Acta Ophthalmologica Scandinavica* 73:323–332, 1995.

Mares-Perlman, J., et al. "Diet and Nuclear Lens Opacities." *American Journal of Epidemiology* 141(4):322–334, 1995.

Potter, A. R. "Reducing Vitamin A Deficiency: Could Save the Eyesight and Lives of Countless Children." *British Medical Journal* 314:317–318, 1 February 1997.

Schalch, W. "Carotenoids in the Retina—A Review of Their Possible Role in Preventing or Limiting Damage Caused by Light and Oxygen." In: *Free Radicals and Aging*. (Basel, Switzerland: Birkhauser Verlag, 1992), pp. 280–298.

Tavani, A., et al. "Food and Nutrient Intake and Risk of Cataract." *Annals of Epidemiology* 6:41–46, 1996.

Taylor, A. "Effects of Nutrition on Cataract and Macular Degeneration" (Beyond Nutrition: New Views on the Function and Health Effects of Vitamins)." *New York Academy of Sciences*, 10:9–12 February 1992.

Taylor, A., et al. "Relations Among Aging, Antioxidant Status, and Cataract." *American Journal of Clinical Nutrition* 62(Suppl.):1439S–1447S, 1995.

White, A. C., et al. "Glutathione Deficiency in Human Disease." *Journal of Nutritional Biochemistry* 5:218–226, May 1994.

Fibrocystic Breast Disease

Berkow, R. (ed.). *The Merck Manual,* 16th ed. (Rahway, NJ: Merck Research Laboratories, 1992).

Boyd, N. F., et al. "Effect of a Low Fat, High Carbohydrate Diet on Symptoms of Cyclical Mastopathy." *Lancet* 2(8603):128–132, 1988.

DeCherney, A. H., and M. I. Pernoll. (eds.). *Current Obstetrics and Gynecology Diagnosis and Treatment* (East Norwalk, CT: Appleton and Lange, 1994), pp. 1118–1119.

Estes, N. C. "Mastodynia Due to Fibrocystic Disease of the Breast Controlled with Thyroid Hormone." *American Journal of Surgery* 142(6):764–766, 1981.

Fibrocystic breast disease. *LE Magazine*, January, 1996. www.lef.org.

Haas, E. M. *Staying Healthy with Nutrition: The Complete Guide to Diet and Nutritional Medicine* (Berkeley, CA: Celestial Arts Publishing, 1992), pp. 67–69, 94–98, 101–102.

Hoffmann, D. *The New Holistic Herbal* (Rockport, MA: Element, 1990), p. 61.

Hoffmann, D. *Therapeutic Herbalism: A Correspondence Course in Phytotherapy.*

Hudson, T. *Gynaecology and Naturopathic Medicine*, 3rd ed. (TR Publications, 1994), ch. 7.

Lark, S. M. *The Woman's Health Companion* (Berkeley, CA: Celestial Arts Publishing, 1995), pp. 113–117, 191.

London, R. S., et al. "The Effect of Alpha-Tocopherol on Premenstrual Symptomatology: A Double-Blind Study." *Journal of the American College of Nutrition* 2(2):115–122, 1983.

Martinez, I., et al. "Thyroid Hormones in Fibrocystic Breast Disease." *European Journal of Endocrinology* 132(6):673–676, 1995.

Meyer, E. C., et al. "Vitamin E and Benign Breast Disease." *Surgery* 107(5):549–551, 1990.

Murray, M. T. *The Complete Book of Juicing.* (Rocklin, CA: Prima Publishing, 1992), pp. 71–72, 123–124, 136, 142–143, 149, 192, 215.

———. *The Healing Power of Herbs,* rev. 2nd ed. (Rocklin, CA: Prima Publishing, 1995), pp. 173–183.

Nagata, C., et al. "Decreased Serum Estradiol Concentration Associated with High Dietary Intake of Soy Products in Premenopausal Japanese Women." *Nutrition and Cancer* 29(3):228–233, 1997.

Ody, P. *The Complete Medicinal Herbal* (London: Dorling Kindersley, 1993), p. 85.

Pizzorno, J. E., and M. T. Murray. *The Textbook of Natural Medicine.* (Seattle: Bastyr University Publications, 1993).

Rhoades, R., and R. Pflanzer. *Human Physiology,* 3rd ed. (Philadelphia: Saunders College Publishing, 1996), p. 385.

Rothman, K. J., et al. "Teratogenicity of High Vitamin A Intake." *New England Journal of Medicine* 333:1369–1373, 1995.

Russell, L. C. "Caffeine Restriction as Initial Treatment for Breast Pain." *Nurse Practitioner* 14(2):36–37, 40, 1989.

Sandaram, G. S., et al. "Serum Hormones and Lipoproteins in Benign Breast Disease." *Cancer Research* 14(9 Pt2):3814–3816, 1981.

Smith, E. Fibrocystic Breast Disease: www.fibrocystic.com.

Stansbury, J. Botanical Therapies for Fibrocystic Breast Disease. *Medical Herbalism* July 31, 1997 9(2): 1, 11–13. www.medherb.com/Therapeutics/Female_-_Botanical_Therapies_for_Fibrocystic_Breast_Disease.

Stoll, B. A. "Macronutrient Supplements May Reduce Breast Cancer Risk: How, When, and Which." *European Journal of Clinical Nutrition* 51(9):573–577, 1997.

Werbach, M. *Healing with Food* (New York: HarperCollins, 1993), pp. 41–45.

Werbach, M., and M. T. Murray. *Botanical Influences on Illness: A Sourcebook of Clinical Research* (Tarzana, CA: Third Line Press, 1994), p. 33.

Zych, F., et al. "Fibrocystic Disease of the Breast and Pituitary-Thyroid Axis Function," *Polski Merkuriusz Lekarski* 1(4):227–228, 1996.

Fibromyalgia Syndrome

Donaldson, M. S., et al. "Fibromyalgia Syndrome Improved Using a Mostly Raw Vegetarian Diet; An Observational Study." *BMC Complementary Alternative Medicine* 1:7, September 2001.

Eisinger, J., et al. "Studies of Transketolase in Chronic Pain." *Journal of Advancement in Medicine* 5(2):105–113, Summer 1992.

Kaartinen, K., et al. "Vegan Diet Alleviates Fibromyalgia Symptoms." *Scandinavian Journal of Rheumatology* 2000;29(5):308–313.

Malic Acid and Fibromyalgia. *Nutritional News,* December 1, 1995. www.immunesupport.com.

Murray, M. *Encyclopedia of Nutritional Supplements* (Rocklin, CA: Prima Publishing, 1996).

Nicolson, G. L. "Relationship to Fibromyalgia Syndrome, Chronic Fatigue Syndrome/M.E. and the Possible Role of Vaccines." www.shirleys-wellness-cafe.com/fibro.htm.

Romano, T., and J. W. Stiller. "Magnesium Deficiency and Fibromyalgia Syndrome." *The Journal of Nutritional Medicine* 4:165–167, 1994.

Russell I. J., et al. "Treatment of Fibromyalgia Syndrome with Super Malic: A Randomized, Double-blind, Placebo-controlled, Crossover Pilot Study." *Journal of Rheumatology,* 22(5):953–958, May 1995.

St. Amand, R. P. "Exploring the Fibromyalgia Connection." *The Vulvar Pain Newsletter* 1, 4–6, Fall 1996.

Wong, C. "Herbs and Supplements for Fibromyalgia." January 30, 2007. www.about.com.

Gallstones and Liver–Gallbladder Congestion

"Does Vitamin C Cause Gallstones?" www.vitamincfoundation.org.

Gustafsson, U., et al. "The Effect of Vitamin C in High Doses on Plasma and Biliary Lipid Composition in Patients with Cholesterol Gallstones: Prolongation of the Nucleation Time." *European Journal of Clinical Investigation* 27:387–391, 1997.

Heaton, K. W., et al. "An Explanation for Gallstones in Normal-Weight Women: Slow Intestinal Transit." *Lancet* 341:8–10, January 2, 1993.

Klawansky, S., and T. C. Chalmers. "Fat Content of Very Low Calorie Diets and Gallstone Formation," *Journal of the American Medical Association* 268(7):873, August 19, 1992.

Lieber, C. S. "Alcoholic Liver Disease: New Insights in Pathogenesis Lead to New Treatments." *Journal of Hepatology.* 32 (1 Suppl):113–128, 2000.

Mercola, J. "Gallbladder Flushes and Cleanses." Mercola.com. www.mercola.com/2002/feb/13/gall_bladder.htm

Moritz, A. "The Amazing Liver and Gallbladder Flush." Ener-chi.com. May 6, 2007.

Ortega, R., et al. "Differences in Diet and Food Habits Between Patients with Gallstones and Controls." *Journal of the American College of Nutrition* 16(1):88–95, 1997.

Simon, J. A. "Ascorbic Acid and Cholesterol Gallstones." *Medical Hypotheses* 40:81–84, 1993.

Simon, J. A., and E. S. Hudes. "Serum Ascorbic Acid and Gallbladder Disease Prevalence Among U.S. Adults." *Archives of Internal Medicine* 160:931–936, 2000.

Simon J. A., et al. "Ascorbic Acid Supplement Use and the Prevalence of Gallbladder Disease." *Journal of Clinical Epidemiology* 51:257–265, 1998.

Tandon, R. K., et al. "Dietary Habits of Gallstone Patients in Northern India: A Case Control Study," *Journal of Clinical Gastroenterology* 22(1):23–27, 1996.

Gout

Balch, P., and J. Balch. *Prescription for Nutritional Healing,* 4th ed. (New York: Avery, 2006).

Blau, L. W. "Cherry Diet Control for Gout and Arthritis." *Texas Report on Biology and Medicine* 8:309–312, 1950.

Choi, H. K., et al. "Purine-Rich Foods, Dairy and Protein Intake, and the Risk of Gout in Men." *New England Journal of Medicine* (350):1093–1103, March 11, 2004.

Emmerson, B. T. "Effect of Oral Fructose on Urate Production." *Annals of the Rheumatic Diseases* 33:276, 1974.

Escott-Stump, S. *Nutrition and Diagnosis-Related Care.* (Philadelphia: W. B. Saunders, 1988).

Gout. University of Maryland Medical Center. www.umm.edu/altmed/articles/gout-000070.htm.

Gout. www.niams.nih.gov/health_info/Gout/gout_ff.asp.

Krause, M., and L. Mahan. *Food, Nutrition and Diet Therapy* (Philadelphia: W. B. Saunders, 1984).

Shils, M., and V. Young. *Modern Nutrition in Health and Disease* (Philadelphia: Lea & Feibiger, 1988).

Stein, H. B., et al. "Ascorbic Acid-induced Uricosuria: A Consequence of Megavitamin Therapy." *Annals of Internal Medicine* 84:385–388, 1976.

Herpes

Balch, P., and J. Balch. *Prescription for Nutritional Healing,* 4th ed. (New York: Avery, 2006).

Chandra, R. K. "Nutrition and Immunity—Basic Considerations. Part I." *Contemporary Nutrition* 11:11, 1986.

Dietary management of Genital Herpes. www.best-herpes-treatments.com.

Griffith, R., et al. "Relations of Arginine-Lysine Antagonism to Herpes Simplex Growth in Tissue Culture." *Chemotherapy* 27:209–213, 1981.

Murray, M. *Encyclopedia of Nutritional Supplements* (Rocklin, CA: Prima Publishing, 1996).

Picozzi, M. "Alternative Treatments for Herpes Offer Real Relief." www.healingdeva.com/herpes.htm.

Rhodes, J. "Human Interferon Action: Reciprocal Regulation by Retinoic Acid and Beta-Carotene." *Journal of the National Cancer Institute* 70:833–837, 1983.

Terezhalmy, G. T., et al. "The Use of Water Soluble Bioflavonoid-Ascorbic Acid Complex in the Treatment of Recurrent Herpes Labialis. Oral Surgery. Oral Medicine." *Oral Pathology* 45:56–62, 1978.

Tsai, Y., et al. "Antiviral Properties of Garlic: In Vitro Effects of Influenza B, Herpes Simplex and Coxsackie Viruses," *Planta Medica* (5):460–461, 1985.

High Blood Pressure (Hypertension)

Abe Y, Umemura S, Sugimoto K, et al. "Effect of Green Tea Rich in Gamma-Aminobutyric Acid on Blood Pressure of Dahl Salt-Sensitive Rats," *American Journal of Hypertension* 8:74–79, 1995. In: Mitscher L, Dolby V. *The Green Tea Book* (Garden City Park, NY: Avery Publishing Group, 1998).

Appel, L. J., et al. "A Clinical Trial of the Effects of Dietary Patterns on Blood Pressure." *New England Journal of Medicine* 36:1117–1124, 17 April 1997.

Aviram, M., and L. Dornfeld. "Pomegranate Juice Consumption Inhibits Serum Angiotensin Converting Enzyme Activity and Reduces Systolic Blood Pressure. *Atherosclerosis*. (1):195–198, September, 2001, on www.lef.org/protocols/heart_circulatory/high_blood_pressure_refs.htm.

Borok, G. "Nutritional Aspects of Hypertension." *South African Medical Journal* 76:125–126, 5 August 1989.

"Diets Rich in Omega-3 Fatty Acids May Lower Blood Pressure." American Heart Association, 06/06/2007. www.americanheart.org/presenter.jhtml?identifier=3048211.

Douglass, J. M., et. al. "Effects of a Raw Food Diet on Hypertension and Obesity." *Southern Medical Journal* 78(7):841–844, July 1985.

Duffy, S. J., et al. "Treatment of Hypertension with Ascorbic Acid." *Lancet* 354(9195):2048–2049, December 11, 1999, on www.lef.org/protocols/heart_circulatory/high_blood_pressure_refs.htm.

Gordon, L. "Exercise and Salt Restriction May be Enough for Mildly High BP." *Medical Tribune 8*, 21 December 1995.

Henry, J. P., and P. Stephens-Larson. "Reduction of Chronic Psychosocial Hypertension in Mice by Decaffeinated Tea," *Hypertension* 6(3):437–444, 1984. In: Mitscher, L., and V. Dolby. *The Green Tea Book* (Garden City Park, NY: Avery Publishing Group, 1998).

High blood pressure. "The Green Pharmacy Herbal Handbook." www.mothernature.com/Library/Bookshelf/Books/41/65.cfm.

Ignarro, L. J., et al. "Pomegranate Juice Protects Nitric Oxide Against Oxidative Destruction and Enhances the Biological Actions of Nitric Oxide." *Nitric Oxide* 2006 Apr 18. www.lef.org/protocols/heart_circulatory/high_blood_pressure_refs.htm.

Lardinois, C. K. "Nutritional Factors and Hypertension," *Archives of Family Medicine* 4:707–713, August 1995.

"Magnesium Lowers Blood Pressure," *Nutrition Week* 7, 24 May 1996.

National Institutes of Health. The DASH Eating Plan. www.nhlbi.nih.gov/health/public/heart/hbp/dash.

Osborne, C. G., et al. "Evidence for the Relationship of Calcium to Blood Pressure." *Nutrition Reviews* 54(12):365–381, December 1996.

Pauletto, P., et al. "Blood Pressure, Serum Lipids, and Fatty Acids in Populations on a Lake-Fish Diet or a Vegetarian Diet in Tanzania." *Lipids* 31:S309–S312, 1996 (Suppl.).

Rosanoff, A. "Magnesium and Hypertension." *Clinical Calcium*. 15(2):255–260, February 2005.

Solzback, U., et al. "Vitamin C Improves Endothelial Dysfunction of Epicardial Coronary Arteries in Hypertensive Patients." *Circulation* 96(5):1513–1519, 2 September 1997.

Stensvold, I., et al. "Tea Consumption. Relationship to Cholesterol, Blood Pressure, and Coronary and Total Mortality," *Preventive Medicine* 21:546–553, 1992. In: Mitscher, L., and V. Dolby. *The Green Tea Book* (Garden City Park, NY: Avery Publishing Group, 1998).

Superka, H. R., et al. "Effects of Cessation of Caffeinated-Coffee Consumption on Ambulatory and Resting Blood Pressure in Men." *American Journal of Cardiology* 73: 780–784, 15 April 1994.

Tattelman, E. "Health Effects of Garlic." *American Family Physician*. 72(1):103–106, July 1, 2005, on www.lef.org/protocols/heart_circulatory/high_blood_pressure_refs.htm.

Touyz, R. M., et al. "The 2004 Canadian Recommendations for the Management of Hypertension: Part III: Lifestyle Modifications to Prevent and Control Hypertension." *Canadian Journal of Cardiology*. 20(1):55–59, January 2004, on www.lef.org/protocols/heart_circulatory/high_blood_pressure_refs.htm.

"What Is High Blood Pressure?" National Heart, Lung, and Blood Institute. www.nhlbi.nih.gov/health/dci/Diseases/Hbp/HBP_WhatIs.html.

Hypoglycemia

Alchemical Medicine Research and Teaching Association. "Condition: Hypoglycemia. Body System: Endocrine System." IBIS: Integrative BodyMind Information System, Version 1.2, 1994. Gaia Multimedia, Inc.

Anderson, R. A. "Nutritional Factors Influencing the Glucose/Insulin System: Chromium." *Journal of the American College of Nutrition* 16(5):404–410, October 1997.

Haas, E. M. *Staying Healthy with Nutrition* (Berkeley, CA: Celestial Arts, 1992).

Hoffmann, D. *The Herbal Handbook: A User's Guide to Medical Herbalism.* (Rochester, NY: Healing Arts Press, 1988).

Hypoglycemia: http://www.faqs.org/health/Sick-V2/Hypoglycemia.html.

"Hypoglycemia." MayoClinic.com. www.mayoclinic.com/print/hypoglycemia/DS00198/DSECTION=all&METHOD=print.

Mercola, J. "Caffeine Plus Sugar Can Fool the Brain." Mercola.com. http://www.mercola.com/1997/archive/caffeine_and_sugar.htm.

———. "Lower Your Grains and Lower Your Insulin Levels! A Novel Way to Treat Hypoglycemia." Mercola.com. http://www.mercola.com/article/carbohydrates/lower_your_grains.htm.

Pitchford, P. *Healing with Whole Foods: Oriental Traditions and Modern Nutrition.* (Berkeley, CA: North Atlantic Books, 1993).

Pizzorno, J. E., and M. T. Murray. *The Textbook of Natural Medicine.* (Seattle: Bastyr University Publications, 1992), 1–7.

Rieske, K. "Scientific Proof Carbohydrates Cause Disease." http://www.mercola.com/display/PrintPage.aspx?docid=30114&PrintPage=yes.

Rutherford, W. J. "Hypoglycemia and Endurance Exercise: Dietary Considerations." *Nutrition and Health* 6(4):173–181, 1990.

Werbach, M. R. *Nutritional Influences on Illness.* (New Canaan, CT: Keats Publishing, 1987).

Indigestion

Al-Yahya, M. A., et al. "Gastroprotective Activity of Ginger Zingiber Officinale Rosc. in Albino Rats." *American Journal of Chinese Medicine* 17(1–2):51–56, 1989.

Aroroa, A., and M. P. Sharma. "Use of Banana in Non-ulcer Dyspepsia." *Lancet* 355, March 1990.

Colbin, A. *Food and Healing.* (New York: Ballantine Books, 1986).

Elta, G. H., et al. "Comparison of Coffee Intake and Coffee-Induced Symptoms in Patients with Duodenal Ulcer, Nonulcer Dyspepsia, and Normal Controls." *American Journal of Gastroenterology* 85(10):1339–1342, 1990.

Gaia Multimedia, Inc. Interactive BodyMind Information System. http://www.teleport.com/~ibis/ (1994).

Haas, E. M. *Staying Healthy with Nutrition.* (Berkeley, CA: Celestial Arts, 1992).

Hoffmann, D. *The Herbal Handbook: A User's Guide to Medical Herbalism* (Rochester, NY: Healing Arts Press, 1988).

Mahan, K. L., and S. Escott-Stump. *Krause's Food, Nutrition, and Diet Therapy,* 9th ed. (Philadelphia: W. B. Saunders, 1996).

Matthews, G. "Gut Fermentation." *Journal of the Royal Society of Medicine* 85:304–305, May 1992.

Mullan, A., et al. "Food and Nutrient Intakes and Eating Patterns in Functional and Organic Dyspepsia." *European Journal of Clinical Nutrition* 48(2):97–105, February 1994.

Murray, M. T., and J. Pizzorno. *Encyclopedia of Natural Medicine,* 2nd ed. (Rocklin, CA: Prima Publishing, 1998).

Pitchford, P. *Healing with Whole Foods: Oriental Traditions and Modern Nutrition.* (Berkeley, CA: North Atlantic Books, 1993).

Pizzorno, J., and M. Murray. *The Textbook of Natural Medicine.* (Seattle: Bastyr University Publications, 1992).

Warden, R. A., et al. "Vitamin A Deficiency Exacerbates Methotrexate-Induced Jejunal Injury in Rats." *Journal of Nutrition* 127(5):770–776, May 1997.

Inflammation

Alschuler, L. "Botanical Medicine I, II, III, IV" (lectures). Seattle: Bastyr University, 1998.

Bistrian, B. R., et al. "Cytokines, Muscle Proteolysis, and the Catabolic Response to Infection and Inflammation." *Proceedings of the Society for Experimental Biology and Medicine* 200:220–223, 1992.

Denko, C. W., et al. "Inflammation in Relation to Dietary Intake of Zinc and Copper." *International Journal of Tissue Reactions* 3:73–76, 1981.

Fleck, A. "Clinical and Nutritional Aspects of Changes in Acute-Phase Proteins During Inflammation." *Proceedings of the Nutrition Society* 48:347–354, 1989.

Gaby, A. "Therapeutic Nutrition I, II" (lectures). Seattle: Bastyr University, 1998.

Grimble, R. "Inflammation, Cytokines and Nutrition." *European Journal of Clinical Nutrition* 45:413–417, 1991.

Grimble, R. F. "Nutritional Antioxidants and the Modulation of Inflammation: Theory and Practice." *New Horizons* 2:175–185, 1994.

Grogg, J. L., et al. *Advanced Nutrition and Human Metabolism*, 2nd ed. (New York: West Publishing Co., 1995).

Haas, E. M. *Staying Healthy with Nutrition* (Berkeley, CA: Celestial Arts, 1992).

Hyman, M. "How Does Inflammation Affect Your Weight?" coaches.aol.com/wellness/feature/_a/how-does-inflammation-affect-your-weight/20060620170209990001.

Kirschmann, G. J., and J. D. Kirschmann. *Nutrition Almanac*, 4th ed. (New York: McGraw-Hill, 1996).

Mandel, D. "Safe Solutions for Inflammation." www.bellaonline.com.

Milanino, R., and G. P. Velo. "Multiple Actions of Copper in Control of Inflammation: Studies in Copper-Deficient Rats." *Agents Actions Supplement* 8:209–230, 1981.

Roubenoff, R., et al. "Abnormal Vitamin B_6 Status in Rheumatoid Cachexia. Association with Spontaneous Tumor Necrosis Factor Alpha Production and Markers of Inflammation." *Arthritis and Rheumatism* 38:105–109, 1995.

Tate, G., et al. "Suppression of Acute and Chronic Inflammation by Dietary Gamma Linolenic Acid." *Journal of Rheumatology* 16:729–734, 1989.

Terano, T., et al. "Eicosapentaenoic Acid as a Modulator of Inflammation. Effect on Prostaglandin and Leukotriene Synthesis." *Biochemical Pharmacology* 35:779–785, 1986.

Wan, J. M., et al. "Nutrition, Immune Function, and Inflammation: An Overview." *Proceedings of the Nutrition Society* 48: 315–335, 1989.

Influenza

Chandra, R. K., and L. D. McBean. "Zinc and Immunity." *Nutrition* 10(1), 1994.

Halpern, G. M., and C. I. Trapp. "Nutrition and Immunity: Where Are We Standing?" *Allergy and Immunopathology* 21(3):122–126, 1993.

Klenner, F. R. "The Treatment of Poliomyelitis and Other Virus Diseases with Vitamin C." *Southern Medical Journal* 111:210–214, 1949.

Mercola, J. "Flu vaccines." Mercola.com. www.search.mercola.com/Results.aspx?q=Flu%20vaccines.

Nakayama, M., et al. "Inhibition of the Infectivity of Influenza Virus by Black Tea Extract." *Kansenshogaku Zasshi—Journal of the Japanese Association for Infectious Diseases* 68(7): 824–829, 1994. In: Mitscher, L., and V. Dolby. *The Green Tea Book* (Garden City Park, New York: Avery Publishing Group, 1998).

Nakayama, M., et al. "Inhibition of the Infectivity of Influenza Virus by Tea Polyphenols." *Antiviral Research* 21:289–299, 1993.

Pauling, L. *Vitamin C, the Common Cold and the Flu* (San Francisco: W. H. Freeman & Company, 1976) [review].

Scaglione, F., et al. "Efficacy and Safety of the Standardized Ginseng Extract G 115 for Potentiating Vaccination Against Common Cold and/or Influenza Syndrome." *Drugs in Experimental and Clinical Research* 22(2):65–72, 1996.

Shrauzer, G. N. "Selenium and the Immune Response." *The Nutrition Report* 10(3):17, 24, March 1992.

Sunkind, R. "Immunologic Mechanisms and the Role of Nutrition." In: *Principles and Practice of Environmental Medicine* (New York: Plenum Medical Book Company, 1992), pp. 159–172.

Tsai, Y., et al. "Antiviral Properties of Garlic: In Vitro Effects of Influenza B, Herpes Simplex and Coxsackie Viruses." *Planta Medica* (5):460–461, 1985.

Insomnia and Jet Lag

Berry, E. M., and M. Levy. "Foods and Their Effects on Sleep Patterns." *International Clinical Nutrition Review* 7:76–78, April 1987.

Brown, D. J. "Valerian Root: Non-Addictive Alternative for Insomnia and Anxiety." *Quarterly Review of Natural Medicine* 221–224, Fall 1994.

The Burton Goldberg Group (J. Strohecker, exec. ed.). *Alternative Medicine: The Definitive Guide.* (Puyallup, WA: Future Medicine Publishing, 1994), pp. 838–847.

Calbom, C., and J. Calbom. *Sleep Away the Pounds* (New York: Warner, 2006).

Comperatore, C. A., et al. "Melatonin Efficacy in Aviation Missions Requiring Rapid Deployment and Night Operations." *Aviation, Space, and Environmental Medicine* 67(6):520–524, June 1996.

Foster, S. "A Good Night's Sleep." Supplement to *Herb Companion* 73–74, June/July 1995.

"Halcion vs. Valerian in the Treatment of Insomnia." *American Journal of Natural Medicine* 2:7–9, May 1995.

Insomnia. www.nhlbi.nih.gov/health/dci/Diseases/inso/inso_whatis.html.

Murray, M. T. *Encyclopedia of Nutritional Supplements.* (Rocklin, CA: Prima Publishing, 1996).

Phillips, F., et al. "Isocaloric Diet Changes and Electroencephalographic Sleep." *Lancet* 723–725, October 18, 1975.

Pitchford, P. *Healing with Whole Foods: Oriental Traditions and Modern Nutrition* (Berkeley, CA: North Atlantic Books, 1993).

Porter, J. M., and J. A. Home. "Bed-Time Food Supplements and Sleep: Effects of Different Carbohydrate Levels." *Electroencephalography and Clinical Neurophysiology* 51:426–433, 1981.

Menopause

Bolton, J. L., et al. "Role of Quinoids in Estrogen Carcinogenesis." *Chemical Research Toxicology* 11(10):1113–1127, 1998.

Genant, H. K., et al. "Low-dose Esterified Estrogen Therapy: Effects on Bone, Plasma Estradiol Concentrations, Endometrium, and Lipid Levels." *Archives of Internal Medicine* 157(22), 1997.

Gleason S. "Menopause: It's Not a Disease: Natural Approaches to a Change of Life." *Good Medicine* 8–10, Spring 1994.

Hunt, C. D., et al. "Metabolic Responses of Postmenopausal Women to Supplemental Dietary Boron and Aluminum During Usual and Low Magnesium Intake: Boron, Calcium, and Magnesium Absorption and Retention and Blood Mineral Concentrations." *American Journal of Clinical Nutrition* 65:803–813, 1997.

Menopause. The Canadian Women's Health Network. www.cwhn.ca/resources/faq/menopause.html.

Mercola, J. "Soy Supplements Fail to Help Menopause Symptoms." Mercola.com.www.mercola.com/1999/archive/soy_fails_to_help_menopause.htm.

Murray, M. T. "Essential Fatty Acid Supplementation." In: Murray, M. T. *Encyclopedia of Nutritional Supplements.* (Rocklin, CA: Prima Publishing, 1996).

Muti, P., et al. "Estrogen Metabolism and Risk of Breast Cancer: A Prospective Study of the 2:16 Alpha-hydroxyestrone Ratio in Premenopausal and Postmenopausal Women." *Epidemiology* 11(6):635–640, 2000.

Shoman, M. "Soy's Thyroid Dangers." www.thyroid.about.com/cs/soyinfo/a/soy.htm.

Torgerson, D. J., et al. "Alcohol Consumption May Influence Onset of the Menopause." *British Medical Journal* 315–318, July 19, 1997.

Wahlqvist, M. L. "Phytoestrogens: Emerging Multifaceted Plant Compounds." *Medical Journal of Australia* 167:119–120, August 4, 1997.

Menstrual Disorders

Bagga, D., et al. "Effects of a Very Low Fat, High Fiber Diet on Serum Hormones and Menstrual Function: Implications for Breast Cancer Prevention." *Cancer* 76(3):2491–2496, December 15, 1995.

Campbell, E. M., et al. "Premenstrual Symptoms in General Practice Patients: Prevalence and Treatment." *Journal of Reproductive Medicine* 42(10):637–646, October 1997.

Chan, W. Y., and J. C. Hill. "Determination of Menstrual Prostaglandin Levels in Non-Dysmenorrheic Subjects." *Prostaglandins* 15(2):365–375, February 1978.

Deutch, B. "Menstrual Pain in Danish Women Correlated with Low Omega-3 Polyunsaturated Fatty Acid Intake." *European Journal of Clinical Nutrition* 49(7):508–516, July 1995.

Downing, I., et al. "Uptake of [3H]-Arachidonic Acid by Human Endometrium: Differences Between Normal and Menorrhagic Tissue." *Prostaglandins* 26:55–69, 1983.

Ermans, S. J. "Menarche and Beyond: Do Eating and Exercise Make a Difference?" *Pediatric Annals* 26(2 Supplement):S137–S141, February 1997.

Fowler, G. C., et al. "Menstrual Irregularities: A Focused Evaluation." *Patient Care* 155–164, 15 April 1994.

Gladstar, R. *Herbal Healing for Women.* (New York: Fireside, 1993).

Hoffmann, D. *The New Holistic Herbal.* (Rockport, MA: Element, 1990).

Kjerulff, K. H., et al. "Chronic Gynecological Conditions Reported by U.S. Women: Findings from the National Health Interview Survey, 1984 to 1992." *American Journal of Public Health* 86(2):195–199, February 1996.

Lark, S. "What Are Menstrual Cramps?" www.healthy.net/scr/Article.asp?Id=1374&xcntr=3.

Lewis, S. J., et al. "Lower Serum Oestrogen Concentrations Associated with Faster Intestinal Transit." *British Journal of Cancer* 76(3):395–400, 1997.

Murray, M. T. *The Complete Book of Juicing.* (Rocklin, CA: Prima Publishing, 1992), p. 462.

Murray, M. T., and J. Pizzorno. *The Encyclopedia of Natural Medicine,* 2nd ed. (Rocklin, CA: Prima Publishing, 1998).

"Nutrients to Ease Monthly Distress." www.mothernature.com/Library/Bookshelf/Books/10/84.cfm.

Penland, J. G., and P. E. Johnson. "Dietary Calcium and Manganese Effects on Menstrual Cycle Symptoms." *American Journal of Obstetrics and Gynecology* 168(5):1417–1423, May 1993.

Taussig, S., and R. Batkin. "Bromelain: The Enzyme Complex of Pineapple (*Ananas comosus*) and Its Clinical Application: An Update." *Journal of Ethnopharmacology* 22:191–203, 1988. Cited in Murray, M. T., *The Complete Book of Juicing,* pp. 40–41.

Migraine Headaches

Alchemical Medicine Research and Teaching Association. "Condition: Headache, Vascular. Body System: Nervous System." IBIS: Integrative BodyMind Information System, Version 1.2, 1994. Gaia Multimedia, Inc.

Bic, Z., et al. "In Search of the Ideal Treatment for Migraine Headache." *Medical Hypotheses* 50:1–7, 1998.

Colbin, A. *Food and Healing.* (New York: Ballantine Books, 1986), pp. 264–266.

Diener, H. C., et al. "Efficacy and Safety of 6.25 Mg t.i.d. Feverfew CO_2-extract (MIG-99) in Migraine Prevention—A Randomized, Double-blind, Multicentre, Placebo-controlled Study." *Cephalalgia* 25(11):1031–1041, November 2005.

Federation of American Societies for Experimental Biology [FASEB]. "Analysis of Adverse Reactions to Monosodium Glutamate (MSG)" (Bethesda, MD: Life Sciences Research Office, FASEB, 1995).

Haas, E. M. *Staying Healthy with Nutrition.* (Berkeley, CA: Celestial Arts, 1992).

Hanington, E. "Diet and Migraine." *Journal of Human Nutrition* 34:175–180, 1980.

Hoffmann, D. *The New Holistic Herbal,* 3rd ed. (Rockport, MA: Element Books, 1992).

Holzhammer, J. and C. Wober. "[Alimentary Trigger Factors That Provoke Migraine and Tension-Type Headache]" [in German]. *Schmerz* 20 (2): 151–159, 2006.

Hughes, E. C., et al. "Migraine: A Diagnostic Test for Etiology of Food Sensitivity by a Nutritionally Supported Fast and Confirmed by Long-Term Report." *Annals of Allergy* 55(1):28–32, July 1985.

Johnson, B. S., et al. "Efficacy of Feverfew: A Prophylactic Treatment of Migraine." *British Medical Journal* 291:569–574, August 1985.

Lauritzen, M. "Pathophysiology of the Migraine Aura. The Spreading Depression Theory." *Brain* 117 (1): 199–210, 1994.

Low Tyramine Headache Diet. National Headache Foundation, October 2004. Retrieved on 2006-10-12.

Mansfield, I. E., et al. "Food Allergy and Adult Migraine: Double-Blind and Mediator Confirmation of an Allergic Etiology." *Annals of Allergy* 55(2):126–129, August 1985.

Marcus, D. A., et al. "A Double-Blind Provocative Study of Chocolate as a Trigger of Headache." *Cephalalgia* 17(8):855–862, December 1997.

Mauskop, A., et al. "Deficiency in Serum Ionized Magnesium but Not Total Magnesium in Patients with Migraines. Possible Role of Ica2+/IMg2+ Ratio." *Headaches* 33(3):135–138, March 1993.

———. "Intravenous Magnesium Sulfate Rapidly Alleviates Headaches of Various Types." *Headache* 36(3):154–160, March 1996.

McCaren, T., et al. "Amelioration of Severe Migraine by Fish Oil." *American Journal of Clinical Nutrition* 41(4):874, April 1985.

Mercola, J. "Many Migraine Sufferers Undertreated—What Can You Do for Migraines?" www .mercola.com/2001/sep/29/migraine_treatment.htm.

Murray, M. T., and J. Pizzorno. *Encyclopedia of Natural Medicine,* 2nd ed. (Rocklin, CA: Prima Publishing, 1998).

Peatfield, R. C. "Relationship Between Food, Wine, and Beer—Precipitated Migrainous Headaches." *Headache* June 35(6):355–357, 1995.

Peikert, A., et al. "Prophylaxis of Migraine with Oral Magnesium: Results from a Prospective, Multi-center, Placebo-controlled and Double-blind Randomized Study." *Cephalalgia* 16 (4): 257–263, 1996.

Pitchford P. *Healing with Whole Foods: Oriental Traditions and Modern Nutrition.* (Berkeley, CA: North Atlantic Books, 1993).

Rozen, T. D., et al. "Open Label Trial of Coenzyme Q10 as a Migraine Preventive." *Cephalalgia* 22(2):137–141, March 2002.

Sándor, P. S., et al. "Efficacy of Coenzyme Q10 in Migraine Prophylaxis: A Randomized Controlled trial." *Neurology* 64: 713–715, 2005.

Schwerzmann, M., et al. "Percutaneous Closure of Patent Foramen Ovale Reduces the Frequency of Migraine Attacks." *Neurology* 62 (8): 1399–1401, 2004.

Werbach, M. R. *Nutritional Influences on Illness.* (New Canaan, CT: Keats Publishing, 1987).

Multiple Sclerosis

Agranoff, B., and D. Goldberg. "Diet and the Geographical Distribution of Multiple Sclerosis." *Lancet* 2:1061, 1974.

Alter, M. "Multiple Sclerosis and Nutrition." *Archives of Neurology* 31:262–272, 1974.

Alternative Medicine and Health.com. "Multiple Sclerosis." http://alternative-medicine-and-health.com/conditions/msclerosis.htm.

Bates, D., et al. "Polyunsaturated Fatty Acids in Treatment of Acute Remitting Multiple Sclerosis." *British Medical Journal* 2:1390–1391, 1978.

Elian, M., and G. Dean. "Multiple Sclerosis Among the United Kingdom–Born Children of Immigrants from the West Indies." *Journal of Neurological Neurosurgery and Psychiatry* 50:327–332, 1987.

Farinotti, M., et al. "Dietary Interventions for Multiple Sclerosis." Cochrane Database of Systematic Reviews (online) (1): CD004192, 2007.

Hayes, C. E., et al. "Vitamin D and Multiple Sclerosis." *Proceedings of the Society of Experimental Biology and Medicine* 216(1):21–27, 1997.

Hutter, C. D., and P. Laing. "Multiple Sclerosis: Sunlight, Diet, Immunology and Aetiology." *Medical Hypotheses* 46(2):67–74, 1996.

Islam, T., et al. "Childhood Sun Exposure Influences Risk of Multiple Sclerosis in Monozygotic Twins." *Neurology* 69:381–388, 2007.

Kruzel, T. "Multiple Sclerosis and Alternative Medicine." American Association of Naturopathic Physicians. www.healthy.net/scr/Article.asp?Id=729&xcntr=2.

Lauer, K. "Environmental Associations with the Risk of Multiple Sclerosis: The Contribution of Ecological Studies." *Acta Neurological Scandinavica Supplement* 161: 77–88, 1995.

----. "The Risk of Multiple Sclerosis in the USA in Relation to Sociographic Features: A Factor-Analytic Study." *Journal of Clinical Epidemiology* 47(1):43–48, 1994.

Manley, P. "Diet in Multiple Sclerosis." *Practitioner* 238(1538):358–363, 1994.

Mercola, J. "Curry Spice May Fight Multiple Sclerosis." Reported in: *Annual Experimental Biology* 2002 Conference New Orleans, April 23, 2002. http://www.mercola.com/2002/may/11/curry.htm.

Messina, V. K., and K. I. Burke. "Position of the ADA: Vegetarian Diets." *Journal of the American Dietetic Association* 97(11): 1317–1321, 1997.

Miller, J., et al. "Double-blind Trial of Linoleate Supplementation of the Diet in Multiple Sclerosis." *British Medical Journal* 765–768, 1973.

Munger, K. L., et al. "Serum 25-hydroxyvitamin D Levels and Risk of Multiple Sclerosis." *Journal of the American Medical Association* 296 (23): 2832–2838, 2006.

National Multiple Sclerosis Society. http://www.nationalmssociety.org.

Rosner, L. J., and S. Ross. *Multiple Sclerosis: New Hope and Practical Advice for People with MS and Their Families,* updated ed. (New York: Fireside, 1992).

Sahelian, R. "Natural Treatment for Multiple Sclerosis (MS)." http://www.raysahelian.com/multiplesclerosis.html.

Stout, T. R. "Multiple Sclerosis: The Blood–Brain Barrier, and New Treatment." web.archive.org/web/20040620134245/www.el-dorado.ca.us/~tstout/articles/multiple-sclerosis.shtml.

Swank, R. L. "Multiple Sclerosis: A Fat-Oil Relationship." *Nutrition* 7(5):368–376, 1991.

----. "Effect of Low Saturated Fat Diet in Early and Late Cases of Multiple Sclerosis." *Lancet* 336(8706): 37–39, 1990.

Swank, R. L., and B. B. Dugan. *The Multiple Sclerosis Diet Book.* (Garden City, NY: Doubleday, 1987).

Swank, R. L., and A. Grimsgaard. "Multiple Sclerosis: The Lipid Relationship." *American Journal of Clinical Nutrition* 48:1387, 1988.

Van der Mei, I. A., et al. "Past Exposure to Sun, Skin Phenotype, and Risk of Multiple Sclerosis: Case-control Study." *BMJ* 327 (7410): 316, 2003.

Weil, A. *Eight Weeks to Optimum Health.* (New York: Alfred A. Knopf, 1997), pp. 47–52, 84. This book contains a very inspiring story of a woman's recovery from MS disability on pp. 146–148.

Osteoarthritis

Altman, R. D., and K. C. Marcussen. *Arthritis and Rheumatism* 44(11):2531–2538, November 2001.

Arabelovic, S., and T. E. McAlindon. *Current Rheumatology Reports* 7(1):29–35, March 2005.

Arthritis Foundation. "The Facts About Arthritis." www.arthritis.org/resources/gettingstarted/default.asp.

----. "Common Therapies to Consider." www.arthritis.org/common-therapies-to-consider.php.

Bobacz, K., et al. *Arthritis and Rheumatism* 48(9) 2501, September 2003.

Brien, S., et al. "Bromelain as a Treatment for Osteoarthritis: A Review of Clinical Studies." *Evidence-Based Complementary and Alternative Medicine.* eCAM. 1 (3): 251–257, 2004.

Christensen, R. *Osteoarthritis Cartilage.* 13(1):20–27, January 2005.

De Filippis, L., et al. *Reumatismo* 56(3):169–184, July–September 2004.

Felson, D. T. "Weight and Osteoarthritis." *American Journal of Clinical Nutrition* 63 (Suppl):430S–432S, 1996.

Flynn, M., et al. "The Effect of Folate and Cobalamin on Osteoarthritic Hands." *Journal of the American College of Nutrition* 13(4):351–356, 1994.

McAlindon, T. E., et al. "Do Antioxidant Micronutrients Protect Against the Development and Progression of Knee Osteoarthritis?" *Arthritis and Rheumatism* 39:648–656, 1996.

Maltz G. "Get to the Joint: Exercise Benefits Osteoarthritis Patients." *Family Practice News* 20, February 15, 1995.

Murray, M. T., and J. Pizzorno. *Encyclopedia of Natural Medicine,* 2nd ed. (Rocklin, CA: Prima Publishing, 1998).

"Osteoarthritis." Wikipedia. http://en.wikipedia.org/wiki/Osteoarthritis#_note-o

"Osteoarthritis: Complementary and Alternative Medicine." MayoClinic.com. http://www.mayoclinic.com/health/osteoarthritis/DS00019/DSECTION=11.

Pizzorno, J. E. "Natural Medicine Approach to Treating Osteoarthritis." *Alternative and Complementary Therapies* 93–95, January/February 1995.

Poolsup, N., et al. "Glucosamine Long-term Treatment and the Progression of Knee Osteoarthritis: Systematic Review of Randomized Controlled Trials." *Annals of Pharmacotherapy* 39 (6): 1080–1087, 2005.

Srivastava, K. C., and T. Mustafa. "Ginger (*Zingiber officinale*) in Rheumatism and Muscoloskeletal Disorders," *Medical Hypotheses* 39:342–348, 1992.

"Study Links Low Selenium Levels with Higher Risk of Osteoarthritis." UNC news release. Retrieved June 22, 2007.

Vasishta, V. G., et al. Rotational Field Magnetic Resonance (RFQMR) in Treatment of Osteoarthritis of the Knee Joint, *Indian Journal of Aerospace Medicine*, 48 (2), 1–7, 2004.

"Vitamin D Deficits Affect Osteoarthritis." *Nutrition Report* 14(7):54, September–October 1996.

Wilhelmi, G. "Fasting Followed by Vegetarian Diet in Patients with Rheumatoid Arthritis." *Rheumatology* 52(3):174–179, May–June 1993.

Wong, C. "SAMe." www.altmedicine.about.com

Osteoporosis

Abelow, B. J., et al. "Cross-cultural Association Between Dietary Animal Protein and Hip Fracture: A Hypothesis." *Calcified Tissue International* 50 (1): 14–18, 1992.

American Academy of Pediatrics Committee on School Health. "Soft Drinks in Schools." *Pediatrics* 113 (1 Pt 1): 152–154, 2004.

Bellantoni, M. F. "Osteoporosis Prevention and Treatment." *American Family Practice* 54(3):986–992, September 1, 1996.

Bischoff-Ferrari, H. A., et al. "Estimation of Optimal Serum Concentrations of 25-hydroxyvitamin D for Multiple Health Outcomes." *American Journal of Clinical Nutrition* 84 (1): 18–28, 2006.

Bischoff-Ferrari, H. A., et al. "Fracture Prevention with Vitamin D Supplementation: A Meta-analysis of Randomized Controlled Trials." *JAMA* 293 (18): 2257–2264, 2005.

Bonaiuti, D., et al. "Exercise for Preventing and Treating Osteoporosis in Postmenopausal Women." Cochrane Database of Systematic Reviews (online) (3): CD000333, 2002.

Broe, K. E., et al. "A Higher Dose of Vitamin D Reduces the Risk of Falls in Nursing Home Residents: a Randomized, Multiple-dose Study." *Journal of the American Geriatrics Society* 55 (2): 234–239, 2007.

"Cadmium Exposure and Risk of Breast Cancer: Is There a Relationship?" *Science Daily*, July 14, 2003.

Feskanich, D., et al. "Protein Consumption and Bone Fractures in Women." *American Journal of Epidemiology* 143 (5): 472–479, 1996.

Gaby, A. R. *Preventing and Reversing Osteoporosis* (New York: Prima Lifestyles, 1994).

"A Gluten-Free Diet Improves Osteoporosis in Celiac Patients," *Archives of Internal Medicine* 165(4): 393–399, February 28, 2005. Reported online at Mercola.com. http://www.mercola.com/2005/mar/19/osteoporosis_wheat.htm

Harvard Health Publications. "Osteoporosis: Eight Tips for 2008." January 2008 issue of *Harvard Women's Health Watch*. http://www.health.harvard.edu Reported in: *Medical News Today*. January 4, 2008. http://www.medicalnewstoday.com/articles/92898.php.

Hasling, C., et al. "Calcium Metabolism in Postmenopausal Osteoporotic Women Is Determined by Dietary Calcium and Coffee Intake." *Journal of Nutrition* 112: 1119–1126, 1992.

Holick, M. F. "Resurrection of Vitamin D Deficiency and Rickets." *Journal of Clinical Investigation* 116 (8): 2062–2072, 2006.

Hollenback, K. A., et al. "Cigarette Smoking and Bone Mineral Density in Older Men and Women." *American Journal of Public Health* 83(9):1265–1270, September 1993.

Kessler, G. J., *The Bone Density Diet* (New York: Ballantine, 2000).

Kidd, P. M. "An Integrative Lifestyle: Nutritional Survey for Lowering Osteoporosis Risk," *Townsend Letter for Doctors*, 400–405, May 1992.

Mercola, J. "Women Have Higher Risk of Dying from Osteoporosis Than Breast Cancer." http://www.mercola.com/2002/dec/4/osteoporosis.htm. Reported in: *Canadian Medical Journal* November 12, 2002, p. 167.

Murray, M. T., and J. Pizzorno. *Encyclopedia of Natural Medicine*, 2nd ed. (Rocklin, CA: Prima Publishing, 1998).

National Osteoporosis Foundation. http://www.nof.org.

"Osteoporosis." Wikipedia. http://en.wikipedia.org/wiki/Osteoporosis#_note-6.

"Osteoporosis: Not Just a Woman's Disease." *Journal of Nuclear Medicine* 37 (10):N17, 1996.

Prince, R. L., et al. "Effects of Calcium Supplementation on Clinical Fracture and Bone Structure: Results of a 5-year, Double-blind, Placebo-controlled Trial in Elderly Women." *Archives of Internal Medicine* 166 (8): 869–875, 2006.

Riggs, B. L., and L. J. Melton. "The Prevention and Treatment of Osteoporosis." *New England Journal of Medicine* 327(9):620–627, August 27, 1992.

Staessen, J., et al. "Environmental Exposure to Cadmium, Forearm Bone Density, and Risk of Fractures: Prospective Population Study. Public Health and Environmental Exposure to Cadmium (PheeCad) Study Group." *Lancet* 353 (9159): 1140–1144, April 3, 1999.

Swezey, R. L. "Exercise for Osteoporosis—Is Walking Enough?" *Spine* 21:2809–2813, 1996.

Szule, P., and P. D. Delams. "Is There a Role for Vitamin K Deficiency in Osteoporosis?" *Challenge of Modern Medicine* 24(4):303–307, 1995.

Tang, B. M. P., et al. "Use of Calcium or Calcium in Combination with Vitamin D Supplementation to Prevent Fractures and Bone Loss in People Aged 50 Years and Older: A Meta-analysis." *Lancet* 370: 657–666, 2007.

Tucker, K. L., et al. "Colas, But not Other Carbonated Beverages, Are Associated with Low Bone Mineral Density in Older Women: The Framingham Osteoporosis Study." *American Journal of Clinical Nutrition* 84 (4): 936–942, 2006.

Vikhanski, L. "Magnesium May Slow Bone Loss." *Medical Tribune* 1, July 23, 1993.

Parasitic Infections

The Burton Goldberg Group (J. Strohecker, exec. ed.). *Alternative Medicine: The Definitive Guide.* (Puyallup, WA: Future Medicine Publishing, 1994).

Galland, L., and M. Leem. "*Giardia lamblia* Infection as a Cause of Chronic Fatigue." *Journal of Nutritional Medicine* 1:27, 1990.

Gittleman, A. L. *Natural Healing for Parasites* (New York: Healing WisdomPublications, 1995).

Hemell, O., et al. "Killing of *Giardia lamblia* by Human Milk Lipases: An Effect Mediated by Lipolysis of Milk Lipids. *Journal of Infectious Diseases* 153:715, 1986.

Murray, M. T., and J. Pizzorno. *Encyclopedia of Natural Medicine*, 2nd ed. (Rocklin, CA: Prima Publishing, 1998).

Murray, M. *Encyclopedia of Nutritional Supplements.* (Rocklin, CA: Prima Publishing, 1996), pp. 404–405.

Nesheim, M. C. "Human Nutrition Needs and Parasite Infection." *Parasitology* 107:S7–S18, 1993.

Parasitic Infection: Symptoms and Treatment. www.kitchendoctor.com/healthconditions/parasites/parasites.html.

"Results of Testing for Intestinal Parasites by State Diagnostic Laboratories, United States, 1987." *Morbidity and Mortality Weekly Report* 40(SS–4);25–30, 1992.

Prostate Enlargement, Benign (BPH)

Buck, A. C. "Phytotherapy for the Prostate." *British Journal of Urology* 78:325–336, 1996.

Bush, L. M., et al. "Zinc and the Prostate." Presented at the Annual Meeting of the American Medical Association, 1974.

Durak, I., et al. "Tomato Juice Inhibits Adenosine Deaminase Activity in Human Prostate Tissue from Patient with Prostate Cancer." *Nutrition Research* 23 (9): 1183–1188, September 2003.

Gerber, P. C. "Alternative Medicine: "All Eyes on NIH's Office of Alternative Medicine." *Physician Management* 30–42, March 1994.

Murray, M. "Prostate Enlargement." www.doctormurray.com/conditions/Prostate_Enlargement.asp.

Murray, M. T., and J. Pizzorno. *Encyclopedia of Natural Medicine,* 2nd ed. (Rocklin, CA: Prima Publishing, 1998).

Prostate cancer. ADAM Healthcare Center. www.adam.about.com/reports/000033_2.htm.

Walker, N. *Raw Vegetable Juices.* (Phoenix: Norwalk Press Publishers, 1947).

Psoriasis

Murray, F. "Nutrient Therapy Relieves Skin Ailments; B-complex Vitamins, Omega-3 Fish Oils, Vitamin C and Zinc Help Alleviate Psoriasis and Eczema." *Better Nutrition* April, 1990. www.findarticles.com/p/articles/mi_m0860/is_n4_v52/ai_8830505/pg_2.

Murray, M. T. *The Healing Power of Foods.* (Rocklin, CA: Prima Publishing, 1993).

———. *The Healing Power of Herbs.* (Rocklin, CA: Prima Publishing, 1992).

Murray, M. T., and J. Pizzorno. *The Encyclopedia of Natural Medicine,* 2nd ed. (Rocklin, CA: Prima Publishing, 1998).

Naldi, F. "Dietary Factors and the Risk of Psoriasis: Results of an Italian Case-Controlled Study." *British Journal of Dermatology* 134:101–106, January 1996.

Rackett, S. C. "Diet and Dermatology." *Journal of the American Academy of Dermatology* 29:447–459, September 1993.

Swain, R., et al. "Vitamins as Therapy in the 1990s." *Journal of the American Board of Family Practice* 8:206, May/June 1995.

Respiratory Disorders

Alchemical Medicine Research and Teaching Association. "Condition: Bronchitis, Pneumonia, Sinusitis. Body System: Respiratory System." IBIS: Integrative BodyMind Information System, Version 1.2, 1994. Gaia Multimedia, Inc.

The Burton Goldberg Group (J. Strohecker, exec. ed.). *Alternative Medicine: The Definitive Guide* (Puyallup, WA: Future Medicine Publishing, 1994), pp. 81, 816, 820–823.

DeSole, G., et al. "Vitamin A Deficiency in Southern Ethiopia," *American Journal of Clinical Nutrition* 45(4):780–784, April 1987.

Haas, E. M. *Staying Healthy with Nutrition.* (Berkeley, CA: Celestial Arts, 1992).

Hoffmann, D. *The New Holistic Herbal.* (Rockport, MA: Element Books, Inc., 1992).

McCaleb, R. "Boosting Immunity with Herbs." The Herb Research Foundation: Herb Information Greenpaper. http://www.healthy.net.

Pedersen, M. *Nutritional Herbology: A Reference Guide to Herbs* (Warsaw, IN: 1998).

Pitchford, P. *Healing with Whole Foods: Oriental Traditions aud Modern Nutrition.* (Berkeley, CA: North Atlantic Books, 1993).

Pizzorno, J., and M. T. Murray. *The Textbook of Natural Medicine.* (Seattle: Bastyr University Publications, 1992).

Ryan, R. E. "A Double-Blind Clinical Evaluation of Bromelains in the Treatment of Acute Sinusitis." *Headache* 7:13–27, 1967.

Schwartz, J., and S. Weiss. "Dietary Factors and Their Relation to Respiratory Symptoms." *American Journal of Epidemiology* 132(1): 67–76, July 1990.

Tockman, M. S., et al. "Milk Drinking and Possible Reduction of the Respiratory Epithelium," *Journal of Chronic Diseases* 39 (3):207–209, 1986.

West, C.E., et al. "Epithelial Damaging Virus Infections Affect Vitamin A Status in Chickens," *Journal of Nutrition* 122(2): 333–339, February 1992.

Rheumatoid Arthritis and Other Antoimmune Diseases

Blau, L. W. "Cherry Diet Control for Gout and Arthritis." *Texas Report on Biology and Medicine* 8:309–312, 1950.

Darlington, L. G. "Diet Therapy for Arthritis," *Nutrition and Rheumatic Diseases* 17(2):273–285, May 1991.

Darlington, L. G., and N. W. Ramsey. "Clinical Review of Dietary Therapy for Rheumatoid Arthritis." *British Journal of Rheumatology* 32:507–514, 1993.

Hanninen, O., et al. "Vegan Diet in Physiological Health Promotion." *Acta Physiologica Hungarica* 86(3–4):171–180, 1999.

Heliovaara, M., et al. "Coffee Consumption, Rheumatoid Factor, and the Risk of Rheumatoid Arthritis," *Annals of Rheumatic Diseases* 59(8): 631–635, August 2000.

Kjeldsen-Kragh, J., et al. "Controlled Trial of Fasting and One-year Vegetarian Diet in Rheumatoid Arthritis," *Lancet* 338(8772):899–902, October 12, 1991.

Millen, A., and C. W. M. Wilson. "The Metabolism of Ascorbic Acid in Rheumatoid Arthritis." *Proceedings of the Nutrition Society* 35:8A–9A, 1976.

Muller, H., et al. "Fasting Followed by Vegetarian Diet in Patients with Rheumatoid Arthritis: A Systematic Review." *Scandinavian Journal of Rheumatology* 30(1):1–10, 2001.

Nenonen, M. T., et al. "Uncooked, Lactobacilli-rich, Vegan Food and Rheumatoid Arthritis." *British Journal of Rheumatology* 37(3):274–281, March 1998.

Palmblad, J, et al. "Antirheumatic Effects of Fasting." Nutrition and Rheumatic Disease, *Rheumatic Disease Clinics of North America* 17(2):351–362, May 1991.

Prineas, R. J., et al. "Coffee, Tea and VPB." *Journal of Chronic Diseases* 33:67–72, 1980.

Rheumatoid arthritis. www.MedicineNet.com.

Srivastava, K. C., and T. Mustafa. "Ginger (*Zingiber officinale*) in Rheumatism and Musculoskeletal Disorder." *Medical Hypotheses* 39:342–348, 1992.

Volke, D., and M. Garg. "Dietary N-3 Fatty Acid Supplementation in Rheumatoid Arthritis—Mechanisms, Clinical Outcomes, Controversies, and Future Directions." *Journal of Clinical Biochemical Nutrition* 20:83–97, 1996.

Zurie, R. B., et al. "Gamma-Linolenic Acid Treatment of Rheumatoid Arthritis: A Randomized Placebo-Controlled Trial." *Arthritis and Rheumatism* 39:1808–1817, 1996.

Stress

Andrade, F. H., et al. "Effects of Selenium Deficiency on Diaphragmatic Function After Resistive Loading." *Acta Pfrysiologica Scandinavica* 162:141–148, 1998.

Bagchi, D., et al. "Stress, Diet and Alcohol-Induced Oxidative Subsalicylati. *Journal of Applied Toxicology* 18:2–13, 1998.

Balch, P., and J. Balch. *Prescription for Nutritional Healing,* 4th ed. (New York: Avery, 2006).

Barnes, V. et al. "Stress, Stress Reduction and Hypertension in African Americans: An Updated Review." *Journal of the National Medical Association* 89:464–476, 1997.

Carsia, R. V., and P. L. McIlroy. "Dietary Protein Restriction Stress in the Domestic Turkey (*Meleagris gallopavo*) Induces Hypofunction and Remodeling of Adrenal Steroidogenic Tissue." *General and Comparative Endocrinology* 109:140–153, 1998.

Dess, N. K., et al. "The Interaction of Diet and Stress in Rats: High-Energy Food and Sucrose Treatment." *Journal of Experimental Psychology: Animal Behavior Processes* 24:60–71, 1998.

Frame, L. T., et al. "Calorie Restriction as a Mechanism Mediating Resistance to Environmental Disease." *Environmental Health Perspectives* 106(Suppl 1):313–324, 1998.

Groff, J. L., et al. *Advanced Nutrition and Human Metabolism,* 2nd ed. (San Francisco: West, 1995).

Haas, E. M. *Staying Healthy with Nutrition* (Berkeley, CA: Celestial Arts, 1992).

Heath, J. A., and A. M. Duffy. "Body Condition and the Adrenal Stress Response in Captive American Kestrel Juveniles." *Physiological Zoology* 71:67–73, 1998.

Hobbs, C. *Stress & Natural Healing* (Loveland, Co: Interweave Press, 1997).

Konig, D., et al. "Rationale for a Specific Diet from the Viewpoint of Sports Medicine and Sports Orthopedics: Relation to Stress Reaction and Regeneration," *Orthopade* 26:942–950, 1997.

Larsen, C. R., et al. "Effect of Dietary Selenium on the Response of Stressed and Unstressed Chickens to Escherichia coli Challenge and Antigen." *Biological Trace Element Research* 58:169–176, 1997.

Margen, S. (ed.). *University of California at Berkeley: The Wellness Encyclopedia of Food and Nutrition.* (New York: Rebus, 1992).

Murray, M. T., and J. Pizzorno. *Encyclopedia of Natural Medicine,* 2nd ed. (Rocklin, CA: Prima Publishing, 1998), pp. 379–400.

Schneider, R. H., et al. "Lower Lipid Peroxide Levels in Practitioners of the Transcendental Meditation Program." *Psychosomatic Medicine* 60:38–41, 1998.

Seelig, M. S. "Consequences of Magnesium Deficiency on the Enhancement of Stress Reaction. Preventative and Therapeutic Implications—A Review." *Journal of the American College of Nutrition* 13:429–446, 1994.

Skantze, R. B., et al. "Psychosocial Stress Causes Endothelial Injury in Cynmolgus Monkeys VIa Veta 1-Adrenoceptor Activation," *Atherosclerosis* 136:153–161, 1998.

Takahashi, K., et al. "Influences of Dietary Methionine and Cysteine on Metabolic Responses to Immunological Stress by Escherichia coli Lipopolysaccharide Injection and Mitogenic Response in Broiler Chickens." *British Journal of Nutrition* 78:815–821, 1997.

Toates, F. *Stress: Conceptual and Biological Aspects* (New York: John Wiley & Sons, 1995), p. 31.

Van Straten, M. *Healing Foods* (New York: Barnes & Noble, 1997), pp. 52–54.

Watkins, G. G. "Music Therapy: Proposed Physiological Mechanisms and Clinical Implications." *Clinical Nurse Specialist* 11:43–50, 1997.

Werbach, M. R. *Nutritional Influences on Illness.* (New Canaan, CT: Keats, 1990), pp. 155–163.

Yi, I., and F. K. Stephan "The Effects of Food Deprivation, Nutritive and Non-Nutritive Feeding and Wheel Running on Gastric Stress Ulcers in Rats." *Physiology and Behavior* 63:219–225, 1998.

Tuberculosis

Perez-Guzman, C., et al. "A Cholesterol-Rich Diet Accelerates Bacteriologic Sterilization in Pulmonary Tuberculosis." *Chest* 127: 643–651, 2005.

"TB Surges: Diet Link Still Unclear," *Nutrition Week* 17:6–7, May 1, 1992.

Ulcers

Albert-Puleo, M. "Physiological Effects of Cabbage with Reference to Its Potential as a Dietary Cancer-inhibitor and Its Use in Ancient Medicine." *Journal of Ethnopharmacology* 9(2):261–272, December 1983.

Aldori, W. H., et al. "Prospective Study of Diet and the Risk of Duodenal Ulcer in Men." *American Journal of Epidemiology* 145:42–50, 1997.

Balch, P., and J. Balch. *Prescription for Nutritional Healing,* 4th ed. (New York: Avery, 2006).

The Burton Goldberg Group (J. Strohecker, exec. ed.). *Alternative Medicine: The Definitive Guide* (Puyallup, WA: Future Medicine Publishing, 1994).

Cheney, G. et al. "Anti-Peptic Ulcer Dietary Factor (Vitamin "U") in the Treatment of Peptic Ulcers." *Journal of the American Dietetic Association* 25:668–672, 1950.

Heinerman, J. *Encyclopedia of Healing Juices* (Englewood Cliffs, NJ: Prentice Hall, 1994).

Murray, M. T. "Healing Ulcers Naturally: Natural Therapies Are Less Expensive, More Effective, and Much Safer." www.naturodoc.com/library/lifestyle/ulcers.htm.

Murray, M. T., and J. Pizzorno. *Encyclopedia of Natural Medicine,* 2nd ed. (Rocklin, CA: Prima Publishing, 1998).

Rao, N. M. "Protease Inhibitors from Ripened and Unripened Bananas." *Biochemistry International* 24:13–22, 1991.

Rector, P. L. *Healthy Living.* (Carmel Valley, CA: Healthy Living Publications, 1997).

Tovey, F. L. "Diet and Duodenal Ulcer." *Journal of Gastroenterology and Hepatology* 9:177–185, 1994.

"What I Need to Know About Peptic Ulcers." digestive.niddk.nih.gov/ddiseases/pubs/pepticulcers_ez/#1.

Wilson, J. C. "Phytochemicals: Guardians of Our Health," *Journal of the American Dietetic Association* 97:5199–5204, 1997.

Varicose Veins and Hemorrhoids

Balch, P., and J. Balch. *Prescription for Nutritional Healing,* 4th ed. (New York: Avery, 2006).

Bougelet, C., et al. "Effect of Aescine on Hypoxia-induced Neutrophil Adherence to Umbilical Vein Endothelium." *European Journal of Pharmacology* 345:89–95, 1998.

Gabor, M. "The Pharmacologic Effects of Flavonoids on Blood Vessels." *Angologica* 9:355–374, 1972.

Heinerman, J. *Heinerman's Encyclopedia of Healing Juices.* (Englewood Cliffs, NJ: Prentice Hall, 1994).

Kreysel, H. W., et al. "A Possible Role of Lysosomal Enzymes in the Pathogenesis of Varicosis and the Reduction in Their Serum Activity by Venostatin." *Vasa* 12:377–382, 1983.

Murray, M. T., and J. Pizzorno. *Encyclopedia of Natural Medicine,* 2nd ed. (Rocklin, CA: Prima Publishing, 1998).

Newall, C., et al. *Herbal Medicines: A Guide for Health-Care Professionals* (London: Pharmaceutical Press, 1996), p. 166.

Pittler, M. H., and E. Ernst. "Horse Chestnut Seed Extract for Chronic Venous Insufficiency." Cochrane Database of Systematic Reviews: (online) (1):CD003230, January 25, 2006.

Price, L. "Blackberries: Invasive Weed or Nutritional Powerhouse?" August 24, 2006. www.bastyrcenter .org.

Rose, S. "What Causes Varicose Veins?" *Lancet* 1:32, 1986.

Royer, R. J., and C. L. Schmidt. "Evaluation of Venotropic Drugs by Venous Gas Plethysmography. A Study of Procyanidolic Oligomers." *Sem Hop* 57:2009–2013, 1981 [in French].

Sirtori, C. R. "Aescin: Pharmacology, Pharmacokinetics and Therapeutic Profile," *Pharmacological Research* 44:183–193, 2001.

Taussig, S. "The Mechanism of the Physiological Action of Bromelain." *Medical Hypotheses* 6:99–104, 1980.

Water Retention

Alschuler, L. "Botanical Medicine I, II, III, IV" (lectures). Seattle: Bastyr University, 1998.

Bertuglia, S., et al. "Effect of *Vaccinium myrillus* Anthocyanosides on Ischemia Reperfusion Injury in Hamster Cheek Pouch Microcirculation." *Pharmacological Research* 31:183–187, 1995.

Bouskela, E., and K. A. Donyo. "Effects of Oral Administration of Purified Micronized Flavonoid Fraction on Increased Microvascular Permeability Induced by Various Agents and on Ischemia/Reperfusion in Diabetic Hamsters." *International Journal of Microcirculation Clinical Experiments* 15:293–300, 1995.

Bouskela, E., et al. "Oxidant-Induced Increase in Vascular Permeability Is Inhibited by Oral Administration of S-5682 (Daflon 500 mg) and Alpha-tocopherol." *International Journal of Microcirculation Clinical Experiments* 17 Suppl 1:18–20, 1997.

Edelstein, B. *The Woman Doctor's Medical Guide for Women* (New York: William Morrow, 1982).

Ihme, N., et al. "Leg Oedema Protection from a Buckwheat Herb Tea in Patients with Chronic Venous Insufficiency: A Single-Centre, Randomised, Double-Blind, Placebo-Controlled Clinical Trial." *European Journal of Clinical Pharmacology* 50:443–447, 1996.

Kamimur, M. "[Physiology and Clinical Use of Vitamin E," *Hokkaido Igaku Zasshi* 52:185–188, 1977 [in Japanese].

"Liver Foods." Seattle: Bastyr University Nutrition Clinic, 1998.

McGuire, E. A., and V. R. Young. "Nutritional Edema in a Rat Model of Protein Deficiency." *Journal of Nutrition* 116:1209–1224, 1986.

Mian, E., et al. "Anthocyanides and the Walls of Microvessels: Further Aspects of the Mechanism of Action of Their Protective Effect in Syndromes Due to Abnormal Capillary Fragility." *Minerva Medicine* 68: 565–581, 1977.

Qiao, Y., et al. "Effects of Vitamin E on Vascular Integrity in Cholesterol-fed Guinea Pigs." *Atherosclerosis and Thrombosis* 13:1885–1892, 1993.

Rudakova, I. S., and A. M. Chernukh. "Changes in the State of the Microvascular Bed and in the Extent of Transcapillary Exchange by Preparations with P-Vitamin Activity," *Bibliography Anatomy* 10:273–277, 1969.

Weight Loss

"Appetite and High-Fat Food." *Nutrition Week* 27(12):7, March 29, 1997.

"Aspartame and Dieting." *Nutrition Week* 27(23):7, June 13, 1997.

Centers for Disease Control and Prevention (CDC). "Overweight and Obesity." http://www.cdc.gov/nccdphp/dnpa/obesity/index.htm.

———. National Center for Health Statistics (NCHS). "New CDC Study Finds No Increase in Obesity Among Adults; but Levels Still High." November 28, 2007. http://www.cdc.gov/nchs/pressroom/07 newsreleases/obesity.htm.

Grant, K. E., et al. "Chromium and Exercise Training: Effect on Obese Women." *Medicine and Science in Sports and Exercise* 29(8):992–998, 1997.

Jancin, B. "Whole Grain May Reduce Obesity, Hyperinsulinemia." *Family Practice News* 8, May 15, 1998.

"More Than Half of Adults Classified as Overweight." *Nutrition Week* 28(22):2, June 5, 1998.

Murray, M. T., and J. Pizzorno. *Encyclopedia of Natural Medicine*, 2nd ed. (Rocklin, CA: Prima Publishing, 1998).

NHANES (National Health and Nutrition Examination Survey) Data on the Prevalence of Overweight and Obesity Among Adults—United States, 2003–2004. *The Journal of the American Medical Association* (293):5, February 2, 2005.

"Obesity in Children," *Nutrition Week* (16): 7, April 25, 1997.

"Pantothenic Acid and Weight Loss." *The Nutrition Report* 61, September 1995.

Rossner, S., et al. "Weight Reduction with Dietary Fiber Supplements: Results of Two Double-Blind Studies." *Acta Medica Scandinavia* 22:83–88, 1987.

Singh, R. B., et al. "Association of Low Plasma Concentration of Antioxidant Vitamins, Magnesium, and Zinc with High Body Fat Percent Measured by Bioelectrical Impedance Analysis in Indian Men." *Magnesium Research* 11(1):3–10, 1998.

Whitaker, R. C. "Predicting Obesity in Young Adulthood from Childhood and Parental Obesity." *New England Journal of Medicine*, 337(13):869–873, September 25, 1997.

Index

apples/apple juice: cardiovascular disease, 93; colds, 106; constipation, 117; eye disorders, 154; fibromyalgia syndrome, 163; gallstones, 168; influenza, 202; liver and pancreas function, 168; pesticide residues in, 21
apricot juice, 318
arginine-rich foods, 173
arnica, 65
arthritis (osteoarthritis), 227–32
arthritis (rheumatoid arthritis), 12, 67, 94, 255–61
artichoke/artichoke leaf juice, 159, 315
artificial sweeteners. *See* aspartame (NutraSweet); sucralose (Splenda)
asparagus juice, 62, 137, 159, 245, 282, 289
aspartame (NutraSweet): Alzheimer's disease, 35–36; cancer, 73; influenza, 199; migraine headaches, 219; seizures, 147–48; weight loss, 287
aspirin, 129, 228–29, 271
asthma, 49–53
astragalus, 31, 78, 101, 105
atherosclerosis, 86–93
atopic dermatitis, 141–45, 350
attention deficit disorder (ADD/ADHD), 46, 53–59, 349–50
autoimmune disorders: fibromyalgia syndrome, 159–64, 351; inflammatory bowel disease, 107–14; multiple sclerosis, 222–27; psoriasis, 246–49; rheumatoid arthritis, 12, 67, 94, 255–61; vaccinations and, 108, 199
Awesome Green Smoothie, 327

Baggesen, J. Rand, 89–90
bananas, 272
barberry, 83, 242
Barnett, Lewis B., 148, 149
Beautiful-Bone Solution, 328
Beautiful-Skin Cocktail, 328
Beet-Cucumber Cleansing Cocktail, 328–29
beetroot juice/beetroot greens juice: bowel diseases, 113, 114; cancer, 78; chronic fatigue syndrome, 101; colds, 106; eczema, 145; fibrocystic breast disease, 159; gallstones, 168; high blood pressure, 11, 179; hypoglycemia, 185; influenza, 202; for liver cleanse, 318; psoriasis, 249; seizures, 151
Beet Salad with Lemon-Olive Oil Dressing, 316
beginner's seven-day gallbladder cleanse, 320–21
benign prostatic hyperplasia (BPH), 243–46
berry juices, 62, 93. *See also specific types*
beta-carotene. *See* carotenes/beta-carotene/vitamin A
betaine HCl: indigestion, 190–91; iron absorption, 41; parasitic infections, 241; protein digestion, 37, 123; vitamin B$_{12}$ absorption, 37, 41, 52
bilberry, 274
bioflavonoids: allergies, 30; bladder infections, 62; bruises, 64; bursitis and tendinitis, 69; cancer, 76; colds, 104–5; depression, 130; eczema, 143; herpes, 174; inflammation, 196–97; influenza, 200–201; menopausal symptoms, 210; menstrual disorders, 214; prostate enlargement, 244; respiratory disorders, 252–53; rheumatoid arthritis and autoimmune diseases, 259; stress, 266;

tuberculosis, 268–69; ulcers, 273; varicose veins and hemorrhoids, 277; water retention, 282
biotin, 47
Bircher-Benner, Max, 134
birth control pills, 91, 94
bitter melon juice, 137
blackberry juice, 179, 260, 278
blackberry leaf, 135
black cohosh, 211, 214
black haw bark, 215
black radish, 316
black walnut/black walnut hulls, 83, 242
bladder infections, 59–62
Bladder Tonic, 329
bladderwrack, 288–89
bleeding heart, 65
blood pressure. *See* high blood pressure
blood sugar, 13, 55, 131–32, 134, 262. *See also* hypoglycemia
blueberry juice, 154, 175, 260, 278
body mass index (BMI), 283, 355–56
borage, 101
boron, 235
boswellia serrata, 112, 231
bowel bacteria, 13, 109
bowel diseases, 107–14
boysenberry juice, 117
BPH (benign prostatic hyperplasia), 243–46
breast cancer: animal protein, 73, 156, 157; estrogen metabolism, 75–76, 209; gamma-linolenic acid (GLA), 77; raw juices, 74; refined carbohydrates, 73; soy, 230
broccoli juice, 179
bromelain, 252
bruises, 63–67
brussels sprouts juice, 137
burdock root, 144, 282
bursitis and tendinitis, 67–70
butterbur, 221

cabbage juice: anemia, 43; bowel diseases, 113; cancer, 78; canker sores, 86; diabetes, 137; eczema, 145; indigestion, 191; liver and pancreas function, 168; parasitic infections, 242; ulcerative colitis, 114; ulcers, 11, 274
cabbage leaf poultice, 66
Cabbage Patch Cocktail, 329
caffeine/coffee: alcohol and cigarette cravings, 119–20; anxiety and panic attacks, 46; bladder infections, 60, 61; cardiovascular disease, 91; depression, 128; fibrocystic breast disease, 158; fibromyalgia syndrome, 160; high blood pressure, 178; hypoglycemia, 184; insomnia, 204; menstrual disorders, 212–13; osteoporosis, 235; prostate enlargement, 244; rheumatoid arthritis and autoimmune diseases, 258; seizures, 148; stress, 263–64
calciferol, 148
calcium: ADD/ADHD, 57; constipation, 116; high blood pressure, 178; insomnia, 205; menstrual disorders, 213–14; osteoporosis, 235–36

whole-foods diet: ADD/ADHD, 54; Alzheimer's disease, 34; asthma, 51; eczema, 142; fibrocystic breast disease, 156; fibromyalgia syndrome, 160; indigestion, 188; prostate enlargement, 243; psoriasis, 247; rheumatoid arthritis and autoimmune diseases, 256

willow bark oil, 96

yarrow, 253
yeast infection, 80–84, 98, 256, 348
yellow dock, 43, 282
yucca, 96

zinc: ADD/ADHD, 58; Alzheimer's disease, 37–38; anemia, 42; bladder infections, 62; bursitis and tendinitis, 70; cancer, 78; candidiasis, 83; canker sores, 85; chronic fatigue syndrome, 100–101; colds, 105; diabetes, 136; eczema, 144; herpes, 174; inflammation, 196–97; influenza, 201; osteoporosis, 237; prostate enlargement, 245; respiratory disorders, 253; seizures, 151; ulcers, 274; varicose veins and hemorrhoids, 277; weight loss, 288

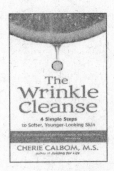
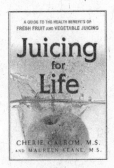
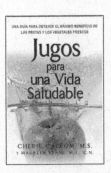